Adolescents with Chronic Kidney Disease

Maha N. Haddad
Erica Winnicki • Stephanie Nguyen
Editors

Adolescents with Chronic Kidney Disease

From Diagnosis to End-Stage Disease

Springer

Editors
Maha N. Haddad, MD
Department of Pediatric Nephrology
UC Davis Medical Center
Sacramento, CA
USA

Stephanie Nguyen, MD, MAS
Department of Pediatrics
UC Davis Children's Hospital
Sacramento, CA
USA

Erica Winnicki, MD
Department of Pediatrics
Division of Nephrology
University of California San Francisco
San Francisco, CA
USA

ISBN 978-3-030-07321-3 ISBN 978-3-319-97220-6 (eBook)
https://doi.org/10.1007/978-3-319-97220-6

Softcover re-print of the Hardcover 1st edition 2019

This Springer imprint is published by the registered company Springer Nature Switzerland AG
The registered company address is: Gewerbestrasse 11, 6330 Cham, Switzerland

To my parents, Najeeb Haddad and Alexandra Sousi, who above all things taught me the noble moral and ethical principles and implanted in me the desire to serve the poor and the needy and the urge to help the sick and the weak, with a loving and merciful heart.

Maha N. Haddad

To my husband Rick and daughters, Anh and Linh, thank you for all your love and support.

Stephanie Nguyen

To all of the adolescents I have had the privilege of caring for and who taught me so much in return, especially F.Z. and M.H.

Erica Winnicki

Preface

Adolescence is an exciting period of transition, sometimes bringing dramatic and turbulent changes especially to those with chronic disease. Physiologic, psychologic, and social demands during adolescence vie for attention with disease management. Parents are unsure of the role they should play in caring for their maturing adolescents and young adults with chronic disease. We hope this text addresses many of the challenges specific to the care of adolescents with chronic kidney disease and is useful to practicing physicians, those in training, and others involved in the care of this unique population.

We would like to extend our thanks to the numerous colleagues who embarked on this adventure with a truly collaborative spirit. Thank you to the medical editors of Springer Publishers, Inc., for their professionalism and guidance. Finally, thank you to our friends and family who exercised patience and have shown us only love and support.

Sacramento, CA, USA — Maha N. Haddad, MD
Sacramento, CA, USA — Stephanie Nguyen, MD, MAS
San Francisco, CA, USA — Erica Winnicki, MD

Contents

Contributors

Nishita Agarwal Berla, PsyD University of California, San Francisco (UCSF) Benioff Children's Hospital, Pediatric Nephrology, San Francisco, CA, USA

Pacific Graduate School of Psychology (PGSP)/Stanford PsyD Consortium, Palo Alto University, Palo Alto, CA, USA

Paul Brakeman, MD PhD Department of Pediatrics, UCSF Benioff Children's Hospital San Francisco, University of California, San Francisco, San Francisco, CA, USA

Jessica Brennan, RN, MS, PNP Division of Transplant, Department of Surgery, University of California, San Francisco, CA, USA

Lavjay Butani, MD, MACM Department of Pediatrics, University of California Davis Medical Center, Sacramento, CA, USA

Eileen Tsai Chambers, MD Department of Pediatrics, Duke University Medical Center, Durham, NC, USA

Annabelle N. Chua, MD Department of Pediatrics, Duke University Medical Center, Durham, NC, USA

Hillary Copp, MD Department of Urology, University of California San Francisco, San Francisco, CA, USA

Emeraghi E. David, BS Department of Pediatrics, Duke University Medical Center, Durham, NC, USA

Maha N. Haddad, M.D. Department of Pediatric Nephrology, UC Davis Medical Center, Sacramento, CA, USA

Kuang-Yu Jen, MD, PhD Department of Pathology and Laboratory Medicine, UC Davis School of Medicine, Sacramento, CA, USA

Arundhati Kale, MD Section of Nephrology, UC Davis Medical Center, Sacramento, CA, USA

Sabrina A. Karczewski, PhD Department of Psychology, Children's Hospital of Orange County (CHOC Children's), Orange, CA, USA

Molly Keane, LCSW, MPH University of California, San Francisco (UCSF) Benioff Children's Hospital, Pediatric Nephrology, San Francisco, CA, USA

Laura M. Kester Adolescent Medicine, UC Davis School of Medicine, Sacramento, CA, USA

Lisa Keung, MS, RD, CSP University of California, San Francisco, CA, USA

Elaine Ku, MD, MAS Department of Medicine and Pediatrics, University of California San Francisco, San Francisco, CA, USA

Jonas Kwok, BA College of Medicine, SUNY Downstate Medical Center, Brooklyn, NY, USA

Marsha Lee, MD UCSF Benioff Children's Hospital Pediatric Dialysis Unit, UCSF Benioff Children's Hospital, Pediatric Nephrology, San Francisco, CA, USA

Mina Matsuda-Abedini, MDCM, FRCPC Hospital for Sick Children, Toronto, ON, Canada

Stephanie Nguyen, MD, MAS Department of Pediatrics, UC Davis Children's Hospital, Sacramento, CA, USA

Aris Oates, MD University of California, San Francisco, CA, USA

Jonathan H. Pelletier, MD Department of Pediatrics, Duke University Medical Center, Durham, NC, USA

Andrew Perry, MD Department of Surgery, University of California, Davis, Sacramento, CA, USA

Kartik Pillutla, MD Department of Pediatrics, Dell Medical School, University of Texas at Austin, Dell Children's Medical Center of Central Texas, Pediatric Nephrology, Austin, TX, USA

Chandrasekar Santhanakrishnan, MD, MPH Department of Surgery, Division of Transplant Surgery, University of California, Davis, Sacramento, CA, USA

Erica Winnicki, MD Department of Pediatrics, Division of Nephrology, University of California San Francisco, San Francisco, CA, USA

Jakub Woloszyn, MD Department of Surgery, University of California, Davis, Sacramento, CA, USA

Chapter 1
Complications of Chronic Kidney Disease in Adolescents

Elaine Ku and Jonas Kwok

Introduction

Definition of CKD

The Kidney Disease Improving Global Outcomes (KDIGO) defines chronic kidney disease (CKD) as "abnormalities of kidney structure or function, present for 3 months, with implications for health, and is classified based on cause, glomerular filtration (GFR) category, and albuminuria (or proteinuria in children) category" [1]. Thus, presence of structural abnormalities, persistently low GFR, or persistent proteinuria for more than 3 months is consistent with a diagnosis of CKD. GFR may be determined by a variety of methods, the most common employed equations of which are based on serum creatinine (SCr). The recommended equation for pediatric patients is the Schwartz "bedside" formula [2], which provides an estimate of the level of kidney function or GFR and is determined by taking 41.3*(height(m)/SCr (mg/dL)). The stages of CKD are shown in Table 1.1.

E. Ku (✉)
Department of Medicine and Pediatrics, University of California San Francisco, San Francisco, CA, USA
e-mail: elaine.ku@ucsf.edu

J. Kwok
College of Medicine, SUNY Downstate Medical Center, Brooklyn, NY, USA
e-mail: Jonas.kwok@pomona.edu

M. N. Haddad et al. (eds.), *Adolescents with Chronic Kidney Disease*,
https://doi.org/10.1007/978-3-319-97220-6_1

Table 1.1 KDIGO stages of chronic kidney disease by eGFR [1]

Stage	eGFR (ml/min/1.73m²)
1	≥90
2	60–89
3a	45–59
3b	30–44
4	15–29
5	≤15
5D	Dialysis or transplant

CKD During Adolescence

Adolescence is a high-risk period for patients with chronic kidney disease (CKD). While the probability of developing end-stage renal disease (ESRD) gradually increases with age in pediatric-onset CKD, a notable decline in survival occurs in puberty and early post-puberty [3]. Mechanisms contributing to the higher rate of progression of CKD in adolescence include higher blood pressures, risk for an imbalance between nephron mass and the filtration demands of growth, and alterations in hormone levels [4].

Adolescence is also unique because patients move from largely passive to more active roles in the management of their care. This period is critical for the development of self-management skills and transition readiness as adolescents prepare for young adulthood. It is not surprising, given the burden of stress on adolescents, that patients 14–16 years old have the highest rates of graft loss among all patients ≤55 years old [5, 6].

A major goal of CKD management in children and adolescents is to delay the onset of ESRD. Children, adolescents, and young adults constitute less than 5% of the ESRD population, and while 10-year survival is 75–80% in pediatric ESRD, the mortality rate is still 30 times higher than their age-matched peers [7]. Given the known average rate of decline in kidney function (approximately 4.3 and 1.5 ml/min per 1.73m^2 per year for glomerular and non-glomerular diagnoses, respectively), many adolescents are likely to see their CKD progress to ESRD during adolescence or young adulthood [3, 8, 9]. In fact, nearly 40% of all pediatric kidney transplants occur in adolescents aged 13–17.

Medical Complications

Growth and Puberty

Puberty is initiated by the gonadotropic hormone axis, which stimulates rapid linear growth, and is characterized clinically by the development of secondary sex characteristics including increased breast size in girls and testicular volume in boys.

However, approximately 80% of growth is already complete by puberty in children [10]. Thus, while compromised accrual of height velocity is most apparent during puberty, prepubertal growth stunting also has a major impact on final height achievement. For children reaching ESRD before or during puberty, the onset of puberty may be delayed by up to 2–2.5 years, and the magnitude of the "growth spurt" that occurs may be substantially reduced [11]. Medications such as steroids that are used to treat the underlying kidney disease can also cause pubertal delay, as it disrupts the hormonal axis for growth [10]. Fortunately, normal onset of puberty is seen in children who are transplanted before 5 years of age [12].

Growth failure in children with CKD is a consequence of a variety of factors, most notably mineral and bone metabolism disorders that occur with CKD [13]. KDIGO guidelines recommend that providers monitor three aspects of bone disease in CKD patients: turnover, mineralization, and volume [14]. Both abnormalities of bone turnover and mineralization increase in prevalence as renal function declines, as measured by GFR. Disruption of the growth hormone-insulin-like growth factor axis, including resistance to growth hormone, also contributes to decreased linear growth [15].

Approximately 45–60% of adults with childhood-onset CKD have short stature [16]. Over one-third of children with CKD were below the 3rd percentile for height upon entry to the North American Pediatric Renal Trials and Collaborative Studies (NAPRTCS) registry [17]. For children with congenital CKD, growth velocity after 2 years of age can normalize to parallel the expected growth velocity, but patients do not necessarily experience "catch-up" growth and may remain persistently shorter than their peers [15, 17, 18]. Findings from the CKiD (Chronic Kidney Disease in Children) study suggest that girls with non-glomerular etiologies of CKD may experience the greatest growth impairment [19]. For adolescents who develop ESRD, this growth failure is associated with higher 5-year mortality [20].

Medical management for growth retardation in adolescents with CKD should focus on the early identification and correction of metabolic derangements, nutritional deficiencies, and hormonal abnormalities [15, 17, 19]. Recombinant human growth hormone (rhGH) has proven to be safe and efficacious, though it is more effective in prepubertal children and during earlier stages of CKD [21, 22]. However, growth hormone is underutilized in the treatment of children with CKD-related growth impairment, in part because patients may be deterred by the prospect of frequent injections [15, 19, 21]. A review of rhGH use in pediatric CKD found that side effects were uncommon in general, although elevated fasting glucose, glucose intolerance, granuloma formation, claudication, hypertension, and worsening of scoliosis are some potential adverse effects [15]. Other adverse effects associated with growth hormone use include decreased kidney function, papilledema with benign intracranial hypertension, or acute rejection in the setting of transplantation [15].

Catch-up growth for children with ESRD is not seen as often in patients on dialysis, but occurs with transplantation, though this growth is attenuated among those who are older at time of transplant and those receiving steroids after transplantation [15, 17].

Adolescence is a critical period for attaining peak bone mass, with 25% of skeletal mass being deposited within the 2 years of peak height velocity [23]. Adolescents are therefore vulnerable to decreased levels of nutritional vitamin D, mineral abnormalities, and alterations in bone accrual, as well as a higher risk of fracture due to relative under-mineralization of bones during this period [24, 25]. Risk of fracture is increased by 2.4- and 3-fold for boys and girls, respectively, compared to their age-matched healthy peers, with boys over 14 years old having the highest incidence of fractures [26]. Advanced pubertal stage, taller stature, and higher serum levels of parathyroid hormone were also associated with greater risk of fractures in the CKiD cohort of children with mild to moderate CKD [26].

Cardiovascular Disease

Traditional risk factors for cardiovascular disease (CVD), including obesity (15%), hypertension (54%), dyslipidemia (45%), and insulin abnormalities (9–19%), all occur at high rates in children and adolescents with CKD [27–29]. Children with CKD are also subject to nontraditional risk factors for CKD, including abnormal mineral metabolism, anemia, chronic inflammation, uremia, and fluid overload [28]. The relationship between disordered mineral metabolism and cardiovascular disease has been described by CKD-MBD (mineral and bone disorder) since the KDIGO consensus in 2009 [14]. Findings such as left ventricular hypertrophy (17–49%), increased carotid intima-media thickness, and vascular calcifications are more prevalent in children with even mild CKD, with still higher rates among those treated with dialysis [28, 30]. Cardiovascular disease still remains the leading cause of death, although this high mortality rate is lower after kidney transplantation [31].

Hypertension, along with albuminuria and low nephron mass, is a major risk factor for the progression of CKD [32]. Hypertension and CKD are intrinsically linked, with worsening of one condition exacerbating the other [28]. Hypertension secondary to increasing intravascular volume and peripheral vascular resistance causes a decline in renal function through intrinsic renal tissue damage and hypoperfusion, thereby triggering renin-angiotensin-aldosterone-system (RAAS) activation, increased salt and volume retention, vasoconstriction, and sympathetic upregulation, resulting in exacerbation of hypertension [32].

Hypertension is extremely common among children with CKD. In CKiD, 54% of the cohort was hypertensive at enrollment, while the NAPRTCS registry found a prevalence of 76.6% [32–34]. Hypertension is associated with the development of target-organ damage in children, and studies suggest the potential for regression of left ventricular hypertrophy through antihypertensive control in children with CKD [35]. In accordance with findings from the CKiD study, KDIGO guidelines recommend pharmacologic antihypertensive treatment for patients with systolic blood pressures above the 90th percentile for age, sex, and height [36]. The 2017 American Academy of Pediatric guidelines, in accordance with results of the ESCAPE trial, recommend hypertensive children with CKD be treated with ACE inhibitors or ARBs – especially in patients with proteinuria [37, 38]. Blood pressure targets in children with CKD are <90th percentile for age, sex, and height or <130/80 mmHg, whichever is lower among adolescents age 13 or older [37]. Ideally, blood pressure should be treated to a mean arterial pressure of <50th percentile on 24-h ambulatory blood pressure monitoring if available [37, 38]. Reduction of salt intake is recommended in the management of hypertension in children with CKD, as decreased intake is associated with reduction in proteinuria and blood pressure [32].

An up to 700-fold increased risk of cardiovascular mortality has been reported for children with ESRD compared to their healthy peers [39]. The US Renal Data System showed that 23% of mortality in children and young adults with childhood-onset ESRD was due to cardiovascular causes and that adolescents with CKD were at higher risk for arrhythmias than younger children [31]. These risk factors have prompted the American Heart Association (AHA) to place pediatric CKD patients in the highest category of cardiovascular risk [40]. However, adolescents with CKD who enter young adulthood may often receive suboptimal preventative CVD care, as measured by cardiovascular risk factor screening and guideline-directed treatment, in spite of the elevated CV risk in this population [41]. The American Heart Association cardiovascular risk management guidelines recommend screening and monitoring of blood pressure, lipids, and glucose, providing dietary counseling, and encouraging smoking cessation and physical activity [40].

Anemia

Anemia is common in childhood CKD, with over 30% of patients meeting National Kidney Foundation Disease Outcomes Quality Initiative criteria [42]. In a recent study, adolescents aged 10–18 in the United States had a high prevalence of anemia. Anemia was especially common among adolescents with long-standing CKD from congenital urological abnormalities [43]. Data from NAPRTCS indicated that the prevalence of anemia increases with progressive CKD stages [44]. The consequences of anemia in adolescents with CKD are numerous, as anemia has been linked to fatigue, depression, sleep disturbances, impaired cognitive function, loss of appetite, decreased exercise tolerance, decreased health-related quality of life in multiple domains, and increased mortality [23, 28, 43, 45].

The etiologies of anemia in CKD are multifactorial, including erythropoietin deficiency, iron deficiency, nutritional deficits, inflammation, hyperparathyroidism, and side effects of medications [23]. For adolescent girls, menstruation may also contribute to anemia. Treatment of anemia in CKD primarily consists of iron supplementation and erythropoietin-stimulating agents (ESAs), as well as management of non-renal complications if present. The 2012 KDIGO guidelines recommend targeting hemoglobin levels of 11–12 g/dl in children receiving ESA therapy [46]. Interestingly, adolescents exhibit the lowest rate of nonadherence (4%) to erythropoietin-stimulating agents among CKD medications [47].

Neurocognition

Adolescents with CKD are at increased risk for neurocognitive deficits compared to their healthy peers. CKD-specific comorbidities that may contribute to neurocognitive sequelae of CKD include anemia, hypertension, and cardiovascular disease [48–50]. While findings have not always been consistent, most of the available literature note either significantly decreased or low-normal scores for academic achievement, executive function, attention regulation, language acquisition, visual-spatial ability, memory, and inhibitory control [48, 49, 51, 52]. These impairments are correlated with worsening disease severity, longer duration of disease, and younger age of onset [53].

Between 21% and 40% of children and adolescents (6–17 years old) with mild to moderate CKD score one or more standard deviations below the average for IQ, academic achievement, attention, or executive functioning [51]. In older children and young adults (8–25 years old), declining renal function is associated with decreased attention, visual-spatial ability, and worse memory [49].

Patients reaching ESRD during childhood have lower IQs compared to their siblings and healthy controls [54]. However, the mode of renal replacement therapy may have different effects on neurocognition. Compared to patients on dialysis, children with renal transplants exhibit comparatively better academic performance and may even achieve normal attention, language, and visual-spatial test scores, with lasting impacts on IQ and educational attainment into adult life [48, 54, 55]. However, the prevalence of patients with CKD who receive special education services in the United States is comparable to the general population [48]. Academic achievement may be further impaired due to frequent absenteeism secondary to outpatient medical visits, hospitalizations, and hemodialysis sessions [48, 55].

In addition to school attainment and performance, neurocognitive deficits in adolescents are also concerning due to their potential influence on work attainment and earning potential. One study found that only 50–75% of adults with pediatric renal transplants were employed as adults [56].

Psychosocial Complications

Quality of Life

The disease burden of CKD is extensive, from systemic consequences and comorbidities, such as disordered bone mineral metabolism and anemia, to its impact on physical and psychosocial development [57]. Similar to adolescents with other chronic diseases, those with CKD often have more behavioral problems, hyperactivity, aggression, anxiety, worry, and depressive symptoms compared to their age-matched peers [57, 58].

A variety of tools have been used to assess health-related quality of life (HRQoL) in adolescents with CKD, and all indicate decreased HRQoL across multiple domains – social, physical, emotional, school function, cognition, pain, and disease-specific (disease burden, symptoms, pain, daily functioning) [45, 59, 60]. Evidence that adolescents and young adults with CKD are "willing to trade considerable life expectancy for perfect health" demonstrates the extent to which CKD disrupts patients' daily lives [59]. Ideally, providers should identify HRQoL issues early in order to improve the social, emotional, and functional outcomes of adolescents with CKD.

Decreased HRQOL has been reported to be associated with changes in physical appearance related to CKD progression and its treatment (stunted growth, edema, and altered body fat distribution from corticosteroid treatment) [57]. Short stature is oft-cited as a major contributor to adolescents' poor quality of life [42, 61]. Delayed puberty in children with CKD also delays adolescents' sexual development, which may influence their self-concept and ability to fit in with their peers. Patients may also feel a lack of normalcy, independence, and ability to socialize and integrate themselves in society [59]. Children on dialysis have been reported to have still lower functional health status than patients who are pre-dialysis [62].

CKD also impacts adolescents' quality of life via its impacts on sleep. The prevalence of sleep disorders in pre-dialysis children and adolescents with CKD is 40–50% and is associated with behavioral deficits, school performance, and decreased HRQoL when present [63]. Data from CKiD indicate that older age, shorter duration of CKD, and glomerular disease are associated with increased daytime sleepiness [63]. Adolescents over 14 years old with measured GFR <50 reported falling asleep two to three times more often during the day than younger children with higher GFRs, and adolescents with CKD also have higher prevalence of restless legs syndrome [42, 61]. Due to disordered hormonal balances and comorbidities, children and adolescents are also at risk for increased body mass index, which is associated with sleep-disordered breathing [63]. Urinary incontinence (mostly bedwetting) in children between 5 and 16 years old is also more common in the presence of CKD and may have lasting effects on adolescents due to the incontinence-related social stigma and lowered self-esteem [64].

Behavioral and emotional disorders in children and adolescents with CKD are common [60]. Depression is more common in children aged 9–18 with CKD stages 1–3 compared to their age-matched peers, with even greater likelihood in adolescents above age 13 [58, 65].

Family and Psychosocial Factors

Compounding patients' personal challenges of living with CKD, patients' families are also at risk for a variety of stressors. Having a child with chronic illness may affect the patient's siblings who may often feel neglected, increase the psychological distress of caretakers by challenging the ability for caretakers to maintain employment, and also contribute to marital strain [53, 66]. Lower socioeconomic status, large families, lack of familial support, and younger patient age are risk factors for poorer psychosocial adjustment and quality of life in the parents of children with CKD [23, 67].

In contrast to patients' self-reported quality of life, which improves with aging, parents tend to report worsening quality of life for their child with increasing age of the patient. While well-adjusted and supportive families can provide a buffer against the negative stressors on the patient and support the transition of patients to adult healthcare systems, low levels of family support are not uncommon and are correlated with worse patient adherence and overall outcomes [57, 68].

Studies have shown that CKD patients with household incomes <$75,000 were more likely to be younger and minorities, lack private insurance, and have mothers with lower education, abnormal birth history, and at least one clinical comorbidity [69]. Patients of low-income families are at higher risk for short stature compared to those with household incomes >$30,000 [69]. Lower maternal education has been associated with lower HRQoL in children with CKD [45]. Socioeconomic factors associated with poorer transition readiness and healthcare utilization in adolescents include younger age, public instead of private insurance, and lack of an individualized education plan (IEP) or 504 plan [70].

Duration of CKD and Its Influence on Quality of Life

Adolescents with CKD can be subdivided into two broad groups. In the first group, adolescents will have onset of their kidney disease during adolescence, often presenting for the first time during their teenage years. Compared to younger children with CKD, these adolescents have a higher incidence of glomerular disease, which is associated with more rapid progression of renal disease [71]. The second group includes adolescent-age patients who have been living with a renal diagnosis for years, often since birth as a result of congenital anomalies of the kidney and urinary tract (CAKUT) [72]. These patients have a much higher incidence of structural urological abnormalities and tend to be anemic and more severely affected by poor growth [17, 43].

CKiD data shows that children who have been living with CKD for a longer duration of time have better physical and emotional functioning compared to those with newer diagnoses [45]. This suggests that adolescents with congenital etiologies of their CKD may be able to better cope with the stressors of CKD, a phenomenon termed "response shift" [45].

Earlier diagnosis does not necessarily mean a more benign patient experience, however. Roumelioti et al. reported that children with long-standing CKD have less energy compared to those who had CKD for less than a quarter of their lives [61]. Children with later onset of CKD, as in adolescence, may have a higher likelihood of achieving normal growth and psychosocial development as a result of having had good health before their CKD diagnosis [53].

The rate of progression of CKD and severity of disease is inversely correlated with self-management ability [23]. Nevertheless, all pediatric CKD patients, regardless of disease severity, report decreased health-related quality of life across physical, social, emotional, and school function domains as assessed by the Pediatric Quality of Life Inventory (PedsQL) and Kidney Disease Quality of Life Instrument (KDQOL) [45, 59, 60].

Transition of Care

Adolescents are at higher risk for complications related to poor self-management and nonadherence [68, 73]. Compared to patients of other age groups with CKD and ESRD, adolescents may struggle with a number of challenges, including the need to fit in with peers, concerns surrounding body and self-image, school or work obligations, and poor recognition of the long-term consequences of their actions, including nonadherence to therapy [23, 74, 75]. Nonadherence in children with CKD has been reported to range from 4% to 22% and is associated with the frequency of medication dosing [47, 76]. As such, healthcare providers should dedicate extra time to adolescents with CKD to ensure that patients are prepared for medical self-management, adherent to therapy, and developing skills needed to navigate their way through adult healthcare systems.

Management of CKD involves keeping track of a list of appointments with nephrologists and other specialists depending on comorbidities, adherence to multiple medications on different dosing schedules, financial and insurance considerations, dietary restrictions, and frequent laboratory monitoring. While the bulk of this responsibility is shouldered by parents in earlier childhood, adolescents around 18–21 years of age are expected to be more self-reliant as they transition to adult care [23, 77]. This transition, compounded by the need to maintain age-appropriate activities and mature physically, sexually, cognitively, and socially, can be challenging in the life of young patients [78]. Ferris and colleagues cite a number of obstacles and challenges faced by adolescents with CKD, including [79]:

- Slower maturation of cognitive function
- Depression, lower socialization skills and self-esteem, and slower achievement of milestones
- Adoption of high-risk behaviors including use of drugs and alcohol and nonadherence to treatment
- Development of personal identity and need for peer recognition
- Overcoming differences in physical appearance including shorter stature and scars from prior surgeries
- Performing school-/work-related tasks in the setting of potential cognitive impairment
- Learning to self-manage medications and appointments
- Transitioning out of the home/loss of parental supervision

A consensus statement endorsed by both the International Society of Nephrology (ISN) and the International Pediatric Nephrology Association (IPNA) states that the transitional years span roughly from 14 to 24 years [78]. This age span underscores the recognition that transitional care should be individualized – not every patient may be ready for transition by 18 or 21 years of age [75, 80]. Transition requires long-term planning, with frequent assessments of readiness beginning as early as ages 12–14, and should involve pediatric and adult physicians, the family, and the patient [75, 81]. Successful transitions between pediatric and adult care may require holistic assessments of patients' ability to self-manage, adhere to medications, and effectively utilize the healthcare system [70].

Ideally, dedicated transition clinics or youth workers should be available to facilitate transitions of care, though most facilities do not have such services [75]. Individualized care based on routine assessments of transition readiness – including emotional maturity, illness stability, availability of developmentally appropriate services, and emotional, physical, and psychological attainment – is essential for optimal transition and transfer of care [78, 79, 80]. Unfortunately, the transition of care from pediatric to adult nephrology is often fragmented, and not all patients may have access to a pediatric nephrologist in the United States [75, 82].

Concluding Thoughts

Chronic kidney disease and its complications have many implications for adolescents. Adolescence is an especially vulnerable stage of life for patients with CKD physically, emotionally, and socially. As a consequence, patients have higher mortality risk, have decreased quality of life, and are subject to the negative consequences of CKD on their growth and neurocognitive outcomes compared to both healthy peers and other CKD age groups. Transition preparation should begin early in adolescence, given the potential for the severe and lasting consequences of inappropriate disease management.

References

1. Kidney Disease: Improving Global Outcomes CWG. KDIGO 2012 clinical practice guideline for the evaluation and management of chronic kidney disease. [Internet]. 2013. [Cited 2018 Feb 17]. Available from: http://www.kdigo.org/clinical_practice_guidelines/pdf/CKD/KDIGO_2012_CKD_ GL.pdf.
2. Mian AN, Schwartz GJ. Measurement and estimation of glomerular filtration rate in children. Adv Chronic Kidney Dis. 2017;24(6):348–56.
3. Ardissino G, Daccò V, Testa S, Bonaudo R, Claris-Appiani A, Taioli E, et al. Epidemiology of chronic renal failure in children: data from the ItalKid project. Pediatrics. 2003;111(4):e382–7.
4. Harambat J, van Stralen KJ, Kim JJ, Tizard EJ. Epidemiology of chronic kidney disease in children. Pediatr Nephrol Berl Ger. 2012;27(3):363–73.

5. NAPRTCS Annual Report. Boston: North American Pediatric Renal Trials and Collaborative Studies [Internet]. 2014. [Cited 2017 Oct 6]. Available from: https://web.emmes.com/study/ped/annlrept/annualrept2014.pdf.
6. Andreoni KA, Forbes R, Andreoni RM, Phillips G, Stewart H, Ferris M. Age-related kidney transplant outcomes: health disparities amplified in adolescence. JAMA Intern Med. 2013;173(16):1524–32.
7. McDonald SP, Craig JC. Long-term survival of children with end-stage renal disease. N Engl J Med. 2004;350(26):2654–62.
8. Furth SL, Abraham AG, Jerry-Fluker J, Schwartz GJ, Benfield M, Kaskel F, et al. Metabolic abnormalities, cardiovascular disease risk factors, and GFR decline in children with chronic kidney disease. Clin J Am Soc Nephrol CJASN. 2011;6(9):2132–40.
9. Furth SL, Cole SR, Moxey-Mims M, Kaskel F, Mak R, Schwartz G, et al. Design and methods of the Chronic Kidney Disease in Children (CKiD) prospective cohort study. Clin J Am Soc Nephrol CJASN. 2006;1(5):1006–15.
10. Haffner D, Zivicnjak M. Pubertal development in children with chronic kidney disease. Pediatr Nephrol. 2017;32(6):949–64.
11. Schaefer F, Seidel C, Binding A, Gasser T, Largo RH, Prader A, et al. Pubertal growth in chronic renal failure. Pediatr Res. 1990;28(1):5.
12. Tainio J, Qvist E, Vehmas R, Jahnukainen K, Hölttä T, Valta H, et al. Pubertal development is normal in adolescents after renal transplantation in childhood. Transplantation. 2011;92(4):404–9.
13. Wesseling-Perry K, Salusky IB. Chronic kidney disease: mineral and bone disorder in children. Semin Nephrol. 2013;33(2):169–79.
14. Kidney Disease: Improving Global Outcomes (KDIGO) CKD-MBD Work Group. KDIGO clinical practice guideline for the diagnosis, evaluation, prevention, and treatment of Chronic Kidney Disease-Mineral and Bone Disorder (CKD-MBD). Kidney Int Suppl. 2009;76(113):S1–130.
15. Greenbaum LA, Warady BA, Furth SL. Current advances in chronic kidney disease in children: growth, cardiovascular, and neurocognitive risk factors. Semin Nephrol. 2009;29(4):425–34.
16. Ingulli EG, Mak RH. Growth in children with chronic kidney disease: role of nutrition, growth hormone, dialysis, and steroids. Curr Opin Pediatr. 2014;26(2):187–92.
17. Rees L, Mak RH. Nutrition and growth in children with chronic kidney disease. Nat Rev Nephrol. 2011;7(11):615–23.
18. Seikaly MG, Salhab N, Gipson D, Yiu V, Stablein D. Stature in children with chronic kidney disease: analysis of NAPRTCS database. Pediatr Nephrol Berl Ger. 2006;21(6):793–9.
19. Rodig NM, McDermott KC, Schneider MF, Hotchkiss HM, Yadin O, Seikaly MG, et al. Growth in children with chronic kidney disease: a report from the chronic kidney disease in children study. Pediatr Nephrol Berl Ger. 2014;29(10):1987–95.
20. Furth SL, Hwang W, Yang C, Neu AM, Fivush BA, Powe NR. Growth failure, risk of hospitalization and death for children with end-stage renal disease. Pediatr Nephrol Berl Ger. 2002;17(6):450–5.
21. Mahan JD, Warady BA, Committee C. Assessment and treatment of short stature in pediatric patients with chronic kidney disease: a consensus statement. Pediatr Nephrol. 2006;21(7):917–30.
22. Hodson EM, Willis NS, Craig JC. Growth hormone for children with chronic kidney disease. In: Cochrane database of systematic reviews [Internet]. Wiley; 2012. [Cited 2017 Oct 4]. Available from: http://onlinelibrary.wiley.com/doi/10.1002/14651858.CD003264.pub3/abstract.
23. Ferris ME, Miles JA, Seamon ML. Adolescents and young adults with chronic or end-stage kidney disease. Blood Purif. 2016;41(1–3):205–10.
24. Maggioli C, Stagi S. Bone modeling, remodeling, and skeletal health in children and adolescents: mineral accrual, assessment and treatment. Ann Pediatr Endocrinol Metab. 2017;22(1):1–5.

25. Kumar J, McDermott K, Abraham AG, Friedman LA, Johnson VL, Kaskel FJ, et al. Prevalence and correlates of 25-hydroxyvitamin D deficiency in the Chronic Kidney Disease in Children (CKiD) cohort. Pediatr Nephrol Berl Ger. 2016;31(1):121–9.
26. Denburg MR, Kumar J, Jemielita T, Brooks ER, Skversky A, Portale AA, et al. Fracture burden and risk factors in childhood CKD: results from the CKiD cohort study. J Am Soc Nephrol JASN. 2016;27(2):543–50.
27. Lilien MR, Groothoff JW. Cardiovascular disease in children with CKD or ESRD. Nat Rev Nephrol. 2009;5(4):229–35.
28. Mitsnefes MM. Cardiovascular disease in children with chronic kidney disease. J Am Soc Nephrol JASN. 2012;23(4):578–85.
29. Saland JM, Pierce CB, Mitsnefes MM, Flynn JT, Goebel J, Kupferman JC, et al. Dyslipidemia in children with chronic kidney disease: a report of the Chronic Kidney Disease in Children (CKiD) study. Kidney Int. 2010;78(11):1154–63.
30. Wesseling-Perry K, Pereira RC, Tseng C-H, Elashoff R, Zaritsky JJ, Yadin O, et al. Early skeletal and biochemical alterations in pediatric chronic kidney disease. Clin J Am Soc Nephrol CJASN. 2012;7(1):146–52.
31. Parekh RS, Carroll CE, Wolfe RA, Port FK. Cardiovascular mortality in children and young adults with end-stage kidney disease. J Pediatr. 2002;141(2):191–7.
32. Gallibois CM, Jawa NA, Noone DG. Hypertension in pediatric patients with chronic kidney disease: management challenges. Int J Nephrol Renov Dis. 2017;10:205–13.
33. Flynn JT, Mitsnefes M, Pierce C, Cole SR, Parekh RS, Furth SL, et al. Blood pressure in children with chronic kidney disease: a report from the chronic kidney disease in children study. Hypertension. 2008;52(4):631–7.
34. Mitsnefes M, Stablein D. Hypertension in pediatric patients on long-term dialysis: a report of the North American Pediatric Renal Transplant Cooperative Study (NAPRTCS). Am J Kidney Dis. 2005;45(2):309–15.
35. Kupferman JC, Aronson Friedman L, Cox C, Flynn J, Furth S, Warady B, et al. BP control and left ventricular hypertrophy regression in children with CKD. J Am Soc Nephrol JASN. 2014;25(1):167–74.
36. Kidney Disease: Improving Global Outcomes CWG. KDIGO clinical practice guideline for the management of blood pressure in chronic kidney disease [Internet]. 2012. [Cited 2018 Feb 18]. Available from: http://kdigo.org/wp-content/uploads/2016/10/KDIGO-2012-Blood-Pressure-Guideline-English.pdf.
37. Flynn JT, Kaelber DC, Baker-Smith CM, Blowey D, Carroll AE, Daniels SR, et al. Clinical practice guideline for screening and management of high blood pressure in children and adolescents. Pediatrics. 2017;140:e20171904.
38. ESCAPE Trial Group, Wühl E, Trivelli A, Picca S, Litwin M, Peco-Antic A, et al. Strict blood-pressure control and progression of renal failure in children. N Engl J Med. 2009;361(17):1639–50.
39. Foley RN, Parfrey PS, Sarnak MJ. Clinical epidemiology of cardiovascular disease in chronic renal disease. Am J Kidney Dis. 1998;32(5):S112–9.
40. Kavey R-EW, Allada V, Daniels SR, Hayman LL, McCrindle BW, Newburger JW, et al. Cardiovascular risk reduction in high-risk pediatric patients: a scientific statement from the American Heart Association Expert Panel on Population and Prevention Science; the Councils on Cardiovascular Disease in the Young, Epidemiology and Prevention, Nutrition, Physical Activity and Metabolism, High Blood Pressure Research, Cardiovascular Nursing, and the Kidney in Heart Disease; and the Interdisciplinary Working Group on Quality of Care and Outcomes Research: endorsed by the American Academy of Pediatrics. Circulation. 2006;114(24):2710–38.
41. Hooper DK, Williams JC, Carle AC, Amaral S, Chand DH, Ferris ME, et al. The quality of cardiovascular disease care for adolescents with kidney disease: a Midwest pediatric nephrology consortium study. Pediatr Nephrol Berl Ger. 2013;28(6):939–49.

42. Wong CJ, Moxey-Mims M, Jerry-Fluker J, Warady BA, Furth SL. CKiD (CKD in children) prospective cohort study: a review of current findings. Am J Kidney Dis Off J Natl Kidney Found. 2012;60(6):1002–11.
43. Gerson A, Hwang W, Fiorenza J, Barth K, Kaskel F, Weiss L, et al. Anemia and health-related quality of life in adolescents with chronic kidney disease. Am J Kidney Dis. 2004;44(6):1017–23.
44. Becherucci F, Roperto RM, Materassi M, Romagnani P. Chronic kidney disease in children. Clin Kidney J. 2016;9(4):583–91.
45. Gerson AC, Wentz A, Abraham AG, Mendley SR, Hooper SR, Butler RW, et al. Health-related quality of life of children with mild to moderate chronic kidney disease. Pediatrics. 2010;125(2):e349–57.
46. KDIGO clinical practice guideline for anemia in chronic kidney disease. National guideline clearinghouse [Internet]. [Cited 2017 Dec 13]. Available from: https://www.guideline.gov/summaries/summary/38245.
47. Akchurin OM, Schneider MF, Mulqueen L, Brooks ER, Langman CB, Greenbaum LA, et al. Medication adherence and growth in children with CKD. Clin J Am Soc Nephrol. 2014;9(9):1519–25.
48. Gerson A, Butler R, Moxey-Mims M, Wentz A, Shinnar S, Lande MB, et al. Neurocognitive outcomes in children with chronic kidney disease: current findings and contemporary endeavors. Ment Retard Dev Disabil Res Rev. 2006;12:208–15.
49. Ruebner RL, Laney N, Kim JY, Hartung EA, Hooper SR, Radcliffe J, et al. Neurocognitive dysfunction in children, adolescents, and young adults with CKD. Am J Kidney Dis. 2016;67(4):567–75.
50. Lande MB, Mendley SR, Matheson MB, Shinnar S, Gerson AC, Samuels JA, et al. Association of blood pressure variability and neurocognition in children with chronic kidney disease. Pediatr Nephrol. 2016;31(11):2137–44.
51. Hooper SR, Gerson AC, Butler RW, Gipson DS, Mendley SR, Lande MB, et al. Neurocognitive functioning of children and adolescents with mild-to-moderate chronic kidney disease. Clin J Am Soc Nephrol CJASN. 2011;6(8):1824–30.
52. Mendley SR, Matheson M, Shinnar S, Lande M, Gerson AC, Butler R, et al. Duration of chronic kidney disease reduces attention and executive function in pediatric patients. Kidney Int. 2015;87(4):800–6.
53. Ferris ME, Mahan JD. Pediatric chronic kidney disease and the process of health care transition. Semin Nephrol. 2009;29(4):435–44.
54. Gipson DS, Duquette PJ, Icard PF, Hooper SR. The central nervous system in childhood chronic kidney disease. Pediatr Nephrol. 2007;22(10):1703–10.
55. Moreira JM, Soares CMBM, Teixeira AL, Silva ACS e, Kummer AM. Anxiety, depression, resilience and quality of life in children and adolescents with pre-dialysis chronic kidney disease. Pediatr Nephrol. 2015;30(12):2153–62.
56. Bartosh SM, Leverson G, Robillard D, Sollinger HW. Long-term outcomes in pediatric renal transplant recipients who survive into adulthood. Transplantation. 2003;76(8):1195–200.
57. Soliday E, Kool E, Lande MB. Psychosocial adjustment in children with kidney disease. J Pediatr Psychol. 2000;25(2):93–103.
58. Pinquart M, Shen Y. Depressive symptoms in children and adolescents with chronic physical illness: an updated meta-analysis. J Pediatr Psychol. 2011;36(4):375–84.
59. Tong A, Wong G, McTaggart S, Henning P, Mackie F, Carroll RP, et al. Quality of life of young adults and adolescents with chronic kidney disease. J Pediatr. 2013;163(4):1179–1185.e5.
60. Marciano RC, Soares CMB, Diniz JSS, Lima EM, Silva JMP, Canhestro MR, et al. Behavioral disorders and low quality of life in children and adolescents with chronic kidney disease. Pediatr Nephrol. 2011;26(2):281–90.
61. Copelovitch L, Warady BA, Furth SL. Insights from the Chronic Kidney Disease in Children (CKiD) study. Clin J Am Soc Nephrol CJASN. 2011;6(8):2047–53.

62. Gerson AC, Riley A, Fivush BA, Pham N, Fiorenza J, Robertson J, et al. Assessing health status and health care utilization in adolescents with chronic kidney disease. J Am Soc Nephrol. 2005;16(5):1427–32.
63. Stabouli S, Papadimitriou E, Printza N, Dotis J, Papachristou F. Sleep disorders in pediatric chronic kidney disease patients. Pediatr Nephrol. 2016;31(8):1221–9.
64. Dodson JL, Cohn SE, Cox C, Hmiel PS, Wood E, Mattoo TK, et al. Urinary incontinence in the CKiD cohort and health related quality of life. J Urol. 2009;182(4 Suppl):2007–14.
65. Kogon AJ, Matheson MB, Flynn JT, Gerson AC, Warady BA, Furth SL, et al. Depressive symptoms in children with chronic kidney disease. J Pediatr. 2016;168:164–70.e1.
66. Medway M, Tong A, Craig JC, Kim S, Mackie F, McTaggart S, et al. Parental perspectives on the financial impact of caring for a child with CKD. Am J Kidney Dis. 2015;65(3):384–93.
67. Fielding D, Brownbridge G. Factors related to psychosocial adjustment in children with end-stage renal failure. Pediatr Nephrol. 1999;13(9):766–70.
68. Bates CM, Charlton JR, Ferris ME, Hildebrandt F, Hoshizaki DK, Warady BA, et al. Pediatric kidney disease: tracking onset and improving clinical outcomes. Clin J Am Soc Nephrol. 2014;9:1141–3. CJN.00860114
69. Hidalgo G, Ng DK, Moxey-Mims M, Minnick ML, Blydt-Hansen T, Warady BA, et al. Income level and kidney disease severity and progression among children and adolescents with CKD: a report from the Chronic Kidney Disease in Children (CKiD) Study. Am J Kidney Dis Off J Natl Kidney Found [Internet]. 2013;62(6). [Cited 2017 Oct 4]. Available from: https://www.ncbi.nlm.nih.gov/pmc/articles/PMC3840111/.
70. Javalkar K, Fenton N, Cohen S, Ferris M. Socioecologic factors as predictors of readiness for self-management and transition, medication adherence, and health care utilization among adolescents and young adults with chronic kidney disease. Prev Chronic Dis [Internet]. 2014; 11. [Cited 2017 Oct 4]. Available from: https://www.ncbi.nlm.nih.gov/pmc/articles/PMC4093979/.
71. Fathallah-Shaykh SA, Flynn JT, Pierce CB, Abraham AG, Blydt-Hansen TD, Massengill SF, et al. Progression of pediatric CKD of nonglomerular origin in the CKiD cohort. Clin J Am Soc Nephrol CJASN. 2015;10(4):571–7.
72. Zilleruelo G, Andia J, Gorman HM, Strauss J. Chronic renal failure in children: analysis of main causes and deterioration rate in 81 children. Int J Pediatr Nephrol. 1980;1(1):30–3.
73. Koshy SM, Hebert D, Lam K, Stukel TA, Guttmann A. Renal allograft loss during transition to adult healthcare services among pediatric renal transplant patients. Transplantation. 2009;87(11):1733–6.
74. O'Donohue W. Behavioral approaches to chronic disease in adolescence: a guide to integrative care. New York, NY: Springer-Verlag; 2009. 339 p.
75. Watson AR. Problems and pitfalls of transition from paediatric to adult renal care. Pediatr Nephrol Berl Ger. 2005;20(2):113–7.
76. Blydt-Hansen TD, Pierce CB, Cai Y, Samsonov D, Massengill S, Moxey-Mims M, et al. Medication treatment complexity and adherence in children with CKD. Clin J Am Soc Nephrol CJASN. 2014;9(2):247–54.
77. Supporting the Health Care Transition From Adolescence to Adulthood in the Medical Home. Pediatrics. 2011;128(1):182–200.
78. Watson AR, Harden PN, Ferris ME, Kerr PG, Mahan JD, Ramzy MF. Transition from pediatric to adult renal services: a consensus statement by the International Society of Nephrology (ISN) and the International Pediatric Nephrology Association (IPNA). Kidney Int. 2011;80(7):704–7.
79. Ferris ME, Cuttance JR, Javalkar K, Cohen SE, Phillips A, Bickford K, et al. Self-management and transition among adolescents/young adults with chronic or end-stage kidney disease. Blood Purif. 2015;39(1–3):99–104.
80. Bell L. Adolescents with renal disease in an adult world: meeting the challenge of transition of care. Nephrol Dial Transplant. 2007;22(4):988–91.

81. Huang JS, Gottschalk M, Pian M, Dillon L, Barajas D, Bartholomew LK. Transition to adult care: systematic assessment of adolescents with chronic illnesses and their medical teams. J Pediatr. 2011;159(6):994–998.e2.
82. Ku E, Johansen KL, Portale AA, Grimes B, Hsu C. State level variations in nephrology workforce and timing and incidence of dialysis in the United States among children and adults: a retrospective cohort study. BMC Nephrol [Internet]. 2015; 16. [Cited 2017 Oct 8]. Available from: https://www.ncbi.nlm.nih.gov/pmc/articles/PMC4361136/.

Chapter 2
Psychological Aspects and Challenges of Living with Chronic Kidney Disease for Adolescents

Sabrina A. Karczewski, Molly Keane, and Nishita Agarwal Berla

Introduction

While medical management is paramount in treating adolescents with chronic kidney disease (CKD), the importance of a multidisciplinary approach in addressing their psychological needs should not be underestimated. Adolescents with CKD and their families must simultaneously navigate normative developmental stressors while also managing a significant medical regimen burden. These youth tend to exhibit higher rates of medical non-adherence and are at risk of sustaining serious associated consequences including accelerated disease progression, prolonged dialysis, or loss of a kidney transplant. Relatedly, adolescents with CKD are at higher risk for negative psychosocial experiences including elevated symptoms of depression, anxiety, neurocognitive sequelae, sleep disturbance, social stress, family stress, and poorer quality of life. Because these psychological symptoms are also related to medical non-compliance and poorer health outcomes, it is crucial to properly assess and intervene in a timely manner. With incidences of CKD increasing

S. A. Karczewski (✉)
Department of Psychology,
Children's Hospital of Orange County (CHOC Children's), Orange, CA, USA
e-mail: skarczewski@choc.org

M. Keane
University of California, San Francisco (UCSF) Benioff Children's Hospital,
Pediatric Nephrology, San Francisco, CA, USA

N. Agarwal Berla
University of California, San Francisco (UCSF) Benioff Children's Hospital,
Pediatric Nephrology, San Francisco, CA, USA

Pacific Graduate School of Psychology (PGSP)/Stanford PsyD Consortium,
Palo Alto University, Palo Alto, CA, USA

M. N. Haddad et al. (eds.), *Adolescents with Chronic Kidney Disease*,
https://doi.org/10.1007/978-3-319-97220-6_2

and disproportionately effecting vulnerable populations (e.g., low-income and ethnic minority children), it is even more prudent to provide psychosocial support in the clinic setting to promote positive outcomes and multidisciplinary treatment planning [1–7]. In this chapter, we summarize literature on psychological aspects of living with CKD including adherence, psychiatric comorbidities, neurocognitive effects, sleep, quality of life, social functioning and peer relationships, caregiver needs, and transition to adulthood. Our primary aim is to elucidate psychosocial factors that have an impact on CKD management and health outcomes and present support for mental health assessment and intervention embedded in nephrology clinics.

Adherence

As medical interventions for youth with CKD and end-stage renal disease (ESRD) develop and improve over time, adolescents have opportunities to live longer and achieve improved quality of life (QOL) with consistent adherence to complex medical regimens [7, 8]. Although each regimen is personalized to an individual's needs, it is common for youth with CKD to take many medications that are dosed between once and several times per day [9]. A study by So and colleagues found that in their pediatric nephrology clinic, patients took an average of 5.7 medications (SD, 4.8), with increases in those numbers for adolescents who were on dialysis or who had been transplanted [10]. Most youth also require fluid and dietary restrictions including modifications of calorie, protein, fat, phosphorous, calcium, sodium, and potassium intake in order to manage malnutrition, mitigate overnutrition, and prevent other negative health outcomes [9, 11]. As kidney functioning declines, regimen tasks increase in amount and complexity; some patients are prescribed daily self-catheterization, blood pressure tracking, growth hormone injections, peritoneal dialysis, or hemodialysis [4]. Furthermore, regimen expectations are dynamic and fluid as medical teams responding to a patient's changing needs, resulting in changes to dietary recommendations or medication dosages. Adolescents and their families must also attend regular clinic appointments, have labs drawn, and maintain close contact with their medical teams.

Types of Non-adherence

Non-adherence occurs on a spectrum and for many different reasons [12–16]. For example, Rianthavorn and Ettenger describe "accidental non-compliers" whose non-adherence is characterized by forgetting, lack of organization, and insufficient reminders or cueing from family members [17]. In contrast, "invulnerable non-compliers," without immediate physical consequences of missed doses, feel invincible or believe that missing medications is not of concern. Finally, they describe "decisive non-compliers" in which a patient makes an active decision to ignore or avoid taking medication [17]. Lee and colleagues identified additional barriers to adherence (beliefs that the medications have too many side effects, difficulties with pill-swallowing, and not wanting to have others see the medication administration) that were all predictive of non-adherence, missed and late doses, out-of-range serum immunosuppressant levels, organ rejection, and death [18]. While the reasons behind non-adherence inform what intervention will be most effective, the unfortunate consequences of non-adherence are similar across groups.

Consequences of Non-adherence

Non-adherence results in significant consequences that promote poorer medical and psychosocial outcomes for the patient and family. Across pediatric chronic illness populations, medication non-adherence has been associated with higher frequency of emergency room visits and inpatient hospitalizations [19]. In CKD populations, non-adherence may expedite the progression and complications of kidney damage or failure, contribute to poor growth, decrease health-related QOL and psychosocial wellness, or delay transplant listing or activation of transplant status [9, 20]. For those who have had a kidney transplant, failure to follow one's regimen substantially increases the risk of organ rejection, the need to return to dialysis, worsened QOL, increased individual costs, and even death [21, 22].

Historical studies estimate that pediatric non-adherence to dialysis regimens ranges from 17% to 43% [23–25]. In the general pediatric transplant population, studies report 30–70% of youth demonstrate poor adherence [26] with the highest rates of non-adherence occurring in the adolescent age group [27]. Those results have been duplicated in the pediatric renal transplant literature, with studies showing that non-adherence is one of the strongest predictors of acute and chronic rejection [28]. In adolescence, 42% of renal transplant graft losses are due to non-adherence [29], and as a result, adolescents in the United States have the worst 5-year graft survival rates of all age groups (55% deceased donor; 72% living donor) [17].

Risk Factors for Non-adherence

Sociodemographic and Medical Risk Factors

The pediatric CKD literature identifies that one of the most prominent risk factors of poor adherence is being an adolescent [17, 30]. Just as healthy adolescents manage developmental milestones such as seeking autonomy and identity, so too do youth with CKD. However, adolescents with CKD may struggle to balance their propensities toward individuation and sense of invincibility with the reality of needing ongoing support and cooperation from caregiving adults and with the potential long-term health consequences of their choices [17, 31, 32]. In particular, the transition-to-adulthood phase is the most vulnerable time for youth with transplants [12, 32]. Watson demonstrated that 35% of adolescent transplant recipients unexpectedly lost their grafts when they transitioned to an adult transplant care center [33]. Additional risk factors for poorer adherence include living in a single-parent home, low socioeconomic status, and having public insurance [30, 34]. Medical risk factors for non-adherence include longer duration of dialysis treatment, adverse treatment side effects, and renal failure sequelae such as changes in taste or oral aversion that make dietary compliance more challenging [17, 35].

Health Literacy

Health literacy is a construct that has been linked to both adherence and health outcomes in CKD populations. In the general chronic illness literature, poor health literacy has been associated with increased hospitalization, emergency department visits, and non-adherence to preventative appointments and healthcare instructions (e.g., difficulty understanding nutrition or prescription labels, errors in dosing) [36]. Low health literacy among parents predicts worse health outcomes for children with a chronic illness and is more likely to occur in individuals with English as a second language, ethnic and cultural minorities, and lower educational attainment and for those with low socioeconomic status [20, 31]. Preliminary data suggests these concerns extend to pediatric nephrology clinics [37].

Psychological Risk Factors

Psychological challenges constitute additional risk factors for non-adherence among adolescents with CKD. A comprehensive review of literature for the broader chronic illness population showed that patients with depression are three times more likely to be noncompliant with medical treatments than non-depressed patients [38]. Shaw and colleagues demonstrated similar findings in a study of pediatric patients with transplanted kidneys: data showed that 30% of patients who were considered "severely non-adherent" had a diagnosis of major depressive disorder, and more than half had other depressive symptomatology [28]. Other psychological risk factors for non-adherence in adolescents with kidney transplants include excessive anger, anxiety, posttraumatic stress, substance use, cognitive development, and executive functioning [17, 18, 23, 39–41].

Family Environment

Although adolescents show emerging independence in many domains, sustained family involvement remains crucial for youth with chronic illnesses, as it predicts increased adherence to treatment regimens [42]. Low family involvement in the treatment plan, family conflict, and external family stressors are among the documented risk factors for poor adherence in adolescents with CKD [16, 23]. In fact, although it may seem counterintuitive to values of promoting independence in adolescent youth, a study by Zelikovsky and colleagues demonstrated that when parents of adolescent transplant recipients participated in the medical regimen, patients had better adherence than if the adolescents had the sole responsibility [16]. Families can also face adherence barriers including difficulty accessing regimen recommendations (e.g., high-protein diets, time and transportation to multiple clinic visits, out-of-pocket medication/procedure costs), for which families should connect with the multidisciplinary team and social worker to problem-solve these challenges [35].

Assessment and Intervention

Assessment of adherence in the adolescent CKD population is difficult due to the various treatment components involved in the medical regimen and the likelihood that many patients are adhering to some, but not all, recommendations [23]. A multimodal assessment is recommended to balance patient and parent self-report with objective measures such as pill counts or refill rates, blood-level trough monitoring, lab values, and frequency of cancelled or no-show clinic appointments [17, 43]. Additional technology is being studied to more objectively assess adherence such as electronic pill bottles for medication monitoring [44] and the Baxter Procard to track dialysis machine usage [45].

Medical regimen adjustments can be made to address treatment barriers including reduction of dosing frequency and avoiding medications with adverse side effects (e.g., steroid-free protocols) [17]. Although health literacy is an important predictor of adherence, studies show that multicomponent interventions with a targeted behavioral piece are more effective than education interventions, alone, in pediatric chronic illness populations [42, 46]. Collaborating with families to create organizational plans including use of a pillbox, identifying environmental cues (e.g., having a designated medication area in the home), setting alarms and writing reminders, pairing medication administration with a habit activity (e.g., brushing teeth), and tracking appointments or medications on a calendar or app may all be helpful in improving adherence [17]. Clinicians can support parents in cuing, maintaining involvement and monitoring, making behavioral contingency plans in which patients are reinforced for adherence, using organizational strategies, and cooperating with family monitoring.

Because chronic non-adherence likely reflects additional motivational, psychological, and/or family-related problems, patients should be referred to pediatric psychologists to develop evidence-based therapeutic treatment plans [17, 47]. Cognitive behavioral treatment elements such as coping skills instruction, structured problem-solving, and social support interventions are also effective in increasing adherence in pediatric chronic illness populations [42, 48, 49]. Motivational interviewing is an evidence-based intervention that can be used in tandem with other therapies and has shown improvement in health behaviors by focusing on eliciting "change talk" to promote patient-motivated adherence [50, 51]. Additional research supports an adapted version of dialectical behavior therapy for chronic medical illnesses (DBT-CMI) that considers non-adherence as a life-limiting factor and identifies it as its primary treatment target [52, 53].

Psychological Comorbidity

It is well documented that both adults and children with chronic illness have higher prevalence of mental health burden than their healthy peers in symptom areas such as depression, anxiety, and behavior problems [54–58]. Research on adults with CKD suggests much higher rates of depression (20–40%), with even higher prevalence for those on dialysis, and only a fraction are treated with antidepressant medication or psychotherapy [59–64]. The psychological comorbidities within adolescents with CKD have been less studied, but research shows an overall trend of psychological adjustment challenges (e.g., body image, self-esteem), higher levels of depressive symptoms, and mixed results regarding anxiety and behavior concerns. Bakr and colleagues demonstrated that the overall prevalence of psychological disorders in youth with renal failure was 52.6%, with a higher prevalence in patients undergoing dialysis than those who were on pre-dialysis and particularly high rates in those on hemodialysis [65]. They found that common disorders included adjustment disorders (18.4%), depression (10.3%), and anxiety (5.1%). Further, Berney-Martinet and colleagues confirmed overall higher rates of lifetime psychiatric disorders in those with pediatric renal failure but noted even higher prevalence rates among those with a kidney transplant [66]. These psychological symptoms are important to evaluate and address given the evidence, suggesting strong associations between psychological problems and QOL, adherence, and health outcomes [28].

General Emotional Functioning and Adjustment

In the context of increased attention to health, demands for self-care, school absences, and familial stress, general emotional functioning and adjustment have the potential to be more challenging for adolescents with CKD than for their healthy peers [67, 68]. Based on the national Chronic Kidney Disease in Children Study (CKiD), Gerson and colleagues found 20% of youth with CKD reported significant problems in emotional functioning [69]. While some studies suggest an older adolescent age is protective, others note that those diagnosed with CKD in later adolescence have more difficulty adjusting to their diagnosis [69, 70]. CKD sequelae and treatment may result in visible physical changes to adolescents' face and body, as well as physical capabilities, which are often of great importance in their concepts of self-identity and confidence. In particular, growth restriction and edema in adolescents with CKD have been associated with increased stress, lower self-esteem, depression, anxiety, and poor QOL [29, 69, 71–73]. Although research shows that severity of kidney dysfunction may not directly correlate with severity of adolescent psychological concerns [68], studies also suggest that those on dialysis report poorer psychosocial wellness [74].

Depression

A higher point prevalence of depression (10–35%) in adolescents with CKD has been found in comparison with that of the general adolescent population (7.5%) [65, 66, 75–77]. However, in a recent, multi-site study, researchers found similar levels of depression in youth with CKD as in the general population [78]. Subclinical depressive symptoms may be much more widespread and can have an influence on patient QOL and outcomes [23, 24, 79]. For instance, in a study of youth undergoing dialysis, Hernandez and colleagues found that while only 10.5% of youth reported high depressive symptomatology, 43.5% of youth reported some depressive features [75]. Additional subclinical depressive features identified in the literature include guilt, anger, poor self-worth, and bereavement related to organ rejection [40, 68, 75]. Preliminary research notes that a risk factor for elevated depression is recent hospitalization [72], while protective factors are family environment and maternal education [67, 77]. Unfortunately, the stigma of mental health conditions as well as focus on the primary medical condition may prevent families from seeking intervention; in one study, researchers found that fewer than half of parents consulted their nephrologist about concerns of their child having depression [77].

Anxiety

Sparse research has been published on anxiety within the adolescent CKD population, and results are mixed. While some studies report equivalent rates of global anxiety with healthy peers [80, 81], others note higher rates of separation anxiety in youth with CKD [79, 82]. Subclinical manifestations of anxiety described in the literature include anxiety related to illness uncertainty and concerns about current and future health status [39, 68]. Although perhaps not greater in magnitude or frequency than the general population, adolescents receiving hemodialysis appear to have the highest levels of anxiety in the CKD population [81]. Despite disparate research findings, screening for anxiety remains a priority in the CKD population given its association with difficulty with symptom management, tolerance of procedures, non-adherence, medical outcomes, and poorer health-related QOL [55, 79, 81, 83].

Behavioral Concerns

Outcomes research on behavioral domains in adolescents with CKD is also rare, and results are mixed. Several studies show no differences between externalizing behavior among adolescents with CKD and the normal population, and some even suggest risk-taking aggression, and conduct problems may be lower than normative populations [80, 84]. However some studies demonstrate much higher rates of conduct concerns including a Brazilian study listing 54% of CKD participants with parent-reported conduct problems [85]. Some researchers note specific subsets of the CKD population that struggle with externalizing symptoms more than others. For example, Soliday and colleagues found that children with steroid-sensitive nephrotic syndrome (SSNS) were more likely to have clinically significant levels of externalizing (e.g., behavioral) symptoms well after steroid termination than the general population [67]. Further research in these areas is needed in order to clarify whether and in what ways behavioral concerns may be different in the CKD population than others.

Assessment and Intervention

As is true in the general population, adolescents with CKD are likely to respond differently to questions and surveys about their own mental health than their parents might report on their behalf [84]. It is crucial, then, to use multiple informants when assessing psychological comorbidities in order to best ascertain symptoms, severity, and their disruption of social functioning, adherence, and health outcomes. Standard screening for depression is recommended in renal clinics, given that evidence suggests high prevalence and that those struggling with these symptoms may not volunteer them or seek support [77, 86]. Several standardized symptom measures have been validated for use with the pediatric CKD population including the Child Behavior Checklist (CBCL), the Behavioral Assessment System for Children (BASC), Children's Depression Inventory (CDI), Patient Health Questionnaire-9 (PHQ-9), Generalized Anxiety Disorder Screener (GAD-7), PedsQL, Strengths and Difficulties Questionnaire (SDQ), and the Child Health and Illness Profile (CHIP-AE) [84, 87]. When concerning psychological symptoms are identified or suspected, it is recommended to consult a pediatric psychologist or other qualified mental health provider with experience in chronic illness who can provide evidence-based psychotherapy that has shown positive outcomes for adolescents (e.g., cognitive behavioral therapy (CBT), behavioral family systems therapy (BFST), acceptance and commitment therapy (ACT), dialectical behavior therapy (DBT)) [23, 52, 53].

Neurocognitive Considerations

Much of the research on neurocognitive sequelae of pediatric CKD is disparate regarding subpopulations studied (e.g., mild to moderate CKD vs. dialysis vs. transplant), mixed age ranges and demographics, and measures used, making aggregate analysis or cross comparison challenging [88, 89]. As a result the overall literature on neurocognitive outcomes of CKD is mixed. While a full review is beyond the scope of this chapter, an overview of apparent trends in the data is discussed below.

Regarding intelligence, research generally demonstrates that youth with CKD have a somewhat lower IQ quotient than healthy peers, typically falling in the low average to average range, with similar slight disparities spanning across both verbal and visuospatial domains [4, 90–93]. Skills of attention, executive functioning, and memory appear to be the most consistently compromised neurocognitive functions in the pediatric CKD population. Specifically, researchers have found that youth with CKD tend to have low average performance in sustained attention regulation and complex auditory attention as compared to healthy peers' average scores. Similar low to low average areas of deficit include executive functions such as initiation, inhibition, and sustained effort [88, 90, 94]. Additional areas of challenge may include short-term visual and verbal memory, working memory, and facial affect recognition [90, 92, 93]. Studies have also shown somewhat poorer academic achievement in the average to low average range among youth with CKD when compared with healthy peers, specifically in areas of math, spelling, and reading that are likely secondary to additional neurocognitive challenges [88, 91]. This in addition to medical demands may explain their higher incidence of learning difficulties, grade retention, and absenteeism at school [4, 91, 93].

Medical Risk and Protective Factors

The pediatric CKD literature has presented various risk factors for the development and severity of neurocognitive sequelae. Younger age of CKD onset, early age malnutrition, and longer duration of disease have been associated with poorer global neurocognitive functioning [88]. Duration of disease was specifically found to increase the risk of neurocognitive deficits, particularly with regard to inhibitory control, visual vigilance, and attention regulation [95, 96]. Researchers also found that while neurocognitive associations with modality of treatment were mixed (conservative treatment vs. dialysis), severity of renal disease as measured by glomerular filtration rate (GFR) was directly associated with impairments in memory, executive function, emotion identification, and academic achievement [4, 93, 95, 97, 98]. Additionally, proteinuria and hypertension in this population have been associated with lower IQ scores and visual-spatial construction and organization [93, 99]. Interestingly, several studies show partial recovery of neurocognitive deficits after a kidney transplant (when GFR levels have normalized), with specific improvement areas of intellectual functioning, academic functioning, processing speed, and sustained attention [100–102]. However, residual deficits often cause adolescents to remain at a lower cognitive level than peers after transplant, and further research is needed to better understand this phenomenon of why some patients recover neurocognitive function while others do not [88].

Assessment and Intervention

Early identification and treatment of cognitive challenges are beneficial given the progressive nature of CKD, as well as research-driven associations among cognitive impairment, adherence, and school performance [4, 73, 90, 103, 104]. Neurocognitive screenings subsequent to parent or school concerns of verbal, visual, attention, and executive functioning performance are recommended in order to identify even mild deficits, as they can progress with poor kidney functioning and may remain present even with medical treatment. Unfortunately, deficits in these areas of functioning, particularly attention and executive functioning, have negative implications for an adolescent's ability to manage a complex medical regimen and can interfere with academic learning, standardized testing, performance in higher education, and job performance. Through the school district or institution, these authors recommend that care teams advocate for adolescents to obtain 504 plans, individual education plans (IEP), or equivalent written accommodations in order to ensure they receive appropriate and equal access to education in the context of their medical/neurocognitive challenges.

Sleep

Sleep is a particularly important construct in the adolescent developmental stage given its role in supporting brain maturation and psychosocial outcomes. In the context of puberty-driven changes to circadian regulation and more independent sleep hygiene habits, many adolescents do not get enough sleep [105, 106]. Further, sleep deprivation has been shown to have deleterious effects on adolescent regulatory capacities such as those for mood, attention, behavior, and academic performance [106].

For adolescents with CKD, these concerns are compounded, with studies showing 25–58.5% of youth with CKD report sleep disturbance, with higher incidences of complaints among those on dialysis [107–110]. Medical factors may partially explain this phenomenon. For instance, researchers notice a strong connection between GFR and symptoms of fatigue, weakness, and daytime somnolence [7]. Extending these findings to adolescents, Roumellioti and colleagues found a strong correlation between low GFR and sleep disturbance, indicating that the higher the stage of CKD, the more severe the sleep disturbance [111]. Adolescents in the later stages of CKD and/or those who are obese may also experience more arousals, apneas, and limb movements (e.g., restless leg syndrome) [111, 112]. Psychological factors including adjustment to a new diagnosis in adolescence or illness uncertainty may also influence adolescents' abilities to fall asleep [39, 111].

Given the high concurrence of sleep disruptions and depressed mood, poorer cognitive and memory performance, low academic achievement, increased risky behavior, and decreased QOL, regular evaluation and intervention of sleep disturbance are necessary to ensure overall patient wellness [112, 113]. Non-pharmacologic sleep interventions are typically a first-line defense. Educational and organizational problem-solving may include sleep hygiene education and incorporating regular sleep-wake routines [114, 115]. Additional cognitive-behavioral interventions also address unhelpful cognitions about sleep and focus on changing the sleep environment through stimulus control (e.g., only using the bed for sleep) [106, 116].

Quality of Life

Although many definitions of quality of life (QOL) have been proposed in the literature, the unifying theme includes subjective assessment of one's overall satisfaction with life across multiple domains (physical, psychological, social, etc.) [117, 118]. For adolescents with CKD, whose complexity and intensity of treatment and diet plans often correlate to their stage of CKD, the medical demands placed on them can be experienced as intrusive. Furthermore, physiological discomfort from kidney failure, medication and treatment side effects, activity restrictions, chronically invasive procedures (e.g., dialysis), frequency of clinic visits, school absences, and CKD-related cognitive and psychosocial problems can interfere with an adolescent's overall sense of well-being and normalcy [7, 72, 119].

Internationally, the literature is consistent in identifying that youth with CKD report lower QOL than both other chronic illness populations (e.g., diabetes, cardiac conditions, asthma) and healthy controls [70, 79, 120–125]. Many studies demonstrate that adolescents on dialysis report poorer QOL than those receiving other modes of treatment [74, 123, 126]. The literature is mixed regarding whether those on hemodialysis have a different QOL than those on peritoneal dialysis [123, 125]. Most studies find that the QOL for those who have had a transplant is rated more positively, with one study in Zurich finding that adolescents with a functioning transplant rated QOL higher even than healthy controls (e.g., [7, 127]). International data is mixed, though, regarding comparisons of QOL between adolescents on dialysis and those who have had a transplant, potentially reflecting local and cultural differences in subjective perceptions of comparative health and wellness [121, 122, 124, 126, 128–130].

It is no surprise that as kidney function declines, so do patient reports of QOL [74]. Additional specific medical risk factors that promote lower QOL in the CKD population include albumin and hematocrit levels, anemia, short stature, and rejection episodes and hospitalizations [40, 69, 74, 87]. Furthermore, psychological concerns including depression and anxiety and behavioral concerns appear to coexist with and exacerbate low QOL [78, 85, 131]. Frequent assessment of QOL is needed in order to best care for an adolescent's overall wellness, evaluate the current treatment plan, promote intervention to alter treatment, introduce supplemental supports, or problem-solve barriers to comfort.

Social Functioning and Peer Relationships

As adolescents' desire to "fit in" and discover one's identity develops, peer relationships and social support become paramount in shaping their experiences. In the pediatric chronic illness literature, social interaction has been characterized as both an opportunity for resilience and an area for potential challenge [132]. On one hand, positive social support has been shown to greatly improve QOL for adolescents with CKD and can serve as a protective factor against internalizing symptoms (e.g., depression, anxiety) [133]. On the other hand, many adolescents with CKD may have difficulty accessing or developing social support due to well-documented physical changes, poorer body image and self-esteem, and generally feeling different than their peers.

Adolescents with chronic illness have poorer social functioning than their healthy peers, in part because of lack of proximity given the amount of time they spend at medical appointments, procedures, in the hospital, or home-schooled [132, 134]. In the CKD population, several studies have indicated poorer social functioning among youth with CKD than healthy peers, especially for those on dialysis [30, 70, 135]. Garralda and colleagues found that youth on dialysis were the least likely of all pediatric CKD participants to have close social relationships [76].

Adolescents have reported feeling self-conscious or "different" than peers due to physical changes related to CKD (i.e., edema and short stature) that can impact body image, self-esteem, and social functioning [69, 72, 136]. Adolescents recently diagnosed with CKD or with worsening kidney function may need to shift their identity self-perception, adjust to new functional limitations, and cope with vulnerability [70, 137]. Those who have been diagnosed for some time may also feel disconnected from peers and unable to relate given prognostic uncertainty and insecurity [70]. Evidence also demonstrates that youth with CKD are treated differently than healthy peers, a barrier for social engagement. An interview-based study found that adolescents with CKD who had short stature, obesity, and/or appeared younger than their chronological age reported being teased or bullied throughout their childhood and felt as if they were treated differently by teachers [137].

Assessment of social functioning, support, and barriers is needed to prevent the unfortunate long-term effects of poor social functioning into adulthood including lack of close relationships and decreased employment rates [23, 138, 139]. However, data suggests that growth in height and use of growth hormone is associated with improvements in social functioning [140]. Having a transplant after experiencing dialysis may improve associated social barriers due to less time spent in isolation and greater freedom with activity participation (e.g., sports) [23, 30].

Caregiver Adjustment

Many professionals who work within the pediatric chronic illness population note that "the entire family is the patient" due to the undeniable importance of caregivers and family support in maintaining wellness as well as the influence of illness on family functioning. While any chronic illness onset fundamentally increases caregiver stress, advancements made in CKD survival and home-based therapies require parents to take on an additional role as healthcare providers (e.g., peritoneal dialysis, transportation to hemodialysis, feeds at home, catheterization, dressing changes) [23, 67, 85, 141–143]. Parents of youth with CKD generally report an overall lower QOL, reporting difficulties managing their child's care and higher levels of stress, anxiety, and depression [144, 145], with parents of youth on dialysis reporting the poorest outcomes [146]. Specifically, parents report challenges coping with uncertainty about prognosis and the future, vigilance related to symptom management, and fatigue [147]. Time spent on an adolescent's medical regimen can interfere with a parent's ability to maintain a social support network, engage in self-care, and contribute to family income [141]. Parent adjustment is an area of importance given research in pediatric chronic illness that demonstrates that parent QOL and mental health may have an influence on adolescent psychosocial well-being and medical outcomes [148].

Screening of parent and family wellness at regular intervals can help to identify concerns and trigger linkage with services that can offer respite, support caregiver burnout and mental health, and improve QOL [4]. Little research was found on interventions for caregivers of youth with CKD beyond educational support [144, 149, 150]. However, drawing from the general pediatric chronic illness literature, evidence-based approaches including caregiver problem-solving therapy (PST) and cognitive behavioral therapy (CBT) have been effective at improving caregiver mental health and indirectly reducing child distress (e.g., pain) across studies [151].

Transition to Adulthood

Adolescents and emerging adults must simultaneously manage the developmental transition to adulthood while also navigating the transition to adult healthcare services. Although patients may be considered adults at 18 years of age, this period from 18 to 25 is fraught with ongoing development of social maturity, emotional regulation, delayed gratification, and inhibition of sensation-seeking tendencies [152–155]. The developmental stage of transition to adulthood in a healthy population is a vulnerable one with increases in rates of substance abuse, mental health disorders, suicide, domestic violence, and risky sexual activity [130, 152]. Research demonstrates that this transitional period is an especially fragile time for adolescents and young adults (AYAs) with CKD, given higher rates of cognitive delay and resultant non-adherence, organ rejection, and poorer QOL [12, 32, 33, 156, 157]. There is a spectrum of behaviors observed with some AYAs exhibiting non-adherence due to burnout and invincibility, while others may struggle with a transfer of responsibility and independence that they are not ready for, having taken on the "sick role" for so long in the family [12, 155, 158]. Thus, the roles of the family and care team in this transition are crucial, and literature recommends they start early (ages 10–14 recommended) by scaffolding and offering graded education and responsibility over time [4, 9, 159, 160]. In fact, research demonstrates that environmental structure and supports (e.g., family cohesion and having a 504/individual education plan) are resiliency factors that appear protective in health outcomes for AYAs with CKD [34, 160]. A number of standardized measures and interviews may be useful in addressing both general transition topics and CKD-specific aims [152, 161]: STARx transition-readiness survey [162, 163], the clinician-administered TRxANSITION Scale [164], Transition Health-Care Assessment tool, Transition Readiness Assessment Questionnaire (TRAQ) [165], Healthy and Ready to Work (HRTW) [166], and the Readiness for Transition Questionnaire (RTQ) [167]. Published guidelines for healthcare transition may be useful in framing clinic procedures, timing transfer in accordance with readiness of patient, and guiding families and receiving adult providers regarding areas of challenge, resiliency, and ongoing goals of care [168, 169]. A more comprehensive review of the literature and the recommendations are available in the "Transitioning Care of the Adolescent Patient to Adult Providers" chapter.

Conclusion

Having a diagnosis of CKD during adolescence, regardless of severity or treatment modality, interrupts normative development and is associated with psychosocial stressors for the patient and family. Changes in physical functioning, identity, expectations, and family roles overlaid on the normal challenges of the adolescent developmental period convey additional stress on the patient and family system. Although adherence to medical regimen is crucial to the preservation of renal health, many adolescents and families struggle with the educational, organizational, and motivational components of good adherence. Adjustment challenges and depression are the most common psychological comorbidities for adolescents with CKD, and they are more likely to demonstrate comparative challenges with neurocognitive abilities. Additionally, adolescents with CKD may experience decreased growth rates, sleep disturbances, and social challenges that contribute to poorer overall QOL. Given these factors' potential interference with treatment adherence and QOL, these authors recommend a strong mental health provider presence in pediatric nephrology clinics, particularly for those patients who are on dialysis or are considering transplant. Pediatric psychologists can perform data-driven assessments and can apply evidence-based therapies that promote improved adherence, psychosocial well-being, family functioning, and positive medical outcomes. Further research is needed in adapting and applying these approaches to the CKD population in time- and cost-effective methods that reach as many youth as possible (e.g., dialysis clinic-based services, adolescent therapeutic groups).

References

1. Sinha A, Srivastava RN. Chronic kidney disease. In: Pediatric nephrology. 6th ed. New Delhi: Jaypee brothers medical publishers (P) ltd; 2016; 374–413.
2. United States Renal Data System. 2016 USRDS annual data report: Epidemiology of kidney disease in the United States. Bethesda, MD: National Institutes of Health, National Institute of Diabetes and Digestive and Kidney Diseases; 2016.
3. Choi AI, Rodriguez RA, Bacchetti P, Bertenthal D, Hernandez GT, O'Hare AM. White/black racial differences in risk of end-stage renal disease and death. Am J Med. 2009;122(7):672–8.
4. Massengill SF, Ferris M. Chronic kidney disease in children and adolescents. Pediatr Rev. 2014;35(1):16–29.
5. Harambat J, van Stralen KJ, Kim JJ, Tizard EJ. Epidemiology of chronic kidney disease in children. Pediatr Nephrol. Springer-Verlag. 2012;27(3):363–73.
6. Yach D, Stuckler D, Brownell KD. Epidemiologic and economic consequences of the global epidemics of obesity and diabetes. Nat Med. 2006;62(6)
7. Jayaraman R, Van der Voort J. Principles of management of chronic kidney disease. Paediatr Child Health (Oxford) [Internet]. 2010 [cited 2017 May 31];20(6):291–6. Available from: http://www.sciencedirect.com/science/article/pii/S175172221000079X.
8. Griffin KJ, Elkin TD. Non-adherence in pediatric transplantation: a review of the existing literature. Pediatr Transplant [Internet]. 2001 [cited 2017 May 31];5(4):246–9. Available from: http://doi.wiley.com/10.1034/j.1399-3046.2001.005004246.x.
9. Akchurin OM, Schneider MF, Mulqueen L, Brooks ER, Langman CB, Greenbaum LA, et al. Medication adherence and growth in children with CKD. Clin J Am Soc Nephrol [Internet]. 2014 [cited 2017 May 31];9(9):1519–25. Available from: http://www.ncbi.nlm.nih.gov/pubmed/24970873.
10. So T-Y, Bradley Layton J, Bozik K, Farrington E, Gipson PE, Gibson K, et al. Cognitive pharmacy services at a pediatric nephrology and hypertension clinic. Ren Fail [Internet]. 2011 [cited 2017 May 31];33(1):19–25. Available from: http://www.tandfonline.com/doi/full/10.3109/0886022X.2010.536291.

11. Levitt R, Zaritsky JJ, Mak RH. Nutritional challenges in pediatric chronic kidney disease. In: Pediatric kidney disease [Internet]. Berlin: Springer Berlin Heidelberg; 2016 [cited 2017 May 31]. p. 1477–505. Available from: http://link.springer.com/10.1007/978-3-662-52972-0_56.
12. Diaz-Gonzalez de Ferris ME. Adolescents and emerging adults with chronic kidney disease: their unique morbidities and adherence issues. Blood Purif [Internet]. 2011 [cited 2017 May 31];31(1–3):203–8. Available from: http://www.ncbi.nlm.nih.gov/pubmed/21228591.
13. Hanghøj S, Boisen KA. Self-reported barriers to medication adherence among chronically ill adolescents: a systematic review. J Adolesc Heal [Internet]. 2014 [cited 2017 May 31];54(2):121–38. Available from: http://www.sciencedirect.com/science/article/pii/S1054139X1300462X.
14. Simons LE, McCormick ML, Mee LL, Blount RL. Parent and patient perspectives on barriers to medication adherence in adolescent transplant recipients. Pediatr Transplant [Internet]. 2009 [cited 2017 May 31];13(3):338–47. Available from: http://doi.wiley.com/10.1111/j.1399-3046.2008.00940.x.
15. Vasylyeva T L., Singh R, Sheehan C, Chennasamudram SP, Hernandez AP. Self-reported adherence to medications in a pediatric renal clinic: psychological aspects. Rypma B, editor PLoS One [Internet] 2013 [cited 2017 May 31];8(7):e69060. Available from: http://dx.plos.org/10.1371/journal.pone.0069060.
16. Zelikovsky N, Schast AP, Palmer J, Meyers KEC. Perceived barriers to adherence among adolescent renal transplant candidates. Pediatr Transplant [Internet]. 2008 [cited 2017 May 31];12(3):300–8. Available from: http://doi.wiley.com/10.1111/j.1399-3046.2007.00886.x.
17. Rianthavorn P, Ettenger RB. Medication non-adherence in the adolescent renal transplant recipient: a clinician's viewpoint. Pediatr Transplant [Internet]. 2005 [cited 2017 May 31];9(3):398–407. Available from: http://doi.wiley.com/10.1111/j.1399-3046.2005.00358.x.
18. Lee JL, Eaton C, Gutierrez-Colina AM, Devine K, Simons LE, Mee L, et al. Longitudinal stability of specific barriers to medication adherence. J Pediatr Psychol [Internet]. 2014 [cited 2017 May 31];39(7):667–76. Available from: https://academic.oup.com/jpepsy/article-lookup/doi/10.1093/jpepsy/jsu026.
19. McGrady ME, Hommel KA. Medication adherence and health care utilization in pediatric chronic illness: a systematic review. Pediatrics [Internet]. 2013 [cited 2017 May 31];132(4) 730–40. Available from: http://pediatrics.aappublications.org/content/132/4/730.short.
20. Chironda G, Bhengu B. Contributing factors to non-adherence among chronic kidney disease (CKD) patients: a systematic review of literature. Med Clin Rev [Internet]. 2016 [cited 2017 May 31];2(4). Available from: http://medical-clinical-reviews.imedpub.com/contributing-factors-to-nonadherence-among-chronic-kidney-disease-ckdpatients-a-systematic-review-of-literature.php?aid=17499.
21. Butler JA, Roderick P, Mullee M, Mason JC, Peveler RC. Frequency and impact of nonadherence to immunosuppressants after renal transplantation: a systematic review. Transplantation [Internet]. 2004;77(5):769–76. Available from: http://content.wkhealth.com/linkback/openurl?sid=WKPTLP:landingpage&an=00007890-200403150-00025.
22. Pinsky BW, Takemoto SK, Lentine KL, Burroughs TE, Schnitzler MA, Salvalaggio PR. Transplant outcomes and economic costs associated with patient noncompliance to immunosuppression. Am J Transplant [Internet]. 2009 [cited 2017 May 31];9(11):2597–606. Available from: http://doi.wiley.com/10.1111/j.1600-6143.2009.02798.x.
23. Pai ALH, Ingerski LM. Psychosocial adjustment and adherence of children and adolescents on dialysis. In: Pediatric dialysis [Internet]. Boston: Springer US; 2012 [cited 2017 May 31]. p. 593–605. Available from: http://link.springer.com/10.1007/978-1-4614-0721-8_30
24. Simoni JM, Asarnow JR, Munford PR, Koprowski CM, Belin TR, Salusky IB. Psychological distress and treatment adherence among children on dialysis. Pediatr Nephrol [Internet]. 1997 [cited 2017 May 31];11(5):604–6. Available from: http://link.springer.com/10.1007/s004670050346.
25. Hudson J, Fielding D, Jones S, McKendrick T. Adherence to medical regime and related factors in youngsters on dialysis. Br J Clin Psychol [Internet]. 1987 [cited 2017 May 31];26(1):61–2. Available from: http://doi.wiley.com/10.1111/j.2044-8260.1987.tb00725.x.

26. Lefkowitz DS, Fitzgerald CJ, Zelikovsky N, Barlow K, Wray J. Best practices in the pediatric pretransplant psychosocial evaluation. Pediatr Transplant [Internet]. 2014 [cited 2017 May 31];18(4):327–35. Available from: http://doi.wiley.com/10.1111/petr.12260.
27. Stone D, Banerjee M, Dupuis J, Leleszi J, Allasio D, Singh TP. Association of parental pretransplant psychosocial assessment with post-transplant morbidity in pediatric heart transplant recipients. Pediatr Transplant [Internet]. 2006 [cited 2017 May 31];10(5):602–7. Available from: http://onlinelibrary.wiley.com/doi/10.1111/j.1399-3046.2006.00543.x/full.
28. Shaw RJ, Palmer L, Blasey C, Sarwal M. A typology of non-adherence in pediatric renal transplant recipients. Pediatr Transplant [Internet]. 2003 [cited 2017 May 31];7(6):489–93. Available from: http://doi.wiley.com/10.1046/j.1397-3142.2003.00117.x.
29. Kelly DA. Current issues in pediatric transplantation. Pediatr Transplant [Internet]. 2006 [cited 2017 May 31];10(6):712–20. Available from: http://doi.wiley.com/10.1111/j.1399-3046.2006.00567.x.
30. Brownbridge G, Fielding DM. Psychosocial adjustment and adherence to dialysis treatment regimes. Pediatr Nephrol [Internet]. 1994 [cited 2017 May 31];8(6):744–9. Available from: http://link.springer.com/10.1007/BF00869109.
31. Ferris ME, Patel UD, Massengill S, Gipson D, Conley W, Layton JB, et al. Pediatric chronic kidney disease in North Carolina. N C Med J [Internet]. 2008 [cited 2017 May 31];69(3):208–14. Available from: http://www.ncbi.nlm.nih.gov/pubmed/18751354.
32. Kaspar CDW, Bholah R, Bunchman TE. A review of pediatric chronic kidney disease. Blood Purif [Internet]. 2016 [cited 2017 May 31];41(1–3):211–7. Available from: http://www.ncbi.nlm.nih.gov/pubmed/26766175.
33. Watson AR. Non-compliance and transfer from paediatric to adult transplant unit. Pediatr Nephrol [Internet]. 2000 [cited 2017 May 31];14(6):0469–72. Available from: http://link.springer.com/10.1007/s004670050794.
34. Javalkar K, Fenton N, Cohen S, Ferris M. Socioecologic factors as predictors of readiness for self-management and transition, medication adherence, and health care utilization among adolescents and young adults with chronic kidney disease. Prev Chronic Dis [Internet]. 2014 [cited 2017 May 31];11:E117. Available from: http://www.ncbi.nlm.nih.gov/pubmed/25010999.
35. Terrill CJ. Nutrition and the pediatric patient with CKD. Nephrol Nurs J [Internet]. 2007 [cited 2017 May 31];34(1) 77–82. Available from: http://search.proquest.com/openview/c7db52beaa51e019dff4fa1c57c36d09/1?pq-origsite=gscholar&cbl=45638.
36. Benyon K. Health literacy. InnovAiT Educ Inspir Gen Pract [Internet]. 2014 [cited 2017 May 31];7(7):437–40. Available from: http://ino.sagepub.com/lookup/doi/10.1177/1755738014532627.
37. Rak EC, Hooper SR, Belsante MJ, Burnett O, Layton B, Tauer D, et al. Caregiver word reading literacy and health outcomes among children treated in a pediatric nephrology practice. Clin Kidney J [Internet]. 2016 [cited 2017 May 31];9(3):510–5. Available from: https://academic.oup.com/ckj/article-lookup/doi/10.1093/ckj/sfw015.
38. DiMatteo MR, Haskard-Zolnierek KB, Martin LR. Improving patient adherence: a three-factor model to guide practice. Health Psychol Rev [Internet]. 2012 [cited 2017 May 31];6(1):74–91. Available from: http://www.tandfonline.com/doi/abs/10.1080/17437199.2010.537592.
39. Maikranz JM, Steele RG, Dreyer ML, Stratman AC, Bovaird JA. The relationship of hope and illness-related uncertainty to emotional adjustment and adherence among pediatric renal and liver transplant recipients. J Pediatr Psychol [Internet]. 2006 [cited 2017 May 31];32(5):571–81. Available from: https://academic.oup.com/jpepsy/article-lookup/doi/10.1093/jpepsy/jsl046.
40. Muehrer RJ, Becker BN. Life after transplantation: new transitions in quality of life and psychological distress. Semin Dial. Blackwell Science Inc. 2005;18:124–31.
41. Lansing AH, Berg CA. Topical review: adolescent self-regulation as a foundation for chronic illness self-management. J Pediatr Psychol [Internet]. 2014 [cited 2017 May 31];39(10):1091–6. Available from: https://academic.oup.com/jpepsy/article-lookup/doi/10.1093/jpepsy/jsu067.

42. Kahana SY, Frazier TW, Drotar D. Preliminary quantitative investigation of predictors of treatment non-adherence in pediatric transplantation: a brief report. Pediatr Transplant [Internet]. 2008 [cited 2017 May 31];12(6):656–60. Available from: http://doi.wiley.com/10.1111/j.1399-3046.2007.00864.x.
43. Apostolou A, Karagiozoglou-Lampoudi T. Dietary adherence in children with chronic kidney disease: a review of the evidence. J Ren Care. 2014;40(2):125–30.
44. Pai ALH, Rausch J, Tackett A, Marsolo K, Drotar D, Goebel J. System for integrated adherence monitoring: real-time non-adherence risk assessment in pediatric kidney transplantation. Pediatr Transplant [Internet]. 2012 [cited 2017 May 31];16(4):329–34. Available from: http://doi.wiley.com/10.1111/j.1399-3046.2012.01657.x.
45. Lee AJ, Kho K, Chia K-S, Oi T-L, Yap C, Foong P-P, et al. Simulating inadequate dialysis and its correction using an individualized patient-derived nomogram. Pediatr Nephrol [Internet]. 2009 [cited 2017 May 31];24(12):2429–38. Available from: http://link.springer.com/10.1007/s00467-009-1241-7.
46. Dean AJ, Walters J, Hall A. A systematic review of interventions to enhance medication adherence in children and adolescents with chronic illness. Arch Dis Child [Internet] 2010;95(9):717–23. Available from: http://adc.bmj.com/cgi/doi/10.1136/adc.2009.175125.
47. Spirito A, Kazak A. Effective and emerging treatments in pediatric psychology [internet]. Oxford University Press, Oxford; 2006 [cited 2017 May 31]. Available from: https://books.google.com/books?hl=en&lr=&id=kl0SDAAAQBAJ&oi=fnd&pg=PR7&dq=Spirito,+A.,+%26+Kazak,+A.+E.+(2006).+Effective+and+emerging+treatments+in+pediatric+psychology.+Oxford+University+Press.&ots=FDc6JRDX2l&sig=L5SLE-Uh_VavsrTKcEW4o6zj5MQ.
48. Graves MM, Roberts MC, Rapoff M, Boyer A. The efficacy of adherence interventions for chronically ill children: a meta-analytic review. J Pediatr Psychol [Internet]. 2010 [cited 2017 May 31];35(4):368–82. Available from: https://academic.oup.com/jpepsy/article-lookup/doi/10.1093/jpepsy/jsp072.
49. La Greca AM, Mackey ER. Type 1 diabetes mellitus. In: Behavioral approaches to chronic disease in adolescence [Internet]. New York: Springer New York; 2009 [cited 2017 May 31]. p. 85–100. Available from: http://link.springer.com/10.1007/978-0-387-87687-0_8
50. Martino S. Motivational interviewing to engage patients in chronic kidney disease management. Blood Purif [Internet]. 2011 [cited 2017 May 31];31(1–3):77–81. Available from: http://www.ncbi.nlm.nih.gov/pubmed/21228571.
51. Gayes LA, Steele RG. A meta-analysis of motivational interviewing interventions for pediatric health behavior change. J Consult Clin Psychol [Internet]. 2014 [cited 2017 May 31];82(3):521–35. Available from: http://doi.apa.org/getdoi.cfm?doi=10.1037/a0035917.
52. Hashim BL, Vadnais M, Miller AL. Improving adherence in adolescent chronic kidney disease: a dialectical behavior therapy (DBT) feasibility trial. Clin Pract Pediatr Psychol [Internet]. 2013 [cited 2017 May 31];1(4):369–79. Available from: http://doi.apa.org/getdoi.cfm?doi=10.1037/cpp0000024.
53. Lois BH, Miller AL. Stopping the nonadherence cycle: the clinical and theoretical basis for dialectical behavior therapy adapted for adolescents with chronic medical illness (DBT-CMI). Cogn Behav Pract. 2017 [cited 2017 May 31];24:405–415 Available from: http://www.sciencedirect.com/science/article/pii/S1077722917300275.
54. Moussavi S, Chatterji S, Verdes E, Tandon A, Patel V, Ustun B. Depression, chronic diseases, and decrements in health: results from the world health surveys. Lancet [Internet]. 2007 [cited 2017 May 31];370(9590):851–8. Available from: http://www.sciencedirect.com/science/article/pii/S0140673607614159.
55. Gandhi B, Cheek S, Campo JV. Anxiety in the pediatric medical setting. Child Adolesc Psychiatr Clin North Am. 2012;21:643–53.
56. Pinquart M, Shen Y. Behavior problems in children and adolescents with chronic physical illness: a meta-analysis. J Pediatr Psychol [Internet]. 2011 1 [cited 2017 May 31];36(9):1003–16. Available from: https://academic.oup.com/jpepsy/article-lookup/doi/10.1093/jpepsy/jsr042.

57. Pinquart M, Shen Y. Anxiety in children and adolescents with chronic physical illnesses: a meta-analysis. Acta Paediatr [Internet]. 2011 [cited 2017 May 31];100(8):1069–76. Available from: https://doi.org/10.1111/j.1651-2227.2011.02223.x.
58. Pinquart M, Shen Y. Depressive symptoms in children and adolescents with chronic physical illness: an updated meta-analysis. J Pediatr Psychol [Internet]. 2011 [cited 2017 May 31];36(4):375–84. Available from: https://academic.oup.com/jpepsy/article-lookup/doi/10.1093/jpepsy/jsq104.
59. Drayer RA, Piraino B, Reynolds CF, Houck PR, Mazumdar S, Bernardini J, et al. Characteristics of depression in hemodialysis patients: symptoms, quality of life and mortality risk. Gen Hosp Psychiatry [Internet]. 2006 [cited 2017 May 31];28(4):306–12. Available from: http://www.sciencedirect.com/science/article/pii/S016383430600048X.
60. Jain N, Trivedi MH, Rush AJ, Carmody T, Kurian B, Toto RD, et al. Rationale and design of the chronic kidney disease antidepressant sertraline trial (CAST). Contemp Clin Trials [Internet]. 2013 [cited 2017 May 31];34(1):136–44. Available from: http://www.sciencedirect.com/science/article/pii/S1551714412002315.
61. Kimmel PL, Cukor D, Cohen SD, Peterson RA. Depression in end-stage renal disease patients: a critical review. Adv Chronic Kidney Dis [Internet]. 2007 [cited 2017 May 31];14(4):328–34. Available from: http://linkinghub.elsevier.com/retrieve/pii/S1548559507000948.
62. Hedayati S, Minhajuddin AT, Toto RD, Morris DW, Rush AJ. Prevalence of major depressive episode in CKD. Am J Kidney Dis [Internet]. 2009 [cited 2017 May 31];54(3):424–32. Available from: http://www.sciencedirect.com/science/article/pii/S0272638609006398.
63. Hedayati S, Minhajuddin AT, Afshar M, Toto RD, Trivedi MH, Rush AJ. Association between major depressive episodes in patients with chronic kidney disease and initiation of dialysis, hospitalization, or death. JAMA [Internet]. 2010 [cited 2017 May 31];303(19):1946. Available from: http://jama.jamanetwork.com/article.aspx?doi=10.1001/jama.2010.619.
64. Young BA, Von Korff M, Heckbert SR, Ludman EJ, Rutter C, Lin EHB, et al. Association of major depression and mortality in stage 5 diabetic chronic kidney disease. Gen Hosp Psychiatry [Internet]. 2010 [cited 2017 May 31];32(2):119–24. Available from: http://www.sciencedirect.com/science/article/pii/S0163834309002461.
65. Bakr A, Amr M, Sarhan A, Hammad A, Ragab M, El-Refaey A, et al. Psychiatric disorders in children with chronic renal failure. Pediatr Nephrol [Internet]. 2007 [cited 2017 May 31];22(1):128–31. Available from: http://link.springer.com/10.1007/s00467-006-0298-9.
66. Berney-Martinet S, Key F, Bell L, Lépine S, Clermont M-J, Fombonne E. Psychological profile of adolescents with a kidney transplant. Pediatr Transplant [Internet]. 2009 [cited 2017 May 31];13(6):701–10. Available from: https://doi.org/10.1111/j.1399-3046.2008.01053.x.
67. Soliday E, Kool E, Lande MB. Psychosocial adjustment in children with kidney disease. J Pediatr Psychol [Internet]. 2000 [cited 2017 May 31];25(2):93–103. Available from: https://doi.org/10.1093/jpepsy/25.2.93.
68. Tong A, Henning P, Wong G, McTaggart S, Mackie F, Carroll RP, et al. Experiences and perspectives of adolescents and young adults with advanced CKD. Am J Kidney Dis. 2013;61(3):375–84.
69. Gerson AC, Wentz A, Abraham AG, Mendley SR, Hooper SR, Butler RW, et al. Health-related quality of life of children with mild to moderate chronic kidney disease. Pediatrics. 2010;125(2):e349–57.
70. Tong A, Wong G, McTaggart S, Henning P, Mackie F, Carroll RP, et al. Quality of life of young adults and adolescents with chronic kidney disease. J Pediatr [Internet]. 2013 [cited 2017 May 31];163(4):1179–1185.e5. Available from: http://www.sciencedirect.com/science/article/pii/S0022347613005313.
71. Korus M, Stinson JN, Pool R, Williams A, Kagan S. Exploring the information needs of adolescents and their parents throughout the kidney transplant continuum. 101177/152692481102100107 [Internet]. 2011 [cited 2017 May 31]; Available from: http://journals.sagepub.com/doi/abs/10.1177/152692481102100107.

72. Selewski DT, Massengill SF, Troost JP, Wickman L, Messer KL, Herreshoff E, et al. Gaining the patient reported outcomes measurement information system (PROMIS) perspective in chronic kidney disease: a Midwest pediatric nephrology consortium study. Pediatr Nephrol. 2014;29(12):2346–56.
73. Wong CJ, Moxey-Mims M, Jerry-Fluker J, Warady BA, Furth SL. CKiD (CKD in children) prospective cohort study: a review of current findings. Am J Kidney Dis. 2012;60(6):1002–11.
74. Fadrowski J, Cole SR, Hwang W, Fiorenza J, Weiss RA, Gerson A, et al. Changes in physical and psychosocial functioning among adolescents with chronic kidney disease. Pediatr Nephrol [Internet]. 2006 [cited 2017 May 31];21(3):394–9. Available from: http://link.springer.com/10.1007/s00467-005-2122-3.
75. Hernandez EG, Loza R, Vargas H, Jara MF. Depressive symptomatology in children and adolescents with chronic renal insufficiency undergoing chronic dialysis. Int J Nephrol [Internet]. 2011 [cited 2017 May 31];2011:798692. Available from: http://www.ncbi.nlm.nih.gov/pubmed/21941654.
76. Garralda ME, Jameson RA, Reynolds JM, Postlethwaite RJ. Psychiatric adjustment in children with chronic renal failure. J Child Psychol Psychiatry [Internet]. 1988 [cited 2017 May 31];29(1):79–90. Available from: https://doi.org/10.1111/j.1469-7610.1988.tb00691.x.
77. Kogon AJ, Vander Stoep A, Weiss NS, Smith J, Flynn JT, McCauley E. Depression and its associated factors in pediatric chronic kidney disease. Pediatr Nephrol. 2013 [cited 2017 May 31];28(9):1855–61. Available from: http://link.springer.com/10.1007/s00467-013-2497-5.
78. Kogon AJ, Matheson MB, Flynn JT, Gerson AC, Warady BA, Furth SL, et al. Depressive symptoms in children with chronic kidney disease. J Pediatr [Internet]. 2016 [cited 2017 May 31];168:164–170.e1. Available from: http://www.sciencedirect.com/science/article/pii/S0022347615010537.
79. Moreira JM, Bouissou Morais Soares CM, Teixeira AL, Simões e Silva AC, Kummer AM. Anxiety, depression, resilience and quality of life in children and adolescents with pre-dialysis chronic kidney disease. Pediatr Nephrol [Internet]. 2015 [cited 2017 May 31];30(12):2153–62. Available from: http://link.springer.com/10.1007/s00467-015-3159-6.
80. Hooper SR, Duquette PJ, Icard P, Wetherington CE, Harrell W, Gipson DS. Social-behavioural functioning in paediatric chronic kidney disease. Child Care Health Dev [Internet]. 2009 [cited 2017 May 31];35(6):832–40. Available from: https://doi.org/10.1111/j.1365-2214.2009.00992.x.
81. Kilis-Pstrusinska K, Medynska A, Adamczak P, Balasz-Chmielewska I, Grenda R, Kluska-Jozwiak A, et al. Anxiety in children and adolescents with chronic kidney disease – multicenter national study results. Kidney Blood Press Res. 2013;37:579–87.
82. Fukunishi I, Kudo H. Psychiatric problems of pediatric end-stage renal failure. Gen Hosp Psychiatry [Internet]. 1995 [cited 2017 May 31];17(1):32–6. Available from: http://www.sciencedirect.com/science/article/pii/016383439400060Q.
83. Kilicoglu AG, Bahali K, Canpolat N, Bilgic A, Mutlu C, Yalcin O, et al. Impact of end-stage renal disease on psychological status and quality of life. Pediatr Int. 2016;58:1316–21.
84. Gerson AC. Psychosocial issues in children with chronic kidney disease. In: Pediatric kidney disease [internet]. Berlin: Springer Berlin Heidelberg; 2016 [cited 2017 May 31]. p. 1603–24. Available from: http://link.springer.com/10.1007/978-3-662-52972-0_60
85. Marciano RC, Bouissou Soares CM, Diniz JSS, Lima EM, Silva JMP, Canhestro MR, et al. Behavioral disorders and low quality of life in children and adolescents with chronic kidney disease. Pediatr Nephrol [Internet]. 2011 [cited 2017 May 31];26(2):281–90. Available from: http://link.springer.com/10.1007/s00467-010-1683-y.
86. Hedayati S, Yalamanchili V, Finkelstein FO. A practical approach to the treatment of depression in patients with chronic kidney disease and end-stage renal disease. Kidney Int [Internet]. 2012 [cited 2017 May 31];81(3):247–55. Available from: http://www.sciencedirect.com/science/article/pii/S0085253815552915.
87. Gerson AC, Riley A, Fivush BA, Pham N, Fiorenza J, Robertson J, et al. Assessing health status and health care utilization in adolescents with chronic kidney disease. J Am Soc Nephrol

[Internet]. 2005 [cited 2017 May 31];16(5):1427–32. Available from: http://www.ncbi.nlm.nih.gov/pubmed/15772253.
88. Gerson AC, Butler R, Moxey-Mims M, Wentz A, Shinnar S, Lande MB, et al. Neurocognitive outcomes in children with chronic kidney disease: current findings and contemporary endeavors. Ment Retard Dev Disabil Res Rev [Internet]. 2006 [cited 2017 May 31];12(3):208–15. Available from: https://doi.org/10.1002/mrdd.20116.
89. Gipson DS, Ferris ME. A measure of success in kidney transplantations. Pediatr Transplant. 2004 [cited 2017 May 31];8(2):104–5. Available from: https://doi.org/10.1046/j.1399-3046.2003.00149.x.
90. Gipson DS, Hooper SR, Duquette PJ, Wetherington CE, Stellwagen KK, Jenkins TL, et al. Memory and executive functions in pediatric chronic kidney disease. Child Neuropsychol. 2006;12:391–405.
91. Brouhard BH, Donaldson LA, Lawry KW, McGowan KRB, Drotar D, Davis I, et al. Cognitive functioning in children on dialysis and post-transplantation. Pediatr Transplant. 2000;4:261–7.
92. Haavisto A, Korkman M, Holmberg C, Jalanko H, Qvist E. Neuropsychological profile of children with kidney transplants. Nephrol Dial Transplant. 2012;27:2594–601.
93. Hooper SR, Gerson AC, Butler RW, Gipson DS, Mendley SR, Lande MB, et al. Neurocognitive functioning of children and adolescents with mild-to-moderate chronic kidney disease. Clin J Am Soc Nephrol. 2011;6(8):1824–30.
94. Fennell RS, Fennell EB, Carter RL, Mings EL, Klausner AB, Hurst JR. A longitudinal study of the cognitive function of children with renal failure. Pediatr Nephrol [Internet]. 1990 [cited 2017 May 31];4(1):11–5. Available from: http://link.springer.com/10.1007/BF00858429.
95. Slickers J, Duquette P, Hooper SR, Gipson DS. Clinical predictors of neurocognitive deficits in children with chronic kidney disease. Pediatr Nephrol. 2007;22:565–72.
96. Mendley SR, Matheson M, Shinnar S, Lande M, Gerson AC, Butler R, et al. Duration of chronic kidney disease reduces attention and executive function in pediatric patients. Kidney Int. 2015;87(4):800–6.
97. Hartung EA, Kim JY, Laney N, Hooper SR, Radcliffe J, Port AM, et al. Evaluation of neurocognition in youth with CKD using a novel computerized neurocognitive battery. Clin J Am Soc Nephrol. 2016;11:39–46.
98. Johnson RJ, Warady BA. Long-term neurocognitive outcomes of patients with end-stage renal disease during infancy. Pediatr Nephrol. 2013;28(8):1283–91.
99. Wong CJ, Moxey-Mims M, Jerry-Fluker J, Warady BA, Furth SL. CKiD (CKD in children) prospective cohort study: a review of current findings. Am J Kidney Dis [Internet]. 2012 [cited 2017 May 31];60(6):1002–11. Available from: http://www.sciencedirect.com/science/article/pii/S0272638612010578.
100. Icard P, Hooper SR, Gipson DS, de Ferris ME. Cognitive improvement in children with CKD after transplant. Pediatr Transplant. 2010;14(7):887–90.
101. Lawry KW, Brouhard BH, Cunningham RJ. Cognitive functioning and school performance in children with renal failure. Pediatr Nephrol. 1994;8:326–9.
102. Mendley SR, Zelko FA. Improvement in specific aspects of neurocognitive performance in children after renal transplantation. Kidney Int. 1999;56(1):318–23.
103. Gelb SR, Shapiro RJ, Thornton WJL. Predicting medication adherence and employment status following kidney transplant: the relative utility of traditional and everyday cognitive approaches. Neuropsychology [Internet]. 2010 [cited 2017 May 31];24(4):514–26. Available from: https://doi.org/10.1037/a0018670.
104. Stilley CS, Bender CM, Dunbar-Jacob J, Sereika S, Ryan CM. The impact of cognitive function on medication management: three studies. Heal Psychol [Internet]. 2010 [cited 2017 May 31];29(1):50–5. Available from: https://doi.org/10.1037/a0016940.
105. Roberts RE, Roberts CR, Duong HT. Sleepless in adolescence: prospective data on sleep deprivation, health and functioning. J Adolesc [Internet]. 2009 [cited 2017 May 31];32(5):1045–57. Available from: http://www.sciencedirect.com/science/article/pii/S0140197109000335.

106. Dahl RE, Lewin DS. Pathways to adolescent health sleep regulation and behavior. J Adolesc Heal [Internet]. 2002 [cited 2017 May 31];31(6):175–84. Available from: http://www.sciencedirect.com/science/article/pii/S1054139X02005062.
107. Sinha R, Davis ID, Matsuda-Abedini M, DL B, CF L, YS P. Sleep disturbances in children and adolescents with non–dialysis-dependent chronic kidney disease. Arch Pediatr Adolesc Med [Internet]. 2009 [cited 2017 May 31];163(9):850. Available from: https://doi.org/10.1001/archpediatrics.2009.149.
108. Copelovitch L, Warady BA, Furth SL. Insights from the chronic kidney disease in children (CKiD) study. Clin J Am Soc Nephrol [Internet]. 2011 [cited 2017 May 31];6(8):2047–53. Available from: http://www.ncbi.nlm.nih.gov/pubmed/21784815.
109. Stabouli S, Papadimitriou E, Printza N, Dotis J, Papachristou F. Sleep disorders in pediatric chronic kidney disease patients. Pediatr Nephrol [Internet]. 2016 [cited 2017 May 31];31(8):1221–9. Available from: http://link.springer.com/10.1007/s00467-015-3237-9.
110. Davis ID, Greenbaum LA, Gipson D, Wu LL, Sinha R, Matsuda-Abedini M, et al. Prevalence of sleep disturbances in children and adolescents with chronic kidney disease. Pediatr Nephrol [Internet]. 2012 [cited 2017 May 31];27(3):451–9. Available from: http://link.springer.com/10.1007/s00467-011-2010-y.
111. Roumelioti M-E, Wentz A, Schneider MF, Gerson AC, Hooper S, Benfield M, et al. Sleep and fatigue symptoms in children and adolescents with CKD: a cross-sectional analysis from the chronic kidney disease in children (CKiD) study. Am J Kidney Dis [Internet]. 2010 [cited 2017 May 31];55(2):269–80. Available from: http://www.sciencedirect.com/science/article/pii/S0272638609013079.
112. Shochat T, Cohen-Zion M, Tzischinsky O. Functional consequences of inadequate sleep in adolescents: a systematic review. Sleep Med Rev [Internet]. 2014 [cited 2017 May 31];18(1):75–87. Available from: http://www.sciencedirect.com/science/article/pii/S1087079213000440.
113. Clarke G, Harvey AG. The complex role of sleep in adolescent depression. Child Adolesc Psychiatr Clin N Am [Internet]. 2012 [cited 2017 May 31];21(2):385–400. Available from: http://www.ncbi.nlm.nih.gov/pubmed/22537732.
114. Moseley L, Gradisar M. Evaluation of a school-based intervention for adolescent sleep problems. Sleep [Internet] 2009;32(3):334–41. Available from: http://www.ncbi.nlm.nih.gov/pmc/articles/PMC2647787/%0Ahttp://www.ncbi.nlm.nih.gov/pmc/articles/PMC2647787/pdf/aasm.32.3.334.pdf%0Ahttp://www.pubmedcentral.nih.gov/articlerender.fcgi?artid=2647787&tool=pmcentrez&rendertype=abstract.
115. Manber R, Bootzin RR, Acebo C, Carskadon MA. The effects of regularizing sleep-wake schedules on daytime sleepiness. Sleep [Internet]. 1996 [cited 2017 May 31];19(5):432–41. Available from: https://doi.org/10.1093/sleep/19.5.432.
116. Smith MT, Perlis ML. Who is a candidate for cognitive-behavioral therapy for insomnia? Heal Psychol [Internet]. 2006 [cited 2017 May 31];25(1):15–9. Available from: https://doi.org/10.1037/0278-6133.25.1.15.
117. Whoquol Group. The World Health Organization quality of life assessment (WHOQOL): position paper from the World Health Organization. Soc Sci Med [Internet]. 1995 [cited 2017 May 31];41(10):1403–9. Available from: http://linkinghub.elsevier.com/retrieve/pii/027795369500112K.
118. Theofilou P. Quality of life: definition and measurement. Eur J Psychol [Internet]. 2013 [cited 2017 May 31];9(1):150–62. Available from: https://pdfs.semanticscholar.org/e6d3/548eb9a7243f4cac2772cd3577b106596975.pdf.
119. Tjaden LA, Grootenhuis MA, Noordzij M, Groothoff JW. Health-related quality of life in patients with pediatric onset of end-stage renal disease: state of the art and recommendations for clinical practice. Pediatr Nephrol [Internet]. 2016 [cited 2017 May 31];31(10):1579–91. Available from: http://link.springer.com/10.1007/s00467-015-3186-3.

120. Varni JW, Seid M, Kurtin PS. PedsQL™ 4.0: reliability and validity of the pediatric quality of life inventory™ version 4.0 generic core scales in healthy and patient populations. Med Care [Internet]. 2001;39(8):800–12. Available from: http://content.wkhealth.com/linkback/openurl?sid=WKPTLP:landingpage&an=00005650-200108000-00006.
121. McKenna AM, Keating LE, Vigneux A, Stevens S, Williams A, Geary DF. Quality of life in children with chronic kidney disease – patient and caregiver assessments. Nephrol Dial Transplant [Internet]. 2006 [cited 2017 May 31];21(7):1899–905. Available from: https://doi.org/10.1093/ndt/gfl091.
122. Buyan N, Türkmen MA, Bilge I, Baskin E, Haberal M, Bilginer Y, et al. Quality of life in children with chronic kidney disease (with child and parent assessments). Pediatr Nephrol [Internet]. 2010 [cited 2017 May 31];25(8):1487–96. Available from: http://link.springer.com/10.1007/s00467-010-1486-1.
123. Goldstein SL, Gerson AC, Goldman CW, Furth S. Quality of life for children with chronic kidney disease. Semin Nephrol [Internet]. 2006 Mar [cited 2017 May 31];26(2):114–7. Available from: http://linkinghub.elsevier.com/retrieve/pii/S0270929505001853.
124. Kul M, Ebru Çengel-Kültür S, Şenses-Dinç G, Bilginer Y, Uluç S, Baykan H. Quality of life in children and adolescents with chronic kidney disease: a comparative study between different disease stages and treatment modalities. Turk J Pediatr [Internet]. 2013 [cited 2017 May 31];55:493–9. Available from: http://www.turkishjournalpediatrics.org/uploads/pdf_TJP_1244.pdf.
125. Lopes M, Ferraro A, Koch VH. Health-related quality of life of children and adolescents with CKD stages 4–5 and their caregivers. Pediatr Nephrol [Internet]. 2014 [cited 2017 May 31];29(7):1239–47. Available from: http://link.springer.com/10.1007/s00467-014-2769-8.
126. Riaño-Galán I, Málaga S, Rajmil L, Ariceta G, Navarro M, Loris C, et al. Quality of life of adolescents with end-stage renal disease and kidney transplant. Pediatr Nephrol [Internet]. 2009 [cited 2017 May 31];24(8):1561–8. Available from: http://link.springer.com/10.1007/s00467-009-1175-0.
127. Falger J, Landolt MA, Latal B, Rüth EM, Neuhaus TJ, Laube GF. Outcome after renal transplantation. Part II: quality of life and psychosocial adjustment. Pediatr Nephrol [Internet]. 2008 [cited 2017 May 31];23(8):1347–54. Available from: http://link.springer.com/10.1007/s00467-008-0798-x.
128. Goldstein SL, Rosburg NM, Warady BA, Seikaly M, McDonald R, Limbers C, et al. Pediatric end stage renal disease health-related quality of life differs by modality: a PedsQL ESRD analysis. Pediatr Nephrol [Internet]. 20097 [cited 2017 May 31];24(8):1553–60. Available from: http://link.springer.com/10.1007/s00467-009-1174-1.
129. Diseth TH, Tangeraas T, Reinfjell T, Bjerre A. Kidney transplantation in childhood: mental health and quality of life of children and caregivers. Pediatr Nephrol [Internet]. 2011 [cited 2017 May 31];26(10):1881–92. Available from: http://link.springer.com/10.1007/s00467-011-1887-9.
130. Park K-S, Hwang YJ, Cho MH, Ko CW, Ha IS, Kang HG, et al. Quality of life in children with end-stage renal disease based on a PedsQL ESRD module. Pediatr Nephrol [Internet]. 2012 [cited 2017 May 31];27(12):2293–300. Available from: http://link.springer.com/10.1007/s00467-012-2262-1.
131. Kiliś-Pstrusińska K, Medyńska A, Adamczak P, Bałasz-Chmielewska I, Grenda R, Kluska-Jóźwiak A, et al. Anxiety in children and adolescents with chronic kidney disease – multicenter national study results. Kidney Blood Press Res [Internet]. 2013 [cited 2017 May 31];37(6):579–87. Available from: http://www.ncbi.nlm.nih.gov/pubmed/24356548.
132. Pinquart M, Teubert D. Academic, physical, and social functioning of children and adolescents with chronic physical illness: a meta-analysis. J Pediatr Psychol [Internet]. 2012 [cited 2017 May 31];37(4):376–89. Available from: https://doi.org/10.1093/jpepsy/jsr106.
133. Oris L, Seiffge-Krenke I, Moons P, Goubert L, Rassart J, Goossens E, et al. Parental and peer support in adolescents with a chronic condition: a typological approach and developmental

implications. J Behav Med [Internet]. 2016 [cited 2017 May 31];39(1):107–19. Available from: http://link.springer.com/10.1007/s10865-015-9680-z.
134. Medyńska A, Zwolińska D, Grenda R, Miklaszewska M, Szczepańska M, Urzykowska A, et al. Psychosocial aspects of children and families treated with hemodialysis. Hemodial Int [Internet]. 2017 [cited 2017 May 31]; https://doi.org/10.1111/hdi.12526.
135. Brem AS, Brem FS, McGrath M, Spirito A. Psychosocial characteristics and coping skills in children maintained on chronic dialysis. Pediatr Nephrol [Internet]. 1988 [cited 2017 May 31];2(4):460–5. Available from: http://link.springer.com/10.1007/BF00853442.
136. Kelly MM. Children and adolescents with chronic kidney disease: a population at risk for more than just kidney disease. Contin Nurs Educ. 2016;43(1):67–70.
137. Lewis H, Arber S. The role of the body in end-stage kidney disease in young adults: gender, peer and intimate relationships. Chronic Illn. 2015;11(3):184–97.
138. Morton MJS, Reynolds JM, Garralda ME, Postlethwaite RJ, Goh D. Psychiatric adjustment in end-stage renal disease: a follow up study of former paediatric patients. J Psychosom Res [Internet]. 1994 [cited 2017 May 31];38(4):293–303. Available from: http://www.sciencedirect.com/science/article/pii/0022399994900345.
139. Rosenkranz J, Bonzel K-E, Bulla M, Michalk D, Offner G, Reichwald-Klugger E, et al. Psychosocial adaptation of children and adolescents with chronic Ren Fail Pediatr Nephrol [Internet]. 1992 [cited 2017 May 31];6(5):459–63. Available from: http://link.springer.com/10.1007/BF00874014
140. Al-Uzri A, Matheson M, Gipson DS, Mendley SR, Hooper SR, Yadin O, et al. The impact of short stature on health-related quality of life in children with chronic kidney disease. J Pediatr [Internet]. 2013 [cited 2017 May 31];163(3):736–741.e1. Available from: http://www.sciencedirect.com/science/article/pii/S0022347613002928
141. Tong A, Lowe A, Sainsbury P, Craig JC. Parental perspectives on caring for a child with chronic kidney disease: an in-depth interview study. Child Care Health Dev [Internet]. 2010 [cited 2017 May 31];36(4):549–57. https://doi.org/10.1111/j.1365-2214.2010.01067.x
142. Haffner JC, Schurman SJ. The technology-dependent child. Pediatr Clin N Am [Internet]. 2001 [cited 2017 May 31];48(3):751–64. Available from: http://linkinghub.elsevier.com/retrieve/pii/S0031395505703370
143. Heaton J, Noyes J, Sloper P, Shah R. Families' experiences of caring for technology-dependent children: a temporal perspective. Heal Soc Care Community [Internet]. 2005 [cited 2017 May 31];13(5):441–50. https://doi.org/10.1111/j.1365-2524.2005.00571.x
144. Tong A, Lowe A, Sainsbury P, Craig JC. Experiences of parents who have children with chronic kidney disease: a systematic review of qualitative studies. Pediatrics. 2008;121(2):349–60.
145. Aldridge MD. How do families adjust to having a child with chronic kidney failure? A systematic review. Nephrol Nurs J. 2008;35(2):157–62.
146. Reynolds JM, Garralda ME, Jameson RA, Postlethwaite RJ. How parents and families cope with chronic renal failure. Arch Dis Child [Internet]. 1988 [cited 2017 May 31];63(7):821–6. Available from: http://www.ncbi.nlm.nih.gov/pubmed/3415300.
147. Weidebusch S, Konrad M, Foppe H, Reichwald-Klugger E, Schaefer F, Schreiber V, et al. Health-related quality of life, psychosocial strains, and coping in parents of children with chronic renal failure. Pediatr Nephrol. 2010;25:1477–85.
148. Cohen MS, Seren M. Families coping with childhood chronic illness: a research review. Fam Syst Heal [Internet]. 1999 [cited 2017 May 31];17(2):149–64. Available from: https://doi.org/10.1037/h0089879.
149. Gayomali C, Sutherland S, Finkelstein FO. The challenge for the caregiver of the patient with chronic kidney disease. Nephrol Dial Transplant [Internet]. 2008 [cited 2017 May 31];23(12):3749–51. Available from: https://doi.org/10.1093/ndt/gfn577.
150. Finkelstein FO, Wuerth D, Finkelstein SH. Health related quality of life and the CKD patient: challenges for the nephrology community. Kidney Int [Internet]. 2009 [cited 2017 May 31];76(9):946–52. Available from: http://www.sciencedirect.com/science/article/pii/S0085253815541045.

151. Eccleston C, Palermo TM, Fisher E, Law E. Psychological interventions for parents of children and adolescents with chronic illness. Cochrane Database Syst Rev [Internet]. 2012 [cited 2017 May 31];8(8):CD009660. Available from: http://www.ncbi.nlm.nih.gov/pubmed/22895990.
152. Ferris ME, Bell LE. Transitioning the adolescent dialysis patient to adult care. In: Pediatric dialysis [Internet]. Boston: Springer US; 2012 [cited 2017 May 31]. p. 673–88. Available from: http://link.springer.com/10.1007/978-1-4614-0721-8_35
153. Casey BJ, Jones RM, Hare TA. The adolescent brain. Ann N Y Acad Sci. 2008;1124:111–26.
154. Luna B, Padmanabhan A, O'Hearn K. What has fMRI told us about the development of cognitive control through adolescence? Brain Cogn [Internet]. 2010 [cited 2017 May 31];72(1):101–13. Available from: http://www.sciencedirect.com/science/article/pii/S0278262609001596.
155. Bell LE. Adolescents with renal disease in an adult world: meeting the challenge of transition of care. Nephrol Dial Transplant [Internet]. 2007 25 [cited 2017 May 31];22(4):988–91. Available from: https://doi.org/10.1093/ndt/gfl770.
156. Bell LE, Ferris ME, Fenton N, Hooper SR. Health care transition for adolescents with CKD—the journey from pediatric to adult care. Adv Chronic Kidney Dis [Internet]. 2011 [cited 2017 May 31];18(5):384–90. Available from: http://www.sciencedirect.com/science/article/pii/S1548559511000668.
157. Lewis H, Marks SD. Differences between paediatric and adult presentation of ESKD in attainment of adult social goals. Pediatr Nephrol. 2014 [cited 2017 May 31];29(12):2379–85. Available from: http://link.springer.com/10.1007/s00467-014-2864-x.
158. Flume PA. Smoothing the transition from pediatric to adult care: lessons learned. Curr Opin Pulm Med [Internet]. 2009 [cited 2017 May 31];15(6):611–4. Available from: http://content.wkhealth.com/linkback/openurl?sid=WKPTLP:landingpage&an=00063198-200911000-00014.
159. van Staa A, Sattoe JNT, Strating MMH. Experiences with and outcomes of two interventions to maximize engagement of chronically ill adolescents during hospital consultations: a mixed methods study. J Pediatr Nurs [Internet]. 2015 [cited 2017 May 31];30(5):757–75. Available from: http://www.sciencedirect.com/science/article/pii/S088259631500216X.
160. Fenton N, Ferris M, Ko Z, Javalkar K, Hooper SR. The relationship of health care transition readiness to disease-related characteristics, psychosocial factors, and health care outcomes: preliminary findings in adolescents with chronic kidney disease. J Pediatr Rehabil Med. 2015 [cited 2017 May 31];8(1):13–22. Available from: http://content.iospress.com/articles/journal-of-pediatric-rehabilitation-medicine/prm00314.
161. Schwartz LA, Daniel LC, Brumley LD, Barakat LP, Wesley KM, Tuchman LK. Measures of readiness to transition to adult health care for youth with chronic physical health conditions: a systematic review and recommendations for measurement testing and development. J Pediatr Psychol [Internet]. 2014 [cited 2017 May 31];39(6):588–601. Available from: https://doi.org/10.1093/jpepsy/jsu028.
162. Ferris ME, Ferris MT, Viall C, Stewart HD, Fenton N, Haberman C, et al. The self-management and transition to adulthood program "UNC STAR x" instruments and lessons from the field. Int J Child Adolesc Heal [Internet]. 2013 [cited 2017 May 31];6(2):137–47. Available from: http://search.proquest.com/openview/cc6cbb516171accf02f39e71b8b33f0b/1?pq-origsite=gscholar&cbl=2034872.
163. Cohen SE, Hooper SR, Javalkar K, Haberman C, Fenton N, Lai H, et al. Self-management and transition readiness assessment: concurrent, predictive and discriminant validation of the STARx questionnaire. J Pediatr Nurs [Internet]. 2015 [cited 2017 May 31];30(5):668–76. Available from: http://www.sciencedirect.com/science/article/pii/S0882596315001505.
164. Ferris ME, Harward DH, Bickford K, Layton JB, Ferris MT, Hogan SL, et al. A clinical tool to measure the components of health-care transition from pediatric care to adult care: the UNC TR x ANSITION scale. Ren Fail. 2012;34(6):744–753. Available from: https://doi.org/10.3109/0886022X.2012.678171.
165. Sawicki GS, Lukens-Bull K, Yin X, Demars N, Huang I-C, Livingood W, et al. Measuring the transition readiness of youth with special healthcare needs: validation of the TRAQ—transition

readiness assessment questionnaire. J Pediatr Psychol [Internet]. 2011 [cited 2017 May 31];36(2):160–71. Available from: https://doi.org/10.1093/jpepsy/jsp128.
166. Betz C, Redcay G, Tan S. Self-reported health care self-care needs of transition-age youth: a pilot study. Issues Compr Pediatr Nurs [Internet]. 2003 [cited 2017 May 31];26(3):159–81. Available from: http://www.tandfonline.com/doi/full/10.1080/01460860390223880.
167. Gilleland J, Amaral S, Mee L, Blount R. Getting ready to leave: transition readiness in adolescent kidney transplant recipients. J Pediatr Psychol [Internet]. 2012 [cited 2017 May 31];37(1):85–96. Available from: https://doi.org/10.1093/jpepsy/jsr049.
168. Watson AR. Problems and pitfalls of transition from paediatric to adult renal care. Pediatr Nephrol [Internet]. 2005 [cited 2017 May 31];20(2):113–7. Available from: http://link.springer.com/10.1007/s00467-004-1763-y.
169. Watson AR, Warady BA. Transition from pediatric to adult-centered care. Dial Transplant. 2011 [cited 2017 May 31];40(4):156–8. https://doi.org/10.1002/dat.20557.

Chapter 3
Nutritional Considerations for Adolescents with Chronic Kidney Disease

Lisa Keung

Introduction

Adequate nutrition is particularly important in children and adolescents in order to promote optimal growth and development. Even healthy adolescents face nutrition challenges related to peer pressure and perceptions of what is healthy versus non-healthy. Adolescents with chronic kidney disease (CKD) face typical nutritional concerns with the additive stress of multiple possible dietary restrictions related to fluid, sodium, protein, potassium, and phosphorus intake. Anorexia from their underlying disease may make receipt of adequate calories challenging. A comprehensive nutrition assessment is an imperative component of the medical evaluation for all children with CKD, and appropriate nutrition is critical to the child's overall well-being. For this reason, a registered dietitian (RD) is a vital member of the care team for all children with CKD. The RD should be an empathetic and supportive team member able to empower the adolescent and their family with the necessary tools to achieve appropriate nutrition and adhere to the necessary dietary restrictions.

Growth Impairment in CKD

Growth impairment is common in children and adolescents with CKD secondary to multiple factors which may include inadequate nutrition, metabolic acidosis, uremia, anemia, calcium and phosphorus imbalance, renal osteodystrophy,

L. Keung
University of California, San Francisco, CA, USA
e-mail: Lisa.Keung@ucsf.edu

M. N. Haddad et al. (eds.), *Adolescents with Chronic Kidney Disease*,
https://doi.org/10.1007/978-3-319-97220-6_3

insensitivity to the action of growth hormone, and use of high-dose glucocorticoids [1–5]. Growth impairment is described as either short stature or growth failure. Short stature is defined as length/height Z-score < 1.88 or a length/height for age < 3rd percentile, while growth failure is defined as short stature for more than 3 months. One third of children with CKD experience growth failure [6]. Children with CKD are generally 1.5 standard deviations below their healthy counterparts [7]. A useful parameter to consider when evaluating a child's growth is the child's genetic growth potential. The genetic growth potential considers the biological parents' height and determines the child's potential height when she or he is adult-aged. It is calculated as the average of the father's height (in cm) and the mother's height ±13 cm (add if male, subtract if female) [8].

A RD reviews growth parameters and growth history as part of their assessment to determine an appropriate intervention. If the child has inadequate weight gain and/or changes in their weight percentiles, then dietary counseling is necessary [9]. Linear growth is monitored closely to determine if poor weight gain has affected linear growth. When nutritional status is optimized and weight returns to its former track and linear growth remains impaired, then growth hormone replacement therapy may be considered for a child with CKD, assuming other parameters, such as metabolic acidosis and secondary hyperparathyroidism, are well-controlled [10].

On the opposite spectrum, one out of every six children are now overweight or obese placing them at an increased risk of developing chronic kidney disease [11]. Overweight is defined as a BMI or weight/length >85th percentile, while >95th percentile is indicative of obesity. Obesity is strongly associated with hypertension and diabetes which are common causes of end-stage renal disease (ESRD) in adults. Weight management counseling is becoming more common and necessary for children with CKD [12].

Nutrition-Focused History

A dietitian will obtain a diet history from the caregiver and child. There are several ways to obtain the dietary history to get "the big picture" of their intake which will then allow the dietitian to tailor counseling from all aspects (growth, medications, laboratory values, and intake).

Important aspects of the history include questions related to appetite, dietary recall, food frequency, and fluid intake as follows:

- Determine changes in appetite and review when the change in appetite was first noted.
- A 3-day dietary recall is ideal to assess average intake, food variety, and food patterns.
- If unable to obtain a 3-day recall, a 24-h recall will provide insight to average intake.

- Food frequency questions should be focused on protein, sodium, potassium, calcium, and phosphorus as interventions may be required to control these specific nutrients.
- If fluid intake is a concern, then a fluid intake history should also be reviewed as part of the diet history. If unknown, the family/child should be encouraged to track future fluid intake.

Nutrition-Focused Physical Exam

Malnutrition, protein-energy wasting, and micronutrient deficiencies are common concerns in adolescents with CKD as they are with any restrictive diet. Laboratory values should be monitored, but physical exams will also reveal a great deal. A renal RD's physical exam focuses on signs of malnutrition, fluid retention, and micronutrient deficiencies [13].

Below are several methods to identify malnutrition:

- Ask the patient to turn their head from side to side or open and close their jaw. While making those motions, check the temple region for the temporalis muscle. If the area is hollowing, scooping, or has depression, there is likely severe malnutrition. If there is a slight depression, there is likely mild-moderate malnutrition.
- Ask the individual to touch their forefinger to their thumb, and check the fat pad on the back of the hand between the thumb and forefinger. If there is an indentation, there is some form of malnutrition.
- Examine the fat pad of the orbital region which is located right above the cheekbone. If the area appears hollow and has dark circles, loose skin, and/or depressions, some malnutrition may be indicated.
- Lanugo, when fine hairs grow all over the body, can be sign of caloric deficiency.

For fluid retention:

- Examine the fat pad of the orbital region. If the area appears puffy, this may indicate some swelling or fluid retention.
- Examine the jawline. If it appears larger than the rest of their face, fluid may be hiding in this area as well.
- Examine the lower extremities (legs, ankles, and feet). Press a finger into the lower limbs. If it leaves an indentation, there is fluid retention.

For micronutrient deficiency/toxicity:

- Check the color under the eyelids. If it appears pale, this may be a sign of iron or vitamin B12 deficiency.
- Hair should be shiny, smooth, and difficult to pluck. If untrue, this may suggest inadequacy of protein, zinc, biotin, and/or essential fatty acid deficiency.
- If alopecia is present, this may be related to biotin deficiency, vitamin A toxicity, and selenium toxicity.

Nutrition-Focused Laboratory Assessment

An assessment of serum electrolytes, micronutrients, and protein is an important component of the nutrition evaluation and helps to guide dietary recommendations for the individual patient. Commonly encountered electrolyte derangements in adolescents with chronic kidney disease include abnormalities of sodium, potassium, calcium, phosphorus, and acid/base homeostasis. The direction of the abnormality varies depending on the underlying cause of CKD; for example, while adolescents with glomerular causes of CKD commonly have salt and water retention requiring sodium restriction, those with congenital anomalies of the kidney and urinary tract may in fact have excessive salt and water loss in the urine requiring salt supplementation. The first step to managing many of these abnormalities is to alter dietary intake (Tables 3.1, 3.2, and 3.3).

Hypernatremia is typically related to dehydration, while hyponatremia can be caused by overhydration or renal salt wasting. Chronic hyponatremia may lead to delayed growth and development and may require sodium supplementation.

In addition to excessive intake of potassium, hyperkalemia may be related to the use of certain medications including ACE inhibitors (i.e., lisinopril, enalapril), immunosuppressant medications (tacrolimus, cyclosporine, thymoglobulin), and spironolactone. Prevention of hyperkalemia includes dietary restriction (Tables 3.1 and 3.2). Correction of metabolic acidosis is also vital to prevent and manage hyperkalemia. Certain medications can cause hypokalemia, such as furosemide, leading the RD to educate on adding back an appropriate amount of potassium foods.

Serum calcium and phosphorus levels are altered in CKD. If serum calcium is low and 25-OH vitamin D level is adequate, an increase in activated vitamin D may

Table 3.1 Low-potassium foods (<200 mg per serving)

Fruit (serving size)	*Potassium (mg) per serving*
Apple (1 medium or 1 cup)	160
Applesauce (1/2 cup)	90
Blackberries (1/2 cup)	140
Blueberries (1 cup)	130
Cherries (10 or 2 oz)	150
Cranberries, raw, whole (1 cup or 3 oz)	67
Fruit cocktail (1/2 cup)	115
Grapes, seedless (10)	90
Grapefruit (1/2 medium or 4 oz)	170
Kiwi (1/2 medium or 1.3 oz)	126
Mango (1/2 medium or 3.5 oz)	160
Pears, canned (1/2 cup)	90
Peach (1 medium or 3 oz)	198
Pineapple (1/2 cup)	90
Plums, canned in syrup (1/2 cup)	115

Table 3.1 (continued)

Fruit (serving size)	*Potassium (mg) per serving*
Raspberries (1/2 cup)	95
Rhubarb, cooked (1/2 cup)	115
Tangerine (1 medium or 3 oz)	130
Watermelon (1 cup)	175
Vegetables (serving size)	*Potassium (mg) per serving*
Alfalfa sprouts (1/2 cup)	15
Asparagus (4 spears or 2 oz)	130
Bamboo shoots, canned (1/2 cup)	53
Bean sprouts (mung), raw (1 cup)	155
Bean sprouts (soybeans), raw (1/2 cup)	170
Bell pepper (1/2 medium or 2 oz)	106
Broccoli, cooked (1/2 cup or 3.2 oz)	166
Cabbage, raw, red/green (1 cup)	172
Cauliflower, raw (1/2 cup)	150
Carrots raw (1/2 cup)	180
Celery, raw (7.5-in. stalk)	115
Chinese broccoli, boiled (1/2 cup)	115
Collards, boiled (1 cup)	170
Corn, frozen, boiled (1/2 cup)	121
Cucumber, with peel (1/4 or 2-in. piece)	108
Cucumber, without peel (1/4 or 2-in. piece)	75
Eggplant, cooked (1/2 cup)	125
Garlic (4 cloves)	50
Ginger root, raw (1/4 cup)	100
Green beans, fresh, boiled (1/2 cup)	187
Green beans, frozen, boiled (1/2 cup)	85
Lemon grass, raw (2 tablespoons)	70
Lettuce, butter head (1 cup)	141
Lettuce, iceberg (1 cup chopped)	87
Lettuce, loose leaf (1 cup)	148
Lettuce, romaine (1 cup)	162
Mixed vegetables, frozen (1/2 cup)	155
Okra, boiled (1/2 cup)	135
Onion, raw, chopped (1/4 cup)	63
Pepper, chili, green, hot, raw (1 pepper)	153
Radishes (10 or 1.5 oz)	105
Rutabagas, raw (1 cup)	150
Spaghetti squash, baked (1 cup)	181
Summer squash, raw, sliced (1/2 cup)	110
Squash, zucchini, raw, sliced (1/2 cup)	140
Turnip, cooked (1/2 cup)	105
Water chestnuts, canned (1/2 cup)	85

Table 3.2 High-potassium foods (>200 mg per serving)

Fruit (serving size)	*Potassium (mg) per serving*
Apricots (3 medium or 3.5 oz)	315
Avocado (1/4 medium or 1.5 oz)	275
Banana (1medium or 4 oz)	450
Cantaloupe (1/2 cup)	245
Cassava (1/2 cup)	279
Dates, dried (5 medium or 1.4 oz)	350
Guava, medium (90 g)	256
Honeydew (1/2 cup)	230
Orange (1 medium or 4.4 oz)	235
Papaya (1/2 med/5 oz)	390
Pear, fresh (1 medium or 5.5 oz)	210
Plums (2 medium or 4.4 oz)	220
Prunes (5 medium or 1.4 oz)	315
Raisins (1/4 cup or 1.3 oz)	310
Tamarind (1/2 cup)	377
100% fruit juice (1 cup)	300–500
Vegetable (serving size)	*Potassium (mg) per serving*
Artichoke (1/4 medium or 2.5 oz)	265
Beans:	
Kidney, canned (1/2 cup)	330
Lima, canned (1/2 cup)	265
Mung, boiled (1/2 cup)	269
Navy, canned (1/2 cup)	380
Pinto, canned (1/2 cup)	290
Beets, boiled (1/2 cup)	260
Brussels sprouts (1/2 cup)	247
Chard, Swiss, boiled (1/2 cup)	430
Corn, fresh, boiled (1/2 cup)	204
Mushrooms, raw (1/2 cup)	259
Peas, dried, cooked:	
Black-eyed peas (1/2 cup)	240
Chickpeas/garbanzo (1/2 cup)	240
Lentils (1/2 cup)	365
Split peas (1/2 cup)	355
Potatoes, all types, baked with skin (1 small or 4.9 oz)	759
Potatoes, all types, boiled without skin	457
Sweet potatoes, baked with skin (1 medium or 4 oz)	397
Sweet potatoes, boiled or mashed (1/2 cup)	302
Tomato, raw, chopped (1 cup)	273
Tomato puree, canned (1/4 cup)	266
Winter squash, baked (1/2 cup)	450
Yam, baked or boiled (1/2 cup)	456

Table 3.3 Phosphorus management with foods

Food group	Foods recommended (low phos)	Foods not recommended (high phos)
Milk and milk products	Cream cheese	Milk, buttermilk
	Whipped cream	Yogurt
	Butter	Pudding
	Nondairy substitutes	Cheeses, natural and processed
Breads and grains	French bread	Bran (wheat or oat)
	Sourdough bread	Oatmeal
	White bread (that does not contain milk)	Whole-grain breads and cereals (only if phosphorus is not controlled with low dairy intake)
	Corn	Breads made with milk or cheese
Meat and protein foods	Egg white (1.14 mg phosphorus/g protein)	Egg, whole (14 mg phosphorus/g protein)
	Beef (7–8 mg phosphorus/g protein)	Egg, yolk (30 mg phosphorus/g protein)
	Pork (8–10 mg phosphorus/g protein)	Lunch meats or sausages containing milk solids or cheese
	Chicken (6.5–7.5 mg phosphorus/g protein)	Ham (13–16 mg phosphorus/g protein)
	Turkey (6.5–7.5 mg phosphorus/g protein)	Salami (7–18 mg phosphorus/g protein)
	Fish (10–14 mg phosphorus/g protein)	Soy including tofu (12–15 mg phosphorus/g protein)
	Split peas (12 mg phosphorous/g protein)	Beans: Kidney, black, garbanzo, navy, pinto (16–20 mg phosphorus/g protein)
		Lentils, nuts and seeds (20–30 mg phosphorus/g protein)
Fruits	All	None
Vegetables	All	None
Snack foods	Popcorn	Snack foods made with cheese or cheese flavoring
	Pretzels	Candy bars with chocolate and nuts
	Tortilla chips	Milk chocolate candy
	Granola bars	Cola drinks
Main dishes	Soups, casseroles, pasta dishes, and other mixed foods made without cheese and/or milk	Pizza, lasagna, and other casseroles made with cheese, cream- or milk-based soups

be required to encourage absorption of intestinal calcium. Hypercalcemia can occur with hypervitaminosis A or hypervitaminosis D. If hypercalcemia occurs concurrently with hyperphosphatemia, then there is an increased risk for arteriosclerosis to develop [14].

Hyperphosphatemia is common in CKD and should be addressed to prevent bone mineral disorder (BMD). Even in the early stages of CKD when serum phosphorus is normal, recommendations for a phosphate additive-free diet is encouraged. The current US food system contains a number of phosphate additives to improve texture, consistency, emulsification, and longer shelf life [15]. These additives are known to be 100% bioavailable, whereas animal-based phosphorus and plant-based phosphorus (phytates) are only 40–60% and 20–50% bioavailable, respectively. Food manufacturers are not required to list the amount of phosphorus on nutritional labels, and this makes it quite difficult to estimate the amount of phosphorus consumed. With the wide variance of phosphates in processed foods [15, 16], recommending a diet free in phosphate additives would be the first step in phosphorus management.

As noted previously, micronutrient deficiencies are common in patients with CKD, and in general, it is recommended to assess for the following deficiencies: folate, vitamin B12, zinc, vitamin D, and iron. If folate or vitamin B12 is found to be deficient, starting a multivitamin is recommended. A normal multivitamin is avoided once the adolescent has stage 4 CKD or higher. This is because filtration of fat-soluble vitamins is decreased in the setting of severe chronic kidney disease and toxicity can develop over time on a regular multivitamin [17]. For this reason, a renal multivitamin (i.e., Nephro-Vite, Rena-Vite, and Nephrocap) should be started in place of a standard multivitamin when the adolescent has progressed to severe CKD. A renal multivitamin is also started at the initiation of dialysis given increased losses of water-soluble vitamins requiring repletion. Zinc can be included if desired or if zinc deficiency is identified. Vitamin D deficiency is common among those with CKD, and supplementation of vitamin D can be started based on the level of 25-hydroxy vitamin D (Table 3.4).

While albumin is the most commonly used serum marker of nutritional status, it is important to keep in mind that serum albumin may also be low in the setting of glomerular losses, gastrointestinal losses, liver disease, systemic inflammation, and fluid retention therefore not accurately assessing nutritional status [18, 19]. For adolescents on dialysis, another useful marker of nutritional status is the nPCR (normalized protein catabolic rate). This marker is calculated using formal urea kinetic modeling (UKM) or an algebraic equation [20]. The calculation for nPCR is as follows: G (mg/min) = $[(C2 \times V2) - (C1 \times V1)]/T$. In this equation, $C1$ is post-dialysis BUN (mg/dL) and $C2$ is pre-dialysis BUN (mg/dL). $V1$ is post-dialysis total body water (dL; $V1 = 5.8$ dL/kg × post-dialysis weight in kg); $V2$ is pre-dialysis total body water (dL; $V2 = 5.8$ dL/kg × pre-dialysis weight in kg); and T is time (minutes) from the end of the dialysis treatment to the beginning of the following treatment [20].

Several studies have shown that nPCR is a better marker than albumin for weight loss in children on long-term hemodialysis [21–23]. In a study of 44 pediatrics patients, serum albumin, nPCR, and weight trends were assessed in the setting of

Table 3.4 Vitamin D supplementation for serum 25-hydoxy vitamin D deficiency and insufficiency for adolescents

25-OH vitamin D level	Ergocalciferol (vitamin D2) supplementation
<5 ng/mL	50,000 units weekly for 4 weeks and then reduce to 50,000 units twice a month for 2 months
5–15 ng/mL	50,000 units twice a month for 3 months
16–30 ng/mL	50,000 units monthly for 3 months

receiving adequate hemodialysis (defined as a KT/V of 1.3). In the adolescent patients, nPCR <1 g/kg/day was associated with weight loss even while serum albumin trends were >4 g/dL [23]. For adolescents age 13 years and older on hemodialysis, a nPCR >1 g/kg helps to ensure that protein and nutritional status are optimized. Of note, the reference range used for nPCR is not as accurate for children less than 13 years of age because the nitrogen balance is affected by growth and development [23]. Tracking trends of nPCR may still be helpful in the younger patients to assess nutritional status.

Nutrition-Focused Medication History

Medications used to treat the child's underlying disease are routinely reviewed by the RD to determine how they might impact the child's nutrition. In Table 3.5, common medications prescribed to children with CKD are reviewed along with how they may impact electrolytes or nutrition. RDs will tailor their counseling and interventions in consideration of the child's current medications.

Table 3.5 Medications and potential side effects on nutrition

Drug	Potential nutritional side effect
Immunosuppressant	
Cyclosporine	Hyperkalemia, hyperglycemia, hypomagnesemia, hyperlipidemia
Tacrolimus	Hyperkalemia, hyperglycemia, hypomagnesemia, metabolic acidosis, nausea, vomiting, diarrhea
Azathioprine	Nausea, vomiting, pancreatitis, diarrhea
Mycophenolate	Nausea, vomiting, diarrhea, edema, gastritis
Prednisone	Hyperglycemia, sodium/fluid retention, hyperlipidemia, increased appetite, excessive weight gain, Cushing's syndrome, calcium and phosphorus imbalance, gastritis
Sirolimus	Hypertriglyceridemia, hypercholesterolemia, peripheral edema, nausea, diarrhea/constipation, abdominal pain
Phosphate binders	
Sevelamer hydrochloride or Sevelamer carbonate	Hypercalcemia, nausea, vomiting, abdominal pain, constipation/diarrhea, peritonitis
Calcium acetate	Hypercalcemia, nausea, vomiting
Calcium carbonate	Hypercalcemia, hypophosphatemia, abdominal pain, anorexia, constipation, nausea, vomiting
Potassium binders	
Sodium polystyrene sulfonate	Hypernatremia, hypocalcemia, hypokalemia, hypomagnesemia, sodium retention, nausea, vomiting, diarrhea/constipation, anorexia, fecal impaction
Patiromer	Hypokalemia, hypomagnesemia, abdominal distress, constipation/diarrhea, nausea

(continued)

Table 3.5 (continued)

Drug	Potential nutritional side effect
Antihypertensive	
Amlodipine	Hyperphosphatemia
Enalapril	Hyperkalemia
Lisinopril	Hyperkalemia, hyperphosphatemia
Bisoprolol	Hyperphosphatemia
Metoprolol	Hyperphosphatemia
Diuretics	
Furosemide	Hypokalemia, hypomagnesemia, hypocalcemia, hyponatremia,
Appetite stimulants	
Cyproheptadine	Nausea, vomiting, constipation/diarrhea
Dronabinol	Abdominal pain, nausea, vomiting
Megestrol acetate	Nausea, vomiting, constipation, abdominal pain, edema, peripheral edema, adrenal cortical insufficiency

Medications may not always be an obvious cause of electrolyte derangements. In a study conducted by Nelson et al. [24], various types of commonly used medications for adult dialysis patients were examined to determine the content of phosphates. They found 11% of prescription drugs contained phosphate and 89% of those medications were either in the cardiovascular system or central nervous system drug categories. The amount of phosphate in these medications depended on the formulation; as an example, the phosphate content varied from 13.8 to 165.6 mg in a 10 mg tablet of amlodipine. Other common medications containing phosphate included lisinopril, bisoprolol, and metoprolol [24]. Thus, for adolescents on multiple antihypertensive medications, phosphate intake from medications alone could contribute a significant load to their total phosphate intake for the day. Close attention to side effects and additives from medications is warranted and may require medication modifications in discussion with the medical team.

Drug-food interactions are also monitored for by the RD. Patients and caregivers are educated on which foods need to be avoided. For instance, grapefruit and pomegranate are known to increase absorption of tacrolimus and may alter drug levels [25, 26]. It is important that these particular fruits be avoided whether whole, in juices, or in dressings to prevent altered ranges of tacrolimus.

Determining Macronutrient Needs

Energy needs for children and adolescents with chronic kidney disease are generally no different than healthy kids unless the child has additional comorbidities. Typically, CKD causes poor appetite leading children to eat less than their estimated energy requirements. For hemodialysis patients, caloric requirements are equivalent to those of healthy children. In the setting of peritoneal dialysis, caloric intake needs may actually be less given the child will receive some calories via dextrose through peritoneal dialysis fluid [17].

Recommendations for protein intake are based on the stage of CKD. For CKD stages 1 and 2, protein intake is not restricted. For CKD stage 3, protein intake is restricted to 100–140% of the daily recommended intake (DRI), and for CKD stages 4 and 5, protein intake is limited to 100–120% of DRI. When starting dialysis, protein needs are increased secondary to losses of protein and amino acids while on dialysis. Per National Kidney Foundation guidelines [17], adolescents on hemodialysis need DRI + 0.1 g of protein/kg/day, while those on peritoneal dialysis need DRI + 0.15–0.3 g of protein/kg/day.

Fluid management needs to be closely monitored by the RD and medical team. As CKD advances, there is a high probability that fluid restriction will be required. If urine output decreases secondary to a decline in kidney function, fluid limits will be initiated. To determine the appropriate fluid restriction for an individual patient on dialysis, it is necessary to take into account insensible water losses, daily urine output, and dialysis fluid removal. For a child with anuria, the fluid recommendation is determined by limiting their interdialytic weight gain to less than 5% of their estimated dry weight.

Nutrition Interventions

Based on the information collected during the visit, the RD will then provide education and counseling to ensure the adolescent will be able to manage their dietary intake appropriately. Counseling and/or interventions specific to dietary changes necessary to correct any determined electrolyte abnormalities are provided. Additional nutritional interventions depend on whether the adolescent is found to have malnutrition. For a significant proportion of adolescents with CKD, and in particular those on chronic corticosteroids, interventions may instead need to be focused on weight loss and management of obesity.

For those patients with glomerular disease or otherwise at risk for salt and water retention, counseling is geared toward dietary modifications to lower sodium intake. First, it is important to identify food sources – fast food, convenience foods, and/or homemade – and how frequently these items are consumed. To avoid excessive sodium intake, it is recommended that the majority of food choices be homemade. With homemade foods, condiments and sauces containing sodium should be avoided and instead, herbs and spices be used for flavoring to improve palatability. Switching from canned goods to frozen or fresh fruits and vegetables will also lower sodium intake. If unable to make this change, then the patient should consider "no added salt" or "low sodium" alternatives and rinse with water prior to preparation to further lower the sodium content. For protein, it is recommended that they choose fresh protein rather than canned. If the protein is frozen, then the nutrition label should be reviewed for the addition of sodium. Avoidance of deli meat and smoked, cured, and canned meat is recommended.

For those adolescents on immunosuppressive medications like transplant recipients, there are many potential medication side effects that affect their nutrition (Table 3.5). Some common side effects include excessive weight gain, hypertension, fluid retention, and electrolyte abnormalities. A dietitian will counsel on a diet consisting of 2–2.3 g per day of sodium, low-concentrated sweets, low fat, and high-fiber intake. Potassium intake may need to be moderated in setting of hyperkalemia due to medications. In regard to unexpected weight gain with immunosuppression, a heart-healthy diet high in fruits, vegetables, and whole grains provides a variety of micronutrients and helps to satiate appetite. If excessive weight gain occurs and leads to obesity, then caloric intake should be reduced to estimated energy needs to aim for weight maintenance or lower for slow weight loss until BMI <85% percentile [27].

Another dietary approach similar to the heart-healthy diet is a plant-based diet which has been shown in adults to decrease the rate of CKD progression. A diet rich in plants contains smaller amounts of saturated fatty acids, protein, and absorbable phosphorus than meat, generates less acid, and is rich in dietary fibers, polyunsaturated and monounsaturated fatty acids, magnesium, potassium, and iron. One study suggested that increased dietary fiber improves peristalsis and frequency of bowel movements, thereby reducing uremic toxin production, exposure, and absorption [28]. By improving uremia, progression of CKD slows down [28, 29]. The major concern with using this dietary intervention in younger children is the potentially deleterious effect on their growth due to inadequate intake of high biological value (HBV) protein; however, it may be appropriate to use in older adolescents as they are nearly at their growth potential. A dietitian could assess and identify a modified diet that balances plant-based approach while also including enough HBV protein to support linear growth.

Interventions for Adolescents with Malnutrition

Progression of CKD may lead to decreased oral intake and weight loss. If this occurs, the dietitian will further counsel the child and caregiver on a high-calorie diet and feeding practices while still staying within their renal diet parameters. This may focus on small frequent meals and use of caloric beverages over water. For foods, use of oils, sour cream, and cream cheese added to prepared dishes is encouraged to boost caloric intake. Switching to bagels and croissants over sliced bread or preparing foods by frying over baking and broiling may be necessary as well.

Despite these recommendations, dietary changes may not be enough to prevent malnutrition. Discussion with the family regarding use of an appetite stimulant versus a nutritional supplement should be started. Both have their pros and cons and will depend upon the child and family's preferences.

An appetite stimulant can be used to encourage oral intake. There are several types of appetite stimulants which include cyproheptadine, dronabinol, and megestrol acetate. Cyproheptadine hydrochloride is a first-generation antihistamine which was noted for its secondary effect of appetite stimulation [30–32] but cyproheptadine may also cause drowsiness [33]. Megestrol acetate is an alternative to promote appetite [30]. One pediatric study showed a significant improvement in weight and BMI with minimal side effects over an 8-month period [34].

Table 3.6 summarizes the different renal nutrition supplements available in the US market. The formulas are separated based on age group. Four of the five supplements are formulated for adult needs, while Renastart™ is recommended for ages 1–10. Children's micronutrient needs are different from adults, so the adult nutrition formulas will not provide the correct amounts of micronutrients for younger children.

Nepro® and Novasource® Renal are higher in protein compared to the other renal formulas and are designed for oral use in adults receiving dialysis. Suplena® is designed for oral use in setting of chronic kidney disease and thus has a lower protein content than Nepro and Novasource Renal. Renalcal® is a high-calorie, low-protein formula designed for adults with acute renal failure and is not palatable by mouth and recommended for enteral use only. It is lower in protein than the other three adult nutrition formulas. Renalcal does not contain any fat-soluble vitamins including vitamin D. The sodium, potassium, and phosphate content are also lower in Renalcal. Renastart is comparable to Renalcal in that it is lower in protein, but it provides more variety of micronutrients than Renalcal. Renastart is currently available as a powder rather than liquid, so the formula can be concentrated from the standard 1 kcal/mL, 14 g protein/L formula up to a 2 kcal/mL, 32 g protein/L formula if desired. Renastart was designed to supplement a child's oral intake. The formula is whey protein-based and purposely lower in protein, potassium, calcium, phosphorus, and vitamin A to allow for a more liberalized diet for the oral feeder [35, 36].

Since there are a limited number of pediatric renal formulas, a RD is responsible for creating a recipe that fits within a child's nutritional needs. This may include using modular powders to help meet calorie or protein needs based on the renal formula used as the base. Table 3.7 shows the two most commonly used modular powders, Duocal and Beneprotein®.

Table 3.6 Renal nutrition formulas

			Per 1000 mL								
Nutrition supplement	Cost per can	Volume per can	Kcal	Protein (g)	Na (mEq)	K+ (mEq)	Ca (mg)	Mg (mg)	Phos (mg)	Vitamin A (IU)	Vitamin D (IU)
Pediatric											
Renastart	$34.00	400 g	1908	15.8	21.8	5.9	221	105	189	909	420
Adult											
Suplena	$3.00	237 mL	1800	45	35	29.1	1055	211	717	3165	84
Nepro	$3.50	237 mL	1800	81	46	27.2	1060	210	720	3180	85
Novasource Renal	$5.00	250 mL	2000	90.7	41	24	840	197	819	1510	400
Renalcal	$9.25	250 mL	2000	34	4	4	60	20	100	0	0

Table 3.7 Modular nutritional supplements

Modulars	Cost	Volume per Can	Kcal	Protein (g)	Na (mEq)	K+ (mEq)	Ca (mg)	Mg (mg)	Phos (mg)	Vitamin A (IU)	Vitamin D (IU)
Duocal	$32.50	400 g	1960	0	3.5	0.5	0.5	0	0.5	0	0
Beneprotein	$15.99	227 g	989	195	21.1	26	648	0	0	0	0

Conclusion

Nutrition is a vital component in the management of CKD for all age groups in order to optimize their growth and development. The renal dietitian is critical in assessing and optimizing the nutritional status of a child with CKD. Use of the renal dietitian's expertise will allow each child to receive an individualized intervention to achieve optimal growth and development while minimizing the complications and progression of CKD.

References

1. Tonshoff B, Mehls O. Growth retardation in children with chronic renal insufficiency: current aspects of pathophysiology and treatment. J Nephrol. 1995;8:133.
2. Tom A, McCauley L, Bell L, Rodd C, Espinosa P, Yu G, et al. Growth during maintenance hemodialysis: impact of enhanced nutrition and clearance. J Pediatr. 1999;134(4):464–71.
3. Kari J, Gonzalez C, Ledermann S, Shaw V, Rees L. Outcome and growth of infants with severe chronic renal failure. Kidney Int. 2000;57(4):1681–7.
4. Boirie Y, Broyer M, Gagnadoux M, Niaudet P, Bresson J. Alterations of protein metabolism by metabolic acidosis in children with chronic renal failure. Kidney Int. 2000;58(1):236–41.
5. Tonshoff B, Kiepe D, Ciarmatori S. Growth hormone/insulin-like growth factor system in children with chronic renal failure. Pediatr Nephrol. 2005;20(3):279–89.
6. Hamiwka L, Midgley J, Wade A, Martz K, Grisaru S. Outcomes of kidney transplantation in children with nephronophthisis: an analysis of the North American pediatric renal trials and collaborative studies (NAPRTCS) registry. Pediatr Transplant. 2008;12(8):878–82.
7. Massengill S, Ferris M. Chronic kidney disease in children and adolescents. Pediatr Rev. 2014;35(1):16–29.
8. Tanner J, Goldstein H, Whitehouse R. Standards for children's height at ages 2-9 years allowing for height of parents. Arch Dis Child. 1970;45(244):755–62.
9. Legler J, Rose L. Assessment of abnormal growth curves. Am Fam Physician. 1998;58(1):153–8.
10. Mahan J, Warady B. Assessment and treatment of short stature in pediatric patients with chronic kidney disease: a consensus statement. Pediatr Nephrol. 2006;21(7):917–30.
11. Ogden C, Carroll M, Lawman H, Fryar C, Kruszon-Moran D, Kit B, et al. Trends in obesity prevalence among children and adolescents in the United States, 1988–1994 through 2013–2014. JAMA. 2016;315(21):2292.
12. Ding W. Impact of obesity on kidney function and blood pressure in children. World J Nephrol. 2015;4(2):223.
13. Green Corkins K. Nutrition-focused physical examination in pediatric patients. Nutr Clin Pract. 2015;30(2):203–9.
14. Isakova T, Nickolas T, Denburg M, Yarlagadda S, Weiner D, Gutiérrez O, et al. KDOQI US commentary on the 2017 KDIGO clinical practice guideline update for the diagnosis, evaluation, prevention, and treatment of chronic kidney disease–mineral and bone disorder (CKD-MBD). Am J Kidney Dis. 2017;70(6):737–51.
15. Parpia AS, L'Abbe M, Goldstein M, Arcand J, Magnuson B, Darling PB. The impact of additives on the phosphorus, potassium, and sodium content of commonly consumed meat, poultry, and fish products among patients with chronic kidney disease. J Ren Nutr. 2018;28(2):83–90.

16. Carrigan A, Klinger A, Choquette S, Luzuriaga-McPherson A, Bell E, Darnell B, et al. Contribution of food additives to sodium and phosphorus content of diets rich in processed foods. J Ren Nutr. 2014;24(1):13–19.e1.
17. National Kidney Foundation. KDOQI clinical practice guideline for nutrition in children with CKD: 2008 update. Am J Kidney Dis. 2009;53(3):S11–S104.
18. Jones C, Akbani H, Croft D, Worth D. The relationship between serum albumin and hydration status in hemodialysis patients. J Ren Nutr. 2002;12(4):209–12.
19. Kaysen G, Dubin J, Müller H, Mitch W, Rosales L, Levin N, et al. Relationships among inflammation nutrition and physiologic mechanisms establishing albumin levels in hemodialysis patients. Kidney Int. 2002;61(6):2240–9.
20. Srivaths P, Wong C, Goldstein S. Nutrition aspects in children receiving maintenance hemodialysis: impact on outcome. Pediatr Nephrol. 2008;24(5):951–7.
21. Goldstein S, Baronette S, Gambrell T, Currier H, Brewer E. nPCR assessment and IDPN treatment of malnutrition in pediatric hemodialysis patients. Pediatr Nephrol. 2002;17(7):531–4.
22. Orellana P, Juarez-Congelosi M, Goldstein S. Intradialytic parenteral nutrition treatment and biochemical marker assessment for malnutrition in adolescent maintenance hemodialysis patients. J Ren Nutr. 2005;15(3):312–7.
23. Juarez-Congelosi M, Orellana P, Goldstein S. Normalized protein catabolic rate versus serum albumin as a nutrition status marker in pediatric patients receiving hemodialysis. J Ren Nutr. 2007;17(4):269–74.
24. Nelson S, Sarabia S, Christilaw E, Ward E, Lynch S, Adams M, et al. Phosphate-containing prescription medications contribute to the daily phosphate intake in a third of hemodialysis patients. J Ren Nutr. 2017;27(2):91–6.
25. Liu C, Shang Y, Zhang X, Zhang X, Wang B, Wu Z, et al. Co-administration of grapefruit juice increases bioavailability of tacrolimus in liver transplant patients: a prospective study. Eur J Clin Pharmacol. 2009;65(9):881–5.
26. Khuu T, Hickey A, Deng M. Pomegranate-containing products and tacrolimus: a potential interaction. J Heart Lung Transplant. 2013;32(2):272–4.
27. Barlow S. Expert committee recommendations regarding the prevention, assessment, and treatment of child and adolescent overweight and obesity: summary report. Pediatrics. 2007;120(Supplement 4):S164–92.
28. David LA, Maurice CF, Carmody RN, Gootenberg DB, Button JE, Wolfe BE, et al. Diet rapidly and reproducibly alters the human gut microbiome. Nature. 2014;505(7484):559–63.
29. Schulman G, Berl T, Beck G, Remuzzi G, Ritz E, Arita K, et al. Randomized placebo-controlled EPPIC trials of AST-120 in CKD. J Am Soc Nephrol. 2014;26(7):1732–46.
30. Couluris M, Mayer J, Freyer D, Sandler E, Xu P, Krischer J. The effect of cyproheptadine hydrochloride (Periactin) and megestrol acetate (Megace) on weight in children with cancer/treatment-related cachexia. J Pediatr Hematol Oncol. 2008;30(11):791–7.
31. Summerbell C, Youle M, McDonald V, Catalan J, Gazzard B. Megestrol acetate vs cyproheptadine in the treatment of weight loss associated with HIV infection. Int J STD AIDS. 1992;3(4):278–80.
32. Homnick D, Homnick B, Reeves A, Marks J, Pimentel R, Bonnema S. Cyproheptadine is an effective appetite stimulant in cystic fibrosis. Pediatr Pulmonol. 2004;38(2):129–34.
33. Homnick D, Marks J, Hare K, Bonnema S. Long-term trial of cyproheptadine as an appetite stimulant in cystic fibrosis. Pediatr Pulmonol. 2005;40(3):251–6.
34. Hobbs D, Bunchman T, Weismantel D, Cole M, Ferguson K, Gast T, et al. Megestrol acetate improves weight gain in pediatric patients with chronic kidney disease. J Ren Nutr. 2010;20(6):408–13.
35. USA V. Vitaflo usa announces availability of renastart™ formula, a one-of-a-kind medical food for children with kidney disease [Internet]. Bing.com. 2018 [cited 14 April 2017]. Available from: https://www.bing.com/cr?IG=479642C4931A46348FAD012E937C622E&CID=2BD6535D83E66D7B351558D782496C52&rd=1&h=jXPakyfZw22rC

WQrVgW2-_cVFjk947SGLei_3yadmHk&v=1&r=https%3a%2f%2fwww.prnewswire.com%2fnews-releases%2fvitaflo-usa-announces-availability-of-renastart-formula-a-one-of-a-kind-medical-food-for-children-with-kidney-disease-300181473.html&p=DevEx,5039.1

36. Renastart™| Dietary Management of Kidney Disease| Renastart Vitaflo USA [Internet]. Bing.com. 2018 [cited 14 April 2017]. Available from: https://www.bing.com/cr?IG=BBE9C25629B543878096732D8E8D1BFC&CID=2973CFA78D356CF73470C42D8C9A6D6A&rd=1&h=6Kwjg49mxakXgPvk1heFQzI6cJFVvERlZ1a9iK8X0ZI&v=1&r=https%3a%2f%2frenastartusa.com%2frenastart%2fabout-renastart%2f&p=DevEx,5049.1

Chapter 4
Reproductive Health in Adolescent and Young Adult Women with Chronic Kidney Disease

Laura M. Kester

Introduction

Special attention should be given to the reproductive health care and development of adolescent and young adults (AYA) with chronic kidney disease (CKD). Although faced with higher rates of sexual dysfunction and fertility challenges, these AYA have questions about their reproductive health care, engage in sexual behaviors, and are at risk for unplanned pregnancies. Comprehensive care should include reproductive and family planning counseling that informs these AYA of their potential for fertility, risks for pregnancy complications, disease stability factors that promote improved pregnancy outcomes, the importance of unplanned pregnancy prevention, options for delaying pregnancy, as well as practices to prevent the acquisition of sexually transmitted infections.

Reproductive Health in AYA with CKD

The adolescent and young adult (AYA) period is a very significant stage in a young woman's overall reproductive health [1]. For AYA women with chronic kidney disease (CKD), this period is as vital and requires just as much attention, if not more, when compared to their non-affected peers. The presence of CKD during these early reproductive stages can affect the reproductive health of these women in a variety of ways, both physically and emotionally.

L. M. Kester
Adolescent Medicine, UC Davis School of Medicine, Sacramento, CA, USA
e-mail: lkester@ucdavis.edu

M. N. Haddad et al. (eds.), *Adolescents with Chronic Kidney Disease*,
https://doi.org/10.1007/978-3-319-97220-6_4

Sexual Health in AYA with CKD

Women with CKD may face a variety of concerns with sexual health, ovulation, and fertility. Studies have shown that AYA with CKD self-report higher rates of sexual dysfunction than those without CKD. It is believed that the sexual dysfunction is secondary to both psychologic as well as physiologic processes that are further complicated by associated comorbidities [2].

Psychological Effects on Sexual Dysfunction

Psychologically, the presence of a chronic illness can affect an individual's overall confidence level in their abilities to be sexually desirable. This may also expand into fears regarding their ability to perform sexually as well as face apprehensions regarding the safety of their use of contraception. Reports of negative body image have been identified in AYA with CKD prior to initiating dialysis [2]. For those women with CKD that desire future family planning, further angst around fertility potential and viability of future pregnancies can further contribute to psychological impacts on sexual function. In addition, it is important to remember that chronic medical conditions are associated with higher rates of depression which has the potential to further complicate presentations of sexual dysfunction in AYA with CKD.

Physiological Effects on Sexual Dysfunction

Physically, AYA with CKD have high rates of sexual dysfunction. These challenges during sexual activity present as a variety of sexual health concerns including decreased sexual libido, difficulty with sexual arousal, vaginismus, decreased vaginal lubrication, dyspareunia, and orgasmic impairment [3, 4].

For these and other reasons, higher rates of abstinence as well as decreased frequency of intercourse are described in AYA with CKD. Although this is important for providers to know and factor into discussions, counseling, and decision-making, it is equally important that providers recognize that this does not describe all AYA with CKD. It is essential that providers realize that AYA with CKD are engaged in sexual relationships and that attention to their reproductive needs and concerns is crucial. It is imperative for providers to realize that there continues to be a complex, poorly understood relationship between sexual dysfunction, fertility and the perceived risks for pregnancy in AYA with CKD that leads to many questions and unknowns for both patients and providers [5].

Impact and Options for Sexual Dysfunction

There is some evidence to support that individuals on hemodialysis, despite having a high frequency of sexual dysfunction, may not feel an overall dissatisfaction with their sexual life [6]. It is important that we remember that every AYA is experiencing a different situation and that we address each AYA with CKD as an individual seeking to identify the presence and impact of any concerns with sexual dysfunction. For this reason as well as its multifactorial etiology, attempts to treat sexual dysfunction in AYA with CKD must be designed to be patient specific and address all the underlying functional and psychosocial factors contributing to its presentation [2].

Ovulatory and Menstrual Abnormalities

Ovulation and menstrual cycles may also be significantly influenced by the presence of CKD. As kidney function deteriorates, decline in GFR is associated with the progression of menstrual dysfunction. What often initially presents as oligomenorrhea can progress to amenorrhea [5]. Individuals with end-stage renal disease (ESRD) have been identified as having pituitary-gonadal hormone disturbances [7], which may be reversible after kidney transplantation [7, 8].

Studies have shown that in AYA with CKD on dialysis, there is a loss of the necessary pulsatile release of gonadotropin-releasing hormones (GnRH) from the hypothalamus. This pulsatile release is essential for normal stimulation of the cyclic release of luteal hormone (LH) and follicle-stimulating hormone (FSH) from the pituitary. In the absence of normal cyclic changes in LH, these women on dialysis can progress to ovulatory failure. Additionally, they can develop poor stimulation of estrogen production and estrogen feedback, which is essential for endometrial development and stabilization [5, 9]. Some studies have shown that women on dialysis can also have reduced secretion of prolactin which further contributes to difficulties with ovulation [5]. In addition to irregular bleeding, AYA on dialysis have higher rates of premature menopause identified by increased levels of FSH and LH which further increases their risk for infertility. These stimulating hormone levels are usually subthreshold to the levels seen in classic menopausal women [3].

Pregnancy Risks in AYA with CKD

AYA women with CKD fall into a very high-risk population for pregnancy complications. During pregnancy, there are significant changes to the maternal renal physiology from the overall size of the kidney to changes in glomerular and tubular function, plasma flow, and glomerular filtration rate. These changes are significant not only to pregnancy outcomes but pregnancy monitoring for kidney functioning and disease progression. Due to the significant role that a young woman's kidneys play in maternal physiology, women with underlying CKD have worse maternal and fetal outcomes when compared to pregnant AYA without CKD [10]. This is particularly true in AYA women with more advanced renal dysfunction that is poorly controlled and associated with proteinuria and hypertension [11]. These poor outcomes include higher rates of preeclampsia, gestational hypertension (with potential for persistence post pregnancy), preterm delivery, congenital malformations, small for gestational age newborns, and increased rates of neonatal intensive care unit admissions [5, 12]. There have been mixed findings regarding the progression of CKD in women after pregnancy. However, there is reasonable evidence to suggest that AYA with early stage CKD, who have normal blood pressure with minimal to no proteinuria, can have good maternal-fetal outcomes despite being at higher risk than their non-CKD AYA counterparts [12, 13].

Fertility and Family Planning

Advances in prenatal and neonatal care have made pregnancy for AYA with CKD a very real option. However, in light of the high-risk nature of pregnancy in these young women, it is important that they are well counseled on the risks around any pregnancy and the important steps involved in preparing, planning, and monitoring such a pregnancy. Discussions regarding fertility, contraception, and pregnancy risk should begin at the onset of puberty and expand appropriately as the AYA advances in reproductive development. When having these conversations, it is essential that an AYA's cognitive and sexual-reproductive developmental stage is taken into consideration so that appropriate and well-communicated conversations are being held.

Creating the Appropriate Setting

When speaking with all adolescents and young adults about contraception and reproductive health-related concerns, it is essential that we are addressing these young people in a manner in which they understand, where they feel comfortable, and where they feel safe [1]. These dynamics help to build rapport and enhance the openness of these communications. It is also important that we create an environment that supports their confidentiality. This reinforces with the AYA that they can feel comfortable having these personal conversations without concern for judgment or fear that their concerns will not be kept private. These conversations should also include discussions about sexuality, pregnancy prevention, and prevention of sexually transmitted infections [1].

Considerations for Family Planning

Due to the high-risk nature of a pregnancy in an AYA with CKD, these young people must be informed that, if they are interested in becoming pregnant, there are important steps that must be taken to promote a safe and healthy pregnancy for both mother and baby. Although the presence of CKD and progression of kidney disease is commonly associated with increased risk for infertility, it is important to recognize that AYA with CKD can still become pregnant. It is also important to make AYA aware that kidney transplantation and frequent dialysis can increase fertility [14, 15]. However, despite the improvement in fertility, these pregnancies remain high-risk due to high rates of preeclampsia, preterm delivery, cesarean section, and newborns that are small for gestational age. These AYA may struggle with balancing the value of a pregnancy with the risk for complications that such a pregnancy may bring to them or their child, including risk of inheritable genetic disease to the future offspring. For each of these reasons, this is essential that these reproductive areas of care be addressed when examining the health status and desired health outcomes of an AYA with CKD.

Determining the Optimal Timing for Pregnancy

The nephrologist plays an important role in assisting AYA with CKD to determine the most optimal time to attempt conception. This would consist of the time in which the AYA is best able to optimize her overall maternal health and disease control. For these youth and their partner, pre-pregnancy counseling includes disease risk stratification as well as a discussion concerning the many potential pregnancy-associated complications [13]. Many physicians may identify a specific level of renal disease severity for which they would not feel comfortable pursuing a pregnancy. Identification of an AYA's renal disease severity is a large part of the pre-pregnancy planning. This risk assessment includes consideration of the disease etiology, the degree of renal dysfunction and baseline renal function, disease stabilization and the rate of GFR decline, previous obstetric history, and the presence of any other risk factors [5]. Individuals interested in pregnancy may benefit from early establishment of a multidisciplinary team that would consist of nephrologists with expertise in CKD during pregnancy, maternal fetal medicine specialists, pharmacists, and dieticians [13].

Effects of Medications on Fertility, Pregnancy, and Fetal Outcomes

Several of the medications used in management of CKD can have potential harmful outcomes to fertility, pregnancy, and fetal outcomes in AYA of childbearing age. For this reason, AYA should be counseled on the risks of the medications on fertility and during pregnancy. Pregnancy tests should be performed prior to initiating these medications, and appropriate steps should be taken to place AYA on these medications on appropriate forms of contraceptive preventive methods.

Cyclophosphamide, an alkylating agent used in patients with CKD who present with rapidly progressive glomerular disease, is known to have gonadotoxic effects in both male and female AYA with CKD with greater concerns for irreversibility in women. Side effects from this medication can include oligospermia, amenorrhea, and ovarian failure. In addition, cyclophosphamide is known to have teratogenic effects such as skeletal malformations (craniofacial and limb abnormalities), fetal visceral abnormalities, growth restriction, and hematopoietic and neurologic impairment [5]. AYA with CKD being placed on cyclophosphamide should be counseled on available options for fertility preservation.

Angiotensin-converting enzyme (ACE) inhibitors and angiotensin receptor blockers (ARBs) are antihypertensive agents that are frequently used for the management of hypertension in AYA with CKD [16]. These medications carry a known box warning for potential harm to a fetus during the second and third trimesters [16]. Use of these medications is strongly cautioned in women of childbearing age and should be counseled and weighed against risk for pregnancy. These medications lead to alterations in the renin-angiotensin system that is essential for normal fetal kidney development [17]. Use of these medications has been associated with impaired fetal renal function that leads to oligohydramnios during pregnancy. Post-delivery, these infants generally have low blood pressure and anuria that quickly leads to renal failure [17]. Oligohydramnios can increase intrauterine complications such as umbilical cord compression as well as pulmonary hypoplasia, limb contractures, and skeletal malformations. The major outcome for these infants is death [17].

Mycophenolate mofetil (MMF), an immunosuppressive agent, is used after renal transplant in AYA with lupus nephritis to prevent organ rejection. MMF is a known teratogen associated with increased risk for congenital malformations as well as first trimester fetal demise. When a fetus is exposed, MMF causes a teratogenic syndrome that consists of hypoplastic nails, shortened fingers, diaphragmatic hernia, microtia, micrognathia, and cleft lip and palate along with congenital heart defects. AYA interested in pursuing family expansion should be switched to an alternate medication at least 3 months prior to attempts to conceive [5]. AYA being taken off of this medication should still continue contraceptive prevention methods until at least 6 weeks after this medication has been discontinued.

AYA with CKD who are being treated with these medications should undergo routine monitoring of pregnancy, and discontinuation of the medications should occur immediately if pregnancy is detected.

Other Considerations for Family Planning

Genetic testing may be available to assist AYA with CKD to identify risk of transmission of an inheritable disease to their future offspring. AYA with high risk of disease passage may consider prenatal diagnostic testing. These individuals, as well as other

AYA with CKD, may consider alternative options for family planning, including in vitro fertilization combined with preimplantation genetic diagnosis, germ cell donation, or adoption. Some of these processes can require a significant amount of time and planning, so it is imperative that discussions around family planning for AYA with CKD begin early and prior to desire for family expansion [18].

Contraceptive Management

Despite challenges with sexual dysfunction, it is vitally important that we remember that AYA with CKD do undergo sexual development, have sexual desires, and engage in sexual activity. Unplanned pregnancies can occur at any stages of CKD, pre and post renal transplantation. Recognizing the potential for such fertility and the high-risk nature of such pregnancies on both maternal and fetal complications makes it essential that the reproductive health management of these young women is at the forefront of our care. The nephrologist plays an important role in ensuring that the AYA with CKD have all the necessary access to the knowledge and tools required to effectively delay and prevent pregnancy until the chosen time.

Non-hormonal Contraceptives

Copper IUD

The copper IUD is a T-shaped device that functions as a long-acting, non-hormonal form of contraception that is placed within the uterus. These devices function by creating a foreign body reaction within the endometrium that creates a hostile environment that impairs sperm function [19]. Due to the release of copper salts, the copper IUD has an even greater foreign body reaction than that of the hormonal IUD [19]. The copper IUD is approved for 10 years of functioning with a 1-year, typical-use failure rate of 0.8% [19]. See Table 4.2. In addition to contraceptive management, the copper IUD can also be used for emergency contraception within 5 days of an unprotected sexual encounter. This unique attribute is only found in the copper IUD and not the hormonal IUDs. However, it should be noted that AYA with CKD who have undergone kidney transplantation have increased reports of contraceptive failure while using the copper IUD due, in part, to the altered immune response by some transplant immunosuppressive agents that is necessary for the effectiveness of the copper IUD [20].

Progesterone-Only Methods

All hormonal forms of contraception contain a progestin component. It is the progesterone component that is responsible for the contraceptive action.

Levonorgestrel IUD

There is limited data on the best form of contraception for patients with CKD. However, in general, long-acting reversible contraception (LARC) is highly recommended in both teens and patients with chronic illness in whom prevention of unplanned pregnancies is essential. This is because LARCs have been identified as the most effective form and often the safest form of contraception. Compared to other forms of contraception, LARCs have both a high perfect and typical use (Table 4.2). In addition, despite potential initial hesitation with starting these methods, they have been found to have the highest rates of both continuation and satisfaction with AYA patients. The potential for reduction in unplanned pregnancies has been acknowledged by the American College of Obstetrics and Gynecology (ACOG), the American Academy of Pediatrics (AAP), the Centers for Disease Control (CDC), as well as the World Health Organization (WHO). In fact, in 2014, the AAP released a policy statement supporting the initial recommendation of ACOG that LARCs be first choice of contraception [21].

In addition to the foreign body reaction that is also seen in the copper IUD, the hormonal IUDs also release levonorgestrel, a hormone that thickens the cervical mucus that prevents sperm penetration and causes endometrial atrophy [19]. In addition, there is a potential for suppression of follicular development and ovulation after 1 year of use. The levonorgestrel IUD 1-year, typical-use failure rate is 0.2%, which is similar to that of female sterilization. In comparison with the copper IUD, the levonorgestrel IUD has been shown to be effective as well as safe in CKD patients who have undergone renal transplantation [22].

There have been reports of patients on peritoneal dialysis that presented with IUD-related peritonitis, and there is some thought that this may be related to retrograde menstruation, which could indicate potential IUD migration. For this reason, this should be considered in the risk-benefit balance of choosing a contraceptive method [23].

Contraceptive Implant

Nexplanon® is a progestin-only (etonogestrel) device that is implanted into the subdermal aspect of the upper arm. It is approved for 3 years with a high efficacy rate (Table 4.2). Nexplanon® works by inhibiting ovulation through the suppression of the LH surge an event which occurs as early as 8 h after placement. Additionally, the progestin acts by thickening cervical mucus to prevent the sperm penetration.

Progesterone-Only Injectable Contraception

Depot medroxyprogesterone acetate (DMPA) is an injectable form of progesterone-only contraceptive that is administered every 3 months as a single dose of 150 mg of progesterone injected intramuscularly. Because of the higher serum levels of hormone following injection, DMPA functions by suppressing ovulation, unlike other lower dose progesterone methods [19]. In addition, it also works to thin the endometrial lining as well as increase the viscosity of cervical mucous. With perfect use, its efficacy is comparable to that of the intrauterine device. However, due to missed and delayed return appointments resulting in late injections, with typical use, its failure rates are much higher than that of the long-acting forms of contraception. DMPA should be used with caution in individuals with a high risk for osteoporosis and/or fracture. This includes AYA with family history of early osteoporosis and those who are on long-term corticosteroid use, are immobilized, have disorders of bone metabolism, have low weight, or are early in bone acquisition. There is minimal information on the effect of DMPA on renal osteodystrophy.

Progestin-Only Pill

The progestin-only pill (POP) works by causing changes to the cervical mucous and the endometrium that obstruct permeability of sperm. The benefit of the progestin-only pill is that there are few contraindications to its use. Currently, the only absolute contraindication is the presence of active breast cancer. In the United States, the POP is only available containing 0.35 mg of norethindrone. The serum levels of the progesterone peak within 2 h and cervical mucosal changes occurring within 2–4 h of administration [19]. This effect generally lasts for 22 h with a rapid decline thereafter. For this reason, the pill must be taken promptly at the same time each day and must be taken continuously without a hormone-free period. If there is a greater than 3 h delay in administration, then its effectiveness should be considered compromised. The pill should be taken immediately, and a backup option must be used for the next 48 h. It is important to note that POPs do not suppress ovulation and therefore individuals may still ovulate. Due to potential changes in the tubal physiology while on POP, there is the potential for increased tubal transport time of the gametes [19]. In the case of method failure, tubal pregnancies are not prevented as effectively in POP users compared to those on combined oral contraceptive pills (COCP) methods. The use of a POP in an AYA should be weighed carefully with the risk for pregnancy due to a high risk of method failure if strict adherence to pill administration is not maintained (Table 4.2).

Combined Hormonal Contraceptives

As is the case for the progestin-only methods, it is the progestin component that is responsible for the contraceptive action as well as the cause of the majority of its side effect profile. The estrogen component assists in stabilizing the endometrial lining.

Combined Hormonal Transvaginal Contraception

NuvaRing® is a combined hormonal contraceptive (etonogestrel and ethinyl estradiol) that is made in the shape of a soft, flexible, and transparent ring. The ring is inserted into the vaginal canal where the hormone is directly absorbed through the squamous epithelium [19]. It is generally left inserted for a total of 3 weeks and is then removed for 1 week of hormone free period during which an individual has a menstrual cycle. Despite peak serum hormone levels that are actually lower in the vaginal ring (30% for etonogestrel and 40% for ethinyl estradiol) compared to oral contraceptive pills (OCP), the vaginal ring is able to sustain ovulation suppression for 5 weeks with less hormone fluctuation than OCPs [19]. Due to the extended potential for ovulation suppression, the vaginal ring can be used for extended cycling with 4 weeks of placement rather than 3, followed by removal and immediate replacement of a new ring. Similar to the transdermal contraceptive patch, first-pass metabolism is in the gastrointestinal tract rather than through the liver. Studies have shown that the vaginal ring is both highly effective (Table 4.2) and safe in individuals with stable kidney function [24].

Combined Hormonal Transdermal Contraceptive Patch

Xulane® is a transdermal contraceptive patch is a CHC (norelgestromin 150 μg/ethinyl estradiol 35 mcg) that is applied topically once weekly over a 3-week period and is then removed for a week in which the patient has a withdrawal menstrual cycle. This method functions similarly to an OCP but without the daily fluctuations in hormone levels [19]. See Table 4.2 for method effectiveness. There have been studies that show increased risk of pregnancy in users with body weights greater than 198 lb. Therefore, risk of pregnancy should be considered and counseled for overweight and obese patients.

The transdermal patch undergoes first-pass metabolism through the gastrointestinal tract and bypasses the liver. Although there are no specific studies involving CKD patients, it has been associated with decreased RAAS activation and less blunting of the RAAS response to simulated orthostatic stress which may be beneficial in those with underlying CKD [25]. Studies have shown that women on the transdermal patch have higher mean levels of estradiol compared to those on 35 mcg OCPs, which has created controversy as to whether this method increases risk for development of venous thromboembolism (VTE) [19]. However, recent studies have found that for non-smoking women under 40 years of age, there is no significant increased risk for VTE in transdermal patch users compared to 30 mcg OCP.

Combined Oral Contraceptive Pills

Combined oral contraceptive pills (COCP) work through the inhibition of ovulation and suppression of gonadotropin hormones. These mechanisms come in a variety of options that differ in the amount of estrogen and type of progesterone. The majority of CHCs in the United States contain ethinyl estradiol that can range in amount from low dose (20–35 mcg) all the way up to high dose (50 mcg) [19]. Table 4.1 lists contraindications for combined hormonal contraceptives. Similar to the progesterone-only methods, it is the progesterone component that is responsible for the contraceptive function as well as the majority of its side effect profile. The estrogen is responsible for uterine stabilization. These pills must be taken on a daily basis

Table 4.1 Contraindications to combined hormonal contraceptives [26]

Hypertension: systolic blood pressure >160 or diastolic >100 mg Hg or vascular disease
History of or current ischemic heart disease or stroke
History of deep vein thrombosis (DVT) or pulmonary embolism (PE), not receiving anticoagulant therapy *with* high risk for recurrent DVT/PE
History of estrogen-associated DVT/PE
Pregnancy-associated DVT/PE
Idiopathic DVT/PE
Known thrombophilia: antiphospholipid syndrome, active cancer (metastatic, receiving therapy, or within 6 months post clinical remission*), history of recurrent DVT/PE
Deep vein thrombosis (DVT) or pulmonary embolism (PE) on established anticoagulant therapy for at least 3 months *with* high risk for recurrent DVT/PE
Known thrombophilia: antiphospholipid syndrome, active cancer (metastatic, receiving therapy, or within 6 months post clinical remission*), history of recurrent DVT/PE
Acute DVT/PE
Major surgery with prolonged immobilization
Known thrombogenic mutations (e.g., factor V Leiden; prothrombin mutation; protein S, protein C, and antithrombin deficiencies),
Postpartum <21 days (breastfeeding or not)
Severe decompensated cirrhosis
Valvular heart disease complicated with pulmonary hypertension, risk for atrial fibrillation, or history of subacute bacterial endocarditis
Peripartum cardiomyopathy with normal or mildly impaired cardiac function (<6 months) or moderately or severely impaired cardiac function
Systemic lupus erythematosus with positive or unknown antiphospholipid antibodies
Migraine with aura
Current breast cancer
Liver tumor (hepatocellular adenoma or malignant hepatoma)
Solid organ transplantation complicated by graft failure (acute or chronic), rejection, cardiac allograft vasculopathy

* i.e. within 6 months post clinical remission (excluds non-melanoma skin cancers)

Table 4.2 Contraception method effectiveness [26]

Contraceptive method	Percentage of unintended pregnancy in 1 year with typical use
Sterilization:	
Male	0.15%
Female	0.5%
IUD:	
Copper	0.8%
Levonorgestrel	0.2%
Implant	0.05%
Injectable	6%
Transdermal patch	9%
Vaginal ring	9%
Pill	9%
Male condom	18%
Withdrawal	22%
Spermicide	28%

and can be taken to produce monthly menstrual cycles or extended to produce prolonged cycles. In a monthly cycle, the active hormonal pill is taken daily for the first 3 weeks, and a placebo pill is taken for the 4th week, during which a menstrual cycle is induced. In the extended cycling, an active hormonal pill is taken daily for a predetermined amount of time, typically 6, 9, 12, 24, 36, or 48 weeks. The use of extended cycling COCs has the same medical risks and contraindications as the monthly cycles but is otherwise felt to be safe and effective (Table 4.2).

Emergency Contraception

In light of the high risk for AYA to have unplanned and/or unprotected sex, it is important that teens are aware of post-sexual encounter methods to prevent pregnancy. Currently there are five types of emergency contraception available (Table 4.3). When compared, ulipristal acetate has a higher pregnancy prevention rate than levonorgestrel. The same concerns that exist with typical use of the copper IUD exists also for its use as emergency contraception for individuals on immunosuppressive medication.

Recommendations for Contraceptive Use by Medical Condition

The CDC developed the US *Medical Eligibility Criteria for Contraceptive Use* (US MEC) [26]. This document is a collection of recommendations based on the critical appraisal of scientific evidence and expert opinion to provide guidance for the safe selection and use of the various contraceptive methods in a variety of medical

Table 4.3 Emergency contraception [26]

Emergency contraceptive method	Use within hours of unprotected intercourse or contraceptive failure
Levonorgestrel 1.5 mg (Plan B)	72–120 h
Levonorgestrel 0.75 mg, two tablets (Next Choice)[a]	72–120 h
Ethinyl estradiol 100 mcg + levonorgestrel 0.5 mg[b]	72 h
Copper IUD	120 h
Ulipristal acetate 30 mg (Ella)	120 h

[a]Can be administered as two doses separated 12 h apart or as a single dose
[b]Administer two doses of estradiol and levonorgestrel 12 h apart (Yuzpe regimen)

conditions, including recommendations for contraceptive initiation and management. The choice for the most efficacious and safest contraceptive mechanism is described based on a rating scale of 1–4. Level 1 refers to a situation which there is no restricted use for the method in that condition. Level 2 rating refers to a situation in which the advantages of using the method generally outweigh the theoretical or proven risks for its use in that particular condition. A level 3 rating refers to a situation in which the theoretical or proven risks usually outweigh the advantages of using the method for that condition. A level 4 rating refers to a situation in which the method is an unacceptable health risk for the specific condition.

Individuals who have undergone solid organ transplantation in the preceding 2 years are at higher risk for adverse health outcomes during and following pregnancy. These individuals may also be on teratogenic medications as part of the treatment regimen [26], which include immunosuppressive, antihypertensive, and antiviral medications [11]. Special considerations should be taken in determining the choice of contraceptive method for individuals who have undergone solid organ transplant like kidney transplantation. In many of these cases, LARC methods are the preferred contraceptive method due to their high effective rate, assuring prevention of an unplanned pregnancy. Recommendation for the safest contraceptive choice is distinguished between those individuals who have undergone "uncomplicated solid organ transplant" and those that have undergone "complicated solid organ transplant." Complicated solid organ transplant is defined as those transplants that resulted in acute or chronic graft failure, rejection, or cardiac allograft vasculopathy. The choice for the most efficacious and safest contraceptive mechanism for uncomplicated versus complicated solid organ transplant recipients is described based on a rating scale of 1–4 and is listed in Table 4.4 [26].

Patients with systemic lupus erythematosus (SLE) are at higher risk than the general population to development of ischemic heart disease, strokes, and venous thrombus embolisms (VTE). The risk for the development of any of these processes is weighed by the presence or absence of any of the following associated

Table 4.4 Categories of acceptability for contraceptive alternatives in solid organ transplant patients [26]

Contraceptive method	Uncomplicated solid organ transplant: initiation (continuation)	Complicated solid organ transplant: initiation (continuation)
Copper IUD	2 (2)	3 (2)
Levonorgestrel IUD	2(2)	3 (2)
Contraceptive implants	2	2
Depot medroxyprogesterone acetate (DMPA)	2	2
Progestin-only pills (POP)	2	2
Combined hormonal contraceptives (CHC)	2	4

1: No restricted use for the method
2: Advantages of using the method generally outweigh the theoretical or proven risks
3: The theoretical or proven risks usually outweigh the advantages of using the method
4: Use of the method is an unacceptable health risk

features: (1) the presence of positive (or unknown) antiphospholipid antibodies, (2) severe thrombocytopenia, and/or (3) immunosuppressive therapy. The recommendations for which methods could safely be used in these conditions are identified by the 1–4 rating scale listed in Table 4.5 [26].

Hypertensive patients with systolic blood pressures ≥160 mm Hg and diastolic blood pressures ≥100 mm Hg are associated with increased risk factors for cardiovascular disease, including stroke, acute myocardial infarction, and peripheral arterial disease. The safety determination for contraceptive recommendations is based on the presence or absence of other risk factors for cardiovascular disease. In the presence of isolated chronic hypertension, recommendations for the safest form of contraception are based on whether there is vascular disease, how well the hypertension is controlled, and the presence of additional risk factors for cardiovascular disease (i.e., older age, smoking, diabetes, hypertension, low HDL, high LDL, or high triglycerides). Recommendations for which contraceptive method to safely use in each of these conditions are identified on the rating scale of 1–4 and are listed in Table 4.6 [26].

Sexual Transmitted Infection Prevention

AYA are at the greatest risk for sexually transmitted infection (STI) acquisition compared to any other age group. In part, this is due to increased number of sexual partners and increased frequency of unprotected sexual encounters. For this reason, we always recommend two forms of contraception in this age group (i.e., hormonal and barrier) for both pregnancy prevention and prevention of STI exposure. All of

Table 4.5 Categories of acceptability for contraceptive alternatives in systemic lupus erythematosus patients [26]

Contraceptive method	Systemic lupus erythematosus: positive or unknown antiphospholipid antibodies initiation (Continuation)	Systemic lupus erythematosus severe thrombocytopenia initiation (continuation)	Systemic lupus erythematosus immunosuppressive therapy initiation (continuation)	Systemic lupus erythematosus none of the mentioned associated conditions initiation (continuation)
Copper IUD	1 (1)	3 (2)	2 (1)	1 (1)
Levonorgestrel IUD	3	2	2	2
Contraceptive implants	3	2	2	2
Depot medroxyprogesterone acetate (DMPA)	3 (3)	3 (2)	2 (2)	2 (2)
Progestin-only pills (POP)	3	2	2	2
Combined hormonal contraceptives (CHC)	4	2	2	2

1: No restricted use for the method
2: Advantages of using the method generally outweigh the theoretical or proven risks
3: The theoretical or proven risks usually outweigh the advantages of using the method
4: Use of the method is an unacceptable health risk

Table 4.6 Categories of acceptability for contraceptive alternatives in hypertensive patients [26]

Contraceptive method	Hypertension: adequately controlled	Hypertension: systolic 140–159 mm Hg or diastolic 90–99 mm Hg	Hypertension: systolic ≥160 mm Hg or diastolic ≥100 mm Hg	Hypertension: vascular disease	Multiple risk factors for atherosclerotic cardiovascular disease older age, smoking, diabetes, hypertension, low HDL, high LDL, or high triglycerides initiation (continuation)
Copper IUD	1	1	1	1	1
Levonorgestrel IUD	1	1	2	2	2
Contraceptive implants	1	1	2	2	2
Depot medroxyprogesterone acetate (DMPA)	2	2	3	3	3
Progestin-only pills (POP)	1	1	2	2	2
Combined hormonal contraceptives (CHC)	3	3	4	4	3 (4)

1: No restricted use for the method
2: Advantages of using the method generally outweigh the theoretical or proven risks
3: The theoretical or proven risks usually outweigh the advantages of using the method
4: Use of the method is an unacceptable health risk

the 50 states along with the District of Columbia allow a minor to consent to confidential STI screening and treatment. In 18 states, a physician can, but is not required to, inform a minor's parents of the STI services if they feel it is in the minor's best interest. It is particularly important for AYA on contraceptive methods to be reminded that although contraception is prevented by these methods, only barrier methods protect against sexually transmitted infections. Individuals on immunosuppressant medications should be particularly reminded of their risk for STI acquisition. Female AYA may often feel less empowered and assertive if male partner rejects the idea of condom usage. Providers can be helpful in role playing or suggestive statements that these young women can use to advocate for safe-sex practices. Ensuring that both female and male AYA are informed of how to appropriately use a condom to prevent breakage is important. Patients that report discomfort with condoms should be reminded that condoms are available in different forms and come either lubricated or unlubricated. Lubricated condoms may relieve some of the discomfort. Water-based lubricants should be used rather than petroleum-based [19]. Thinner condoms may be more likely to tear [19]. Adolescents should apply condom prior to the initiation of any sexual activity and should never use more than one condom at a time, as the friction can increase the likelihood of tearing. Condoms should always be kept in a cool and dry place with avoidance of exposure to excess heat (wallet >1 month or glove compartment in a car) [19]. If tolerable, latex condoms are preferred due to higher rates of STI prevention. Damaged condoms or condom packages should always be discarded.

Ongoing Reproductive Management

Many factors of an AYA life can change from visit to visit. For AYA with CKD, in addition to managing a chronic illness, they are exploring, questioning, and finding a sense of identity. This development can lead to changes in relationship status, changes in decision to take or adhere to contraceptive methods, changes in sexual status and behaviors, and changes in family planning decisions. It is important that reproductive health be an ongoing management process that is re-evaluated at each visit. We must work to ensure that we are incorporating questions, concerns, and decisions of reproductive health care into our ongoing care multidisciplinary management plans.

References

1. Neinstein LS, Katzman D, Callahan T. Neinstein's adolescent and young adult health care: a practical guide. 6th ed. Philadelphia: Wolters Kluwer; 2016. xxviii. p. 690.
2. Finkelstein FO, Shirani S, Wuerth D, Finkelstein SH. Therapy insight: sexual dysfunction in patients with chronic kidney disease. Nat Clin Pract Nephrol. 2007;3(4):200–7.

3. Ahmed SB, Vitek WS, Holley JL. Fertility, contraception, and novel reproductive technologies in chronic kidney disease. Semin Nephrol. 2017;37(4):327–36.
4. Basok EK, Atsu N, Rifaioglu MM, Kantarci G, Yildirim A, Tokuc R. Assessment of female sexual function and quality of life in predialysis, peritoneal dialysis, hemodialysis, and renal transplant patients. Int Urol Nephrol. 2009;41(3):473–81.
5. Wiles KS, Nelson-Piercy C, Bramham K. Reproductive health and pregnancy in women with chronic kidney disease. Nat Rev Nephrol. 2018;14(3):165–84.
6. Mor MK, Sevick MA, Shields AM, Green JA, Palevsky PM, Arnold RM, et al. Sexual function, activity, and satisfaction among women receiving maintenance hemodialysis. Clin J Am Soc Nephrol. 2014;9(1):128–34.
7. Anantharaman P, Schmidt RJ. Sexual function in chronic kidney disease. Adv Chronic Kidney Dis. 2007;14(2):119–25.
8. Wang GC, Zheng JH, Xu LG, Min ZL, Zhu YH, Qi J, et al. Measurements of serum pituitary-gonadal hormones and investigation of sexual and reproductive functions in kidney transplant recipients. Int J Nephrol. 2010;2010:612126.
9. Matuszkiewicz-Rowinska J, Skorzewska K, Radowicki S, Niemczyk S, Sokalski A, Przedlacki J, et al. Endometrial morphology and pituitary-gonadal axis dysfunction in women of reproductive age undergoing chronic haemodialysis – a multicentre study. Nephrol Dial Transplant. 2004;19(8):2074–7.
10. Hladunewich MA. Chronic kidney disease and pregnancy. Semin Nephrol. 2017;37(4):337–46.
11. Webster P, Lightstone L, McKay DB, Josephson MA. Pregnancy in chronic kidney disease and kidney transplantation. Kidney Int. 2017;91(5):1047–56.
12. Piccoli GB, Attini R, Vasario E, Conijn A, Biolcati M, D'Amico F, et al. Pregnancy and chronic kidney disease: a challenge in all CKD stages. Clin J Am Soc Nephrol. 2010;5(5):844–55.
13. Hladunewich MA, Melamad N, Bramham K. Pregnancy across the spectrum of chronic kidney disease. Kidney Int. 2016;89(5):995–1007.
14. Barua M, Hladunewich M, Keunen J, Pierratos A, McFarlane P, Sood M, et al. Successful pregnancies on nocturnal home hemodialysis. Clin J Am Soc Nephrol. 2008;3(2):392–6.
15. Josephson MA, McKay DB. Women and transplantation: fertility, sexuality, pregnancy, contraception. Adv Chronic Kidney Dis. 2013;20(5):433–40.
16. Pucci M, Sarween N, Knox E, Lipkin G, Martin U. Angiotensin-converting enzyme inhibitors and angiotensin receptor blockers in women of childbearing age: risks versus benefits. Expert Rev Clin Pharmacol. 2015;8(2):221–31.
17. Bullo M, Tschumi S, Bucher BS, Bianchetti MG, Simonetti GD. Pregnancy outcome following exposure to angiotensin-converting enzyme inhibitors or angiotensin receptor antagonists: a systematic review. Hypertension. 2012;60(2):444–50.
18. van Eerde AM, Krediet CT, Rookmaaker MB, van Reekum FE, Knoers NV, Lely AT. Pre-pregnancy advice in chronic kidney disease: do not forget genetic counseling. Kidney Int. 2016;90(4):905–6.
19. Emans SJH, Laufer MR. Emans, Laufer, Goldstein's pediatric & adolescent gynecology. 6th ed. Philadelphia: Wolters Kluwer Health/Lippincott Williams & Wilkins Health; 2011. xviii. p. 585.
20. Zerner J, Doil KL, Drewry J, Leeber DA. Intrauterine contraceptive device failures in renal transplant patients. J Reprod Med. 1981;26(2):99–102.
21. Committee on A. Contraception for adolescents. Pediatrics. 2014;134(4):e1244–56.
22. Ramhendar T, Byrne P. Use of the levonorgestrel-releasing intrauterine system in renal transplant recipients: a retrospective case review. Contraception. 2012;86(3):288–9.
23. Bieber SD, Jefferson JA, Anderson AE. Migration of an intrauterine device and peritonitis in a peritoneal dialysis patient. Clin Nephrol. 2013;80(2):146–50.

24. Paternoster DM, Riboni F, Bertolino M, Garofalo G, Lazzarich E, Surico N, et al. The contraceptive vaginal ring in women with renal and liver transplantation: analysis of preliminary results. Transplant Proc. 2010;42(4):1162–5.
25. Odutayo A, Cherney D, Miller J, Ahmed SB, Lai V, Dunn S, et al. Transdermal contraception and the renin-angiotensin-aldosterone system in premenopausal women. Am J Physiol Ren Physiol. 2015;308(6):F535–40.
26. Curtis KMTN, Jatlaoui TC, Berry-Bibee E, Horton LG, Zapata LB, et al. U.S. medical eligibility criteria for contraceptive use. MMWR Recomm Rep. 2016;65(RR-3):1–104.

Chapter 5
Congenital Anomalies of the Kidney and Urinary Tract in Adolescents

Erica Winnicki and Hillary Copp

Introduction

Congenital anomalies of the kidneys and urinary tract (CAKUT) are most often diagnosed in the prenatal or neonatal period. However, as CAKUT is the most common cause of chronic kidney disease (CKD) in children and adolescents, understanding this spectrum of diagnoses is important in caring for the adolescent with CKD. Additionally, adolescence is an important time period for the patient with CAKUT as puberty is associated with more rapid CKD progression as well as changes in bladder function. This chapter will review the epidemiology and etiology of CAKUT and then focus on means of decreasing CKD progression and optimizing the long-term prognosis for adolescents with CKD due to CAKUT.

Epidemiology

CAKUT are a heterogeneous group of anatomic abnormalities that result in a wide spectrum of clinical manifestations (Table 5.1). CAKUT are common birth defects, with autopsy data suggesting that the prevalence of CAKUT is 3.1% [1]. European registry data reports a birth prevalence of 3.3 per 1000 newborns [2]. Familial clustering is common, suggesting that genetic mechanisms are important in the

E. Winnicki (✉)
Department of Pediatrics, Division of Nephrology, University of California San Francisco, San Francisco, CA, USA
e-mail: erica.winnicki@ucsf.edu

H. Copp
Department of Urology, University of California San Francisco, San Francisco, CA, USA
e-mail: Hillary.copp@ucsf.edu

M. N. Haddad et al. (eds.), *Adolescents with Chronic Kidney Disease*,
https://doi.org/10.1007/978-3-319-97220-6_5

Table 5.1 Spectrum of CAKUT

Renal	
	Renal agenesis/aplasia
	Renal dysplasia: multicystic dysplastic kidney, cystic dysplastic kidney, hypoplastic kidney
	Hydronephrosis
	Ectopic kidney
	Horseshoe kidney
Ureter	
	Ureteropelvic junction obstruction
	Ureterovesical junction obstruction
	Duplex collecting system
	Megaureter
	Vesicoureteral reflux
Bladder	
	Bladder exstrophy
	Neurogenic bladder
Urethra	
	Posterior urethral valves
	Anterior urethral obstruction

pathogenesis [3]. Maternal factors associated with development of CAKUT in the child include diabetes [4, 5], advanced age, white race, kidney disease [5], and use of certain medications during pregnancy (cyclophosphamide, adriamycin, mycophenolate mofetil, antiepileptic drugs, ACE/ARBs, cyclosporine A, dexamethasone) [6, 7].

CAKUT are responsible for the majority of chronic kidney disease and end-stage renal disease (ESRD) in children and adolescents. According to data from the US Renal Data System (USRDS), cystic/hereditary/congenital disorders are listed as the cause of ESRD in 33% of children, making this group of diagnoses the leading cause of ESRD in children in the United States [8]. Renal hypoplasia/dysplasia and congenital obstructive uropathies are the main causes of ESRD within this group of diagnoses. CAKUT are also reported to be the most common cause of pediatric ESRD in other developed countries including Europe, Japan, Australia, and New Zealand [9].

Diagnosis and Presenting/Clinical Features

With the wide use of antenatal ultrasonography, CAKUT are commonly diagnosed during the antenatal period, thereby allowing for appropriate postnatal evaluation and follow-up care. For those not diagnosed in the antenatal period, possible presenting features include urinary tract infections, urinary incontinence, voiding dysfunction, or polyuria; abdominal pain, mass, or distension; and signs and symptoms related to CKD including poor growth/failure to thrive and/or hypertension [15]. For patients with posterior urethral valves (PUV) specifically, the diagnosis is usually suspected on antenatal ultrasonography and confirmed in the early neonatal period by VCUG; however, as many as 25% of patients may have a delayed diagnosis after 1 year of age and present with clinical signs and symptoms related to urinary tract obstruction and CKD [16]. Common presenting signs and symptoms for boys with late presentation of PUV may include diurnal enuresis, poor stream, and urinary retention [17]. CAKUT are diagnosed radiographically. The most commonly used imaging modality of the urinary tract is ultrasound [10], which provides important structural information and specifically allows evaluation of kidney size, presence or absence of renal parenchymal abnormalities, collecting system dilation, and bladder wall thickness.

While a number of grading systems based on ultrasound findings have been proposed to quantify the severity of urinary tract dilation, the most recent proposed grading system based on multidisciplinary consensus is known as the Urinary Tract Dilation (UTD) Classification System. The UTD Classification System uses six categories of ultrasound findings to determine the risk (grade 1–3, low to high risk) of significant urologic pathology. These categories consist of anterior-posterior renal pelvic diameter, calyceal dilatation, renal parenchymal thickness, renal parenchymal appearance, bladder abnormalities, and ureteral abnormalities [11]. For postnatal description of UTD, three groups of risk stratification are used including UTD P1 (low risk), UTD P2 (intermediate risk), and UTD P3 (high risk).

Contrast voiding cystourethrogram (VCUG) is considered the gold standard for diagnosis of vesicoureteral reflux (VUR) and PUV; downsides of this procedure include exposure to radiation and procedure-related distress [12].

Radionuclide renal imaging is important to evaluate for urinary tract obstruction or renal scarring; technitium-99m mercaptoacetyltriglycine (MAG3) is commonly used to evaluate for the former, whereas technetium-99m dimercaptosuccinic acid (DMSA) renal scan is commonly used for the latter; either may be used to evaluate split renal function [13]. MR urography may be used for examination of more complex urogenital anomalies [10].

Urodynamic studies are an important tool for evaluating lower urinary tract dysfunction in children. Uroflowmetry is used as a noninvasive first-line test for children with suspected lower urinary tract dysfunction, whereas invasive urodynamic studies are used when the urinary flow curves from noninvasive testing suggest severe lower urinary tract dysfunction including neuropathic or non-neuropathic detrusor-sphincter dysfunction, obstruction, or certain genitourinary abnormalities [14].

CAKUT are associated with other non-urinary congenital anomalies in about one third of cases [18]. For this reason, a diagnosis of CAKUT requires a thorough history and examination to exclude other associated congenital anomalies. The most commonly associated non-urinary congenital anomalies include musculoskeletal anomalies, digestive system anomalies (such as anal atresia or malrotation), cardiac defects, and central nervous system anomalies (such as spina bifida) [18].

Etiology

The pathogenesis of CAKUT involves a disturbance in normal renal development, with both environmental and genetic factors playing an important role in the development of this diverse spectrum of abnormalities. Evidence for the importance of the environment in CAKUT includes the observations that development of CAKUT is associated with fetal exposure to certain drugs that interfere with normal renal development and the observation that CAKUT is associated with maternal diabetes [19]. There is a strong evidence that genetics are important in the development of CAKUT based on the finding of familial clustering [3], and an increasing number of single genes involved in CAKUT have been identified [20]. The primary single-gene mutations associated with CAKUT are shown in Table 5.2 and include a number of genes known to be important in normal renal development. The most common single genes causing CAKUT that have been identified to date are PAX2 and HNF1B [21]. The PAX2 gene encodes a transcription factor important in the regulation of ureteric budding. Mutations in PAX2 may cause renal coloboma syndrome (renal hypodysplasia, optic nerve coloboma, and hearing loss) but have also been associated with isolated CAKUT and a wide spectrum of phenotypes [22]. Mutations in HNF1B were initially recognized as causing the renal cysts and diabetes syndrome but have now been reported in a wide spectrum of renal manifestations (renal cysts and malformations, renal magnesium wasting, hypocalciuria, impaired renal function) as well as extrarenal manifestations which include gout, hyperparathyroidism, and autism in addition to early-onset diabetes [23].

Treatment/Management

Treatment depends on the type of CAKUT, with surgical interventions reserved for those with significant urinary tract obstruction [PUV, ureteropelvic junction obstruction (UPJ)] or VUR and recurrent urinary tract infections [24]. The bladder may be damaged from obstruction or functional causes, and if bladder dysfunction is present, it should be treated to mitigate ongoing renal injury. Bladder function and the type of bladder dysfunction may change over time and in particular during puberty [25]. For this reason, clinical reassessment including urodynamic studies and changes to bladder management might be indicated, especially during adolescence. Bladder dysfunction and changes in function over time have specifically been noted in boys with PUV. Despite relief of the urethral obstruction in PUV, the majority of boys with PUV have bladder dysfunction [26]. It has been shown that while bladder hypercontractility is often present in infancy, the pattern of bladder dysfunction may change to hypocontractility particularly after puberty [27].

There are a number of methods to manage bladder dysfunction including antimuscarinic agents, chronic intermittent catheterization (CIC), and bladder augmentation. Antimuscarinic agents (like oxybutynin) are used to decrease bladder

Table 5.2 Single-gene causes of human-isolated CAKUT and syndromes with a predominant CAKUT phenotype

Gene symbol	Renal phenotype	Extrarenal phenotype	Human disease [OMIM#]
A. Dominant CAKUT			
BMP4	Renal hypodysplasia	Cleft lip, microphthalmia	Microphthalmia, syndromic 6 [607932][a] Orofacial cleft 11 [600625][a]
EYA1	Multicystic dysplastic kidney, renal aplasia	Deafness, ear malformations, branchial cysts	Anterior segment anomalies with or without cataract [113650] Branchiootic syndrome 1 [602588][a] Branchiootorenal syndrome 1, with or without cataracts [113650][a] Otofaciocervical syndrome [166780][a]
GATA3	Renal dysplasia	Hypoparathyroidism, heart defects, immune deficiency, deafness	Hypoparathyroidism, sensorineural deafness, and renal dysplasia [146255][a]
HNF1B	Renal hypodysplasia, single kidney, horseshoe kidney	Diabetes mellitus (MODY5) hyperuricemia, hypomagnesemia, elevated LFT	Diabetes mellitus, noninsulin-dependent [125853][a] Renal cysts and diabetes syndrome [137920][a]
KAL1[a]	Renal agenesis	Micropenis, bilateral cryptorchidism, anosmia	Hypogonadotropic hypogonadism 1 with or without anosmia (Kallmann syndrome 1) [308700][a]
PAX2	Vesicoureteral reflux, renal hypoplasia	Optic nerve colobomas, hearing loss	Papillorenal syndrome [120330][a] Renal hypoplasia, isolated [191830][a]
RET	Renal agenesis	See OMIM# in the next column	Central hypoventilation syndrome, congenital [209880][a] Medullary thyroid carcinoma [155240][a] Multiple endocrine neoplasia IIA [171400][a] Multiple endocrine neoplasia IIB [162300][a] Pheochromocytoma [171300][a] Renal agenesis [191830][a]
ROBO2	VUR, ureterovesical junction defects	None	Vesicoureteral reflux 2 [610878][a]
SALL1	Renal hypodysplasia, renal agenesis	Limb, ear, anal abnormalities	Townes-Brocks syndrome [107480][a]
SIX1	Renal hypodysplasia, VUR	Deafness, ear defects, branchial cysts	Brachiootic syndrome 3 [608389][a] Deafness, autosomal dominant 23 [605192][a]

(continued)

Table 5.2 (continued)

Gene symbol	Renal phenotype	Extrarenal phenotype	Human disease [OMIM#]
SIX2	Renal hypodysplasia	None	–
SIX5	Renal hypodysplasia, VUR	Deafness, ear defects, branchial cysts	Branchiootorenal syndrome 2 [610896][a]
SOX17	VUR, UPJO	None	Vesicoureteral reflux 3 [613674][a]
TNXB	VUR	Joint hypermobility	Ehlers-Danlos syndrome, autosomal dominant, hypermobility type [130020][a] Ehlers-Danlos syndrome, autosomal recessive, due to tenascin X deficiency [606408][a]
UPK3A	Renal adysplasia	Subtle facial and limb defects	Renal adysplasia [191830][a]
WNT4[b]	Renal hypodysplasia	Female-to-male sex reversal, adrenal dysplasia, lung dysplasia (SERKAL)	Müllerian aplasia and hyperandrogenism [158330][a] SERKAL syndrome [611812][a]
CHD1L	Renal hypodysplasia, VUR, UPJO	None	–
DSTYK	Renal hypodysplasia, UPJO	Epilepsy in 2 out of 7 affected	–
MUC1	Medullary cystic kidney disease type 1	–	MCKD1 – medullary cystic kidney disease type 1 [#174000]
UMOD	Medullary cystic kidney disease type 2	Medullary cystic kidney disease type 2	MCKD2 – medullary cystic kidney disease type2 [#603860] HNFJ2 –hyperuricemic nephropathy, familial juvenile 2 [#6130925],[#613092]
B. Recessive CAKUT			
ACE	Absence or incomplete differentiation of proximal tubules	Pulmonary hypoplasia (Potter sequence), skull abnormalities	Renal tubular dysgenesis [267430][a]
AGT	Similar to *ACE*	Similar to *ACE*	Renal tubular dysgenesis [267430][a]
AGTR1	Similar to *ACE*	Similar to *ACE*	Renal tubular dysgenesis [267430][a]
REN	Similar to *ACE*	Similar to *ACE*	Renal tubular dysgenesis [267430][a]
FGF20	Bilateral renal agenesis	None	–
TRAP1	VUR, renal agenesis	VACTERL association	–

Table 5.2 (continued)

Gene symbol	Renal phenotype	Extrarenal phenotype	Human disease [OMIM#]
FRAS1	Renal agenesis	Cryptophthalmos, nose ear and larynx malformations. Mental retardation and syndactyly manifest occasionally	Fraser syndrome [219000][a]
FREM2	Renal agenesis	Cryptophthalmos, nose ear and larynx malformations. Mental retardation and syndactyly manifest occasionally	Fraser syndrome [219000][a]

Reprinted/adapted by permission from Springer Nature, Pediatric Nephology, Single-gene causes of congenital anomalies of the kidney and urinary tract (CAKUT) in humans, Asaf Vivante et al. (2014)

[a]X-linked recessive

[b]Mode of inheritance can be autosomal dominant or autosomal recessive

overactivity and improve bladder compliance and are considered safe for long-term use in pediatric patients [25]. CIC is indicated for children with incomplete bladder emptying and high bladder pressure [25]. Complications of CIC include urethral injury or stricture and, most commonly, urinary tract infections [28]. If CIC cannot be done through the urethra, creation of a continent catheterizable channel between the bladder and skin using the appendix (Mitrofanoff) or tapered ileum (Monti) [29] is an alternate option. CIC should be performed frequently enough to avoid bladder overfilling which increases the risk of UTI [30]. Nonadherence to CIC is of concern, particularly for adolescents, and would be expected to cause an increase in infectious complications. There is some evidence that catheterization through a continent catheterizable channel may be associated with better adherence as compared to urethral catheterization [30]. While symptomatic UTIs should be treated in patient's performing CIC, it is important to note that CIC leads to bladder colonization, and treatment of asymptomatic bacteriuria is not indicated. Children with small-volume or poorly compliant bladders may require bladder augmentation or urinary diversion [31]. Bladder augmentation is most commonly done using the ileum or sigmoid mucosa; however, ureterocystoplasty is preferable when possible as it avoids the potential complications associated with using GI segments (including stomach) for the bladder augment [32]. These potential complications include metabolic acidosis or alkalosis, calculi, and hematuria-dysuria syndrome. Spontaneous bladder perforation is the most serious potential complication of bladder augmentation and is directly related to nonadherence to intermittent bladder catheterization [33].

Bladder management should always be considered in concert with bowel management, and there is evidence for a neurologic basis in the relationship between bladder and bowel function [34]. A dilated rectum alone will cause abnormal voiding parameters including increased post-void residual [35], and as such, maintenance of normal stooling is an important part of the treatment of bladder dysfunction.

The use of antibiotics to prevent urinary tract infections is controversial. In general, however, continuous antibiotic prophylaxis is not recommended in upper urinary tract obstruction due to the low occurrence of UTIs in this group [36, 37]. The use of continuous antibiotic prophylaxis may be considered in those with high-grade VUR, ureteral dilation, and ureterovesical junction (UVJ) obstruction in order to decrease the risk of febrile UTI [38].

Treatment of the complications of CKD in patients with CAKUT, and in particular those complications known to be associated with disease progression such as hypertension and proteinuria, is also of critical importance. Both proteinuria and hypertension have been shown to be independent risk factors for CKD progression in children with non-glomerular causes of CKD in the Chronic Kidney Disease in Children (CKiD) cohort [39]. ACE inhibitors have long been shown to have renoprotective effects above that of other antihypertensive agents [40, 41]. Specifically in children with CKD due to renal dysplasia, it has been shown that intensive blood pressure control on an antihypertensive regimen that includes an ACE inhibitor confers a benefit in decreasing the rate of CKD progression [42]. For this reason, use of ACE inhibitor therapy should be employed for children with CKD due to CAKUT as treatment for hypertension and/or proteinuria assuming there is no contraindication to their use. Hypoalbuminemia and anemia have also been identified as modifiable risk factors for CKD progression in children with non-glomerular causes of kidney disease [43], and these risk factors should be corrected as well.

Prognosis

Given the heterogeneity with regard to the diagnosis of CAKUT, outcomes for these patients are similarly heterogeneous. Prognosis is dependent on the type of CAKUT, with bilateral renal dysplasia (or dysplasia of a solitary kidney) and bilateral obstructive processes (such as PUV) having the worst prognosis [44]. Patients with renal dysplasia require renal replacement therapy at a significantly younger age than patients with other types of CAKUT [45].

Factors associated with progression of CKD in children with CAKUT include heavy proteinuria, hypertension, and postpubertal age [31, 46]. It is particularly important to note that the rapidity of progression of CKD is often noted to be increased during adolescence [31], with an associated increase in the incidence of renal replacement therapy during this time period [45]. As such, adolescent patients with CAKUT should be followed particularly closely. Factors found to be associated with progression to ESRD specifically in PUV include a nadir serum creatinine at presentation (after a period of bladder decompression of at least several days) of greater than 1 mg/dl and bladder dysfunction [26, 47].

There is conflicting evidence as to whether the presence of VUR impacts progression of CKD in children and adolescents with CAKUT. VUR may predispose children to develop urinary tract infections/pyelonephritis, which may lead to renal scarring [48]. It has been shown that prompt treatment of an acute UTI is important in preventing renal parenchymal inflammation, with one study reporting that 41% of children had renal inflammatory changes by DMSA when treated for UTI within 24 h of the onset of fever versus 72% when therapy was delayed to 3–8 days after fever [49]. However, it can be difficult to distinguish between primary renal damage (related to urinary tract obstruction or dysplasia/hypoplasia preceding the infections) and secondary scarring caused by febrile urinary tract infections, and thus there is some debate as to the relative importance that VUR plays in regard to renal scarring [50, 51]. VUR with UTI but without structural abnormalities in the kidneys does not seem to be an important cause of CKD [48]. In a study of children with moderate CKD due to CAKUT, nearly half of whom had associated VUR, the presence of VUR was not found to be associated with progression of CKD, while it was associated with a more prevalent history of UTIs [46].

Dialysis and Transplant

For adolescents with CAKUT who progress to end-stage renal disease (ESRD), the choice of treatment for ESRD depends on multiple patient factors. Preemptive kidney transplantation (transplantation prior to dialysis initiation) is the ideal treatment for children with ESRD as it is associated with better patient survival compared to any dialysis exposure [52]. Children with CAKUT are more likely to receive a preemptive transplant than those with other causes of ESRD [52]. For those who do not undergo preemptive kidney transplantation, in general, peritoneal dialysis is the preferred dialysis modality. This modality is associated with preservation of residual renal function [53] and may be associated with a survival benefit over hemodialysis, particularly in the first year after dialysis initiation [54].

Kidney transplantation is the treatment of choice for all children with ESRD as transplant confers survival benefits as well as improved health-related quality of life, cognition, and growth compared to maintenance dialysis [55–58]. It is imperative that children with CAKUT undergo a thorough urologic evaluation prior to kidney transplantation. Children with lower urinary tract dysfunction should have the dysfunction managed prior to undergoing kidney transplant using antimuscarinic agents, CIC, or surgery, as appropriate for the particular patient. Children who require bladder reconstructive surgery should ideally undergo this prior to kidney transplantation to achieve a low-pressure bladder reservoir and thereby minimize the risk of injury to the allograft from high filling pressure [31, 32]. Following kidney transplantation, while UTI and VUR rates may be higher for those with significant bladder pathology [31], both allograft and patient survival are superior for patients with CAKUT as compared to other causes of ESRD [45].

References

1. Barakat AJ, Drougas JG. Occurrence of congenital abnormalities of kidney and urinary tract in 13,775 autopsies. Urology. 1991;38(4):347–50.
2. European Surveillance of Congenital Anomalies. Prevalence tables 2011–2015. Ispra: EUROCAT; 2013.
3. Bulum B, Ozcakar ZB, Ustuner E, Dusunceli E, Kavaz A, Duman D, et al. High frequency of kidney and urinary tract anomalies in asymptomatic first-degree relatives of patients with CAKUT. Pediatr Nephrol. 2013;28(11):2143–7.
4. Dart AB, Ruth CA, Sellers EA, Au W, Dean HJ. Maternal diabetes mellitus and congenital anomalies of the kidney and urinary tract (CAKUT) in the child. Am J Kidney Dis. 2015;65(5):684–91.
5. Shnorhavorian M, Bittner R, Wright JL, Schwartz SM. Maternal risk factors for congenital urinary anomalies: results of a population-based case-control study. Urology. 2011;78(5):1156–61.
6. Schreuder MF, Bueters RR, Huigen MC, Russel FG, Masereeuw R, van den Heuvel LP. Effect of drugs on renal development. Clin J Am Soc Nephrol. 2011;6(1):212–7.
7. Sekine T, Miura K, Takahashi K, Igarashi T. Children's toxicology from bench to bed – drug-induced renal injury (1): the toxic effects of ARB/ACEI on fetal kidney development. J Toxicol Sci. 2009;34(Suppl 2):SP245–50.
8. US Renal Data System, USRDS. Annual data report: atlas of chronic kidney disease and end-stage renal disease in the United States. Bethesda: National Institute of Health, National Institute of Diabetes and Digestive and Kidney DIseases; 2015.
9. Harambat J, van Stralen KJ, Kim JJ, Tizard EJ. Epidemiology of chronic kidney disease in children. Pediatr Nephrol. 2012;27(3):363–73.
10. Chung EM, Soderlund KA, Fagen KE. Imaging of the pediatric urinary system. Radiol Clin N Am. 2017;55(2):337–57.
11. Nguyen HT, Benson CB, Bromley B, Campbell JB, Chow J, Coleman B, et al. Multidisciplinary consensus on the classification of prenatal and postnatal urinary tract dilation (UTD classification system). J Pediatr Urol. 2014;10(6):982–98.
12. Agrawalla S, Pearce R, Goodman TR. How to perform the perfect voiding cystourethrogram. Pediatr Radiol. 2004;34(2):114–9.
13. Othman S, Al-Hawas A, Al-Maqtari R. Renal cortical imaging in children: 99mTc MAG3 versus 99mTc DMSA. Clin Nucl Med. 2012;37(4):351–5.
14. Bauer SB, Nijman RJ, Drzewiecki BA, Sillen U, Hoebeke P, International Children's Continence Society Standardization Subcommittee. International Children's Continence Society standardization report on urodynamic studies of the lower urinary tract in children. Neurourol Urodyn. 2015;34(7):640–7.
15. Soliman NA, Ali RI, Ghobrial EE, Habib EI, Ziada AM. Pattern of clinical presentation of congenital anomalies of the kidney and urinary tract among infants and children. Nephrology (Carlton). 2015;20(6):413–8.
16. Kibar Y, Ashley RA, Roth CC, Frimberger D, Kropp BP. Timing of posterior urethral valve diagnosis and its impact on clinical outcome. J Pediatr Urol. 2011;7(5):538–42.
17. Ziylan O, Oktar T, Ander H, Korgali E, Rodoplu H, Kocak T. The impact of late presentation of posterior urethral valves on bladder and renal function. J Urol. 2006;175(5):1894–7. discussion 1897
18. Stoll C, Dott B, Alembik Y, Roth MP. Associated nonurinary congenital anomalies among infants with congenital anomalies of kidney and urinary tract (CAKUT). Eur J Med Genet. 2014;57(7):322–8.
19. dos Santos Junior AC, de Miranda DM, Simoes e Silva AC. Congenital anomalies of the kidney and urinary tract: an embryogenetic review. Birth Defects Res C Embryo Today. 2014;102(4):374–81.

20. Vivante A, Kohl S, Hwang DY, Dworschak GC, Hildebrandt F. Single-gene causes of congenital anomalies of the kidney and urinary tract (CAKUT) in humans. Pediatr Nephrol. 2014;29(4):695–704.
21. Weber S, Moriniere V, Knuppel T, Charbit M, Dusek J, Ghiggeri GM, et al. Prevalence of mutations in renal developmental genes in children with renal hypodysplasia: results of the ESCAPE study. J Am Soc Nephrol. 2006;17(10):2864–70.
22. Bower M, Salomon R, Allanson J, Antignac C, Benedicenti F, Benetti E, et al. Update of PAX2 mutations in renal coloboma syndrome and establishment of a locus-specific database. Hum Mutat. 2012;33(3):457–66.
23. Verhave JC, Bech AP, Wetzels JF, Nijenhuis T. Hepatocyte nuclear factor 1beta-associated kidney disease: more than renal cysts and diabetes. J Am Soc Nephrol. 2016;27(2):345–53.
24. Nef S, Neuhaus TJ, Sparta G, Weitz M, Buder K, Wisser J, et al. Outcome after prenatal diagnosis of congenital anomalies of the kidney and urinary tract. Eur J Pediatr. 2016;175(5):667–76.
25. Woodhouse CR, Neild GH, Yu RN, Bauer S. Adult care of children from pediatric urology. J Urol. 2012;187(4):1164–71.
26. DeFoor W, Clark C, Jackson E, Reddy P, Minevich E, Sheldon C. Risk factors for end stage renal disease in children with posterior urethral valves. J Urol. 2008;180(4 Suppl):1705–8. discussion 1708
27. De Gennaro M, Capitanucci ML, Mosiello G, Caione P, Silveri M. The changing urodynamic pattern from infancy to adolescence in boys with posterior urethral valves. BJU Int. 2000;85(9):1104–8.
28. Wyndaele JJ. Complications of intermittent catheterization: their prevention and treatment. Spinal Cord. 2002;40(10):536–41.
29. Farrugia MK, Malone PS. Educational article: the Mitrofanoff procedure. J Pediatr Urol. 2010;6(4):330–7.
30. Kari J, Al-Deek B, Elkhatib L, Salahudeen S, Mukhtar N, Al Ahmad R, et al. Is mitrofanoff a more socially accepted clean intermittent catheterization (CIC) route for children and their families? Eur J Pediatr Surg. 2013;23(5):405–10.
31. Gonzalez Celedon C, Bitsori M, Tullus K. Progression of chronic renal failure in children with dysplastic kidneys. Pediatr Nephrol. 2007;22(7):1014–20.
32. Pereira PL, Urrutia MJ, Lobato R, Jaureguizar E. Renal transplantation in augmented bladders. Curr Urol Rep 2014;15(8):431. https://doi.org/10.1007/s11934-014-0431-4.
33. Husmann DA. Long-term complications following bladder augmentations in patients with spina bifida: bladder calculi, perforation of the augmented bladder and upper tract deterioration. Transl Androl Urol. 2016;5(1):3–11.
34. Franco I. New ideas in the cause of bladder dysfunction in children. Curr Opin Urol. 2011;21(4):334–8.
35. Chung KL, Chao NS, Liu CS, Tang PM, Liu KK, Leung MW. Abnormal voiding parameters in children with severe idiopathic constipation. Pediatr Surg Int. 2014;30(7):747–9.
36. Islek A, Guven AG, Koyun M, Akman S, Alimoglu E. Probability of urinary tract infection in infants with ureteropelvic junction obstruction: is antibacterial prophylaxis really needed? Pediatr Nephrol. 2011;26(10):1837–41.
37. Roth CC, Hubanks JM, Bright BC, Heinlen JE, Donovan BO, Kropp BP, et al. Occurrence of urinary tract infection in children with significant upper urinary tract obstruction. Urology. 2009;73(1):74–8.
38. Herz D, Merguerian P, McQuiston L. Continuous antibiotic prophylaxis reduces the risk of febrile UTI in children with asymptomatic antenatal hydronephrosis with either ureteral dilation, high-grade vesicoureteral reflux, or ureterovesical junction obstruction. J Pediatr Urol. 2014;10(4):650–4.
39. Fathallah-Shaykh SA, Flynn JT, Pierce CB, Abraham AG, Blydt-Hansen TD, Massengill SF, et al. Progression of pediatric CKD of nonglomerular origin in the CKiD cohort. Clin J Am Soc Nephrol. 2015;10(4):571–7.

40. Jafar TH, Schmid CH, Landa M, Giatras I, Toto R, Remuzzi G, et al. Angiotensin-converting enzyme inhibitors and progression of nondiabetic renal disease. A meta-analysis of patient-level data. Ann Intern Med. 2001;135(2):73–87.
41. Jafar TH, Stark PC, Schmid CH, Landa M, Maschio G, Marcantoni C, et al. Proteinuria as a modifiable risk factor for the progression of non-diabetic renal disease. Kidney Int. 2001;60(3):1131–40.
42. ESCAPE Trial Group, Wuhl E, Trivelli A, Picca S, Litwin M, Peco-Antic A, et al. Strict blood-pressure control and progression of renal failure in children. N Engl J Med. 2009;361(17):1639–50.
43. Warady BA, Abraham AG, Schwartz GJ, Wong CS, Munoz A, Betoko A, et al. Predictors of rapid progression of glomerular and nonglomerular kidney disease in children and adolescents: the Chronic Kidney Disease in Children (CKiD) cohort. Am J Kidney Dis. 2015;65(6):878–88.
44. Sanna-Cherchi S, Ravani P, Corbani V, Parodi S, Haupt R, Piaggio G, et al. Renal outcome in patients with congenital anomalies of the kidney and urinary tract. Kidney Int. 2009;76(5):528–33.
45. Wuhl E, van Stralen KJ, Verrina E, Bjerre A, Wanner C, Heaf JG, et al. Timing and outcome of renal replacement therapy in patients with congenital malformations of the kidney and urinary tract. Clin J Am Soc Nephrol. 2013;8(1):67–74.
46. Ishikura K, Uemura O, Hamasaki Y, Nakai H, Ito S, Harada R, et al. Insignificant impact of VUR on the progression of CKD in children with CAKUT. Pediatr Nephrol. 2016;31(1):105–12.
47. Ansari MS, Gulia A, Srivastava A, Kapoor R. Risk factors for progression to end-stage renal disease in children with posterior urethral valves. J Pediatr Urol. 2010;6(3):261–4.
48. Salo J, Ikaheimo R, Tapiainen T, Uhari M. Childhood urinary tract infections as a cause of chronic kidney disease. Pediatrics. 2011;128(5):840–7.
49. Doganis D, Siafas K, Mavrikou M, Issaris G, Martirosova A, Perperidis G, et al. Does early treatment of urinary tract infection prevent renal damage? Pediatrics. 2007;120(4):e922–8.
50. Coulthard MG. Vesicoureteric reflux is not a benign condition. Pediatr Nephrol. 2009;24(2):227–32.
51. Venhola M, Uhari M. Vesicoureteral reflux, a benign condition. Pediatr Nephrol. 2009;24(2):223–6.
52. Amaral S, Sayed BA, Kutner N, Patzer RE. Preemptive kidney transplantation is associated with survival benefits among pediatric patients with end-stage renal disease. Kidney Int. 2016;90(5):1100–8.
53. Moist LM, Port FK, Orzol SM, Young EW, Ostbye T, Wolfe RA, et al. Predictors of loss of residual renal function among new dialysis patients. J Am Soc Nephrol. 2000;11(3):556–64.
54. Chesnaye NC, Schaefer F, Groothoff JW, Bonthuis M, Reusz G, Heaf JG, et al. Mortality risk in European children with end-stage renal disease on dialysis. Kidney Int. 2016;89(6):1355–62.
55. Rana A, Gruessner A, Agopian VG, Khalpey Z, Riaz IB, Kaplan B, et al. Survival benefit of solid-organ transplant in the United States. JAMA Surg. 2015;150(3):252–9.
56. Jung HW, Kim HY, Lee YA, Kang HG, Shin CH, Ha IS, et al. Factors affecting growth and final adult height after pediatric renal transplantation. Transplant Proc. 2013;45(1):108–14.
57. Groothoff JW. Long-term outcomes of children with end-stage renal disease. Pediatr Nephrol. 2005;20(7):849–53.
58. Goldstein SL, Graham N, Burwinkle T, Warady B, Farrah R, Varni JW. Health-related quality of life in pediatric patients with ESRD. Pediatr Nephrol. 2006;21(6):846–50.

Chapter 6
Rapidly Progressive Glomerulonephritis

Lavjay Butani

Introduction

Rapidly progressive glomerulonephritis (RPGN) is the term given to a subset of patients with glomerulonephritis (GN) who have a rapid decline in renal function over a very short period of time; typically this is defined as a 50% decline in renal function over a 3-month period or less. Histologically, patients with RPGN have evidence of severe glomerular inflammation with extra-capillary cellular proliferation and infiltration of inflammatory cells into the Bowman's space resulting in the formation of crescents in the majority of glomeruli. While there are very limited large-scale data on the epidemiology of RPGN in children, it appears evident that RPGN is very uncommon in children [1]. Nevertheless, data extrapolated from adult patients support the critical importance of early diagnosis and treatment in such patients due to the very high morbidity and mortality associated with them and evidence that supports that early treatment may be associated with improved outcomes.

Clinically, as would be expected, patients with RPGN present with hypertension, edema, hematuria (often gross, but sometimes microscopic), and proteinuria and are noted to have acute kidney injury with significant impairment of their glomerular filtration rate (GFR) [2]. Investigations of diagnostic and prognostic value in the setting of RPGN include serologic studies (complement C3, complement C4, antinuclear antibody, antistreptolysin O antibody, antineutrophilic cytoplasmic antibody [ANCA], and anti-glomerular basement membrane [GBM] antibody) and a renal biopsy that must be analyzed via immunofluorescence staining (IF) and electron microscopy [3]. A renal biopsy with IF staining is of utmost

L. Butani
Department of Pediatrics, University of California Davis Medical Center,
Sacramento, CA, USA
e-mail: lbutani@ucdavis.edu

M. N. Haddad et al. (eds.), *Adolescents with Chronic Kidney Disease*,
https://doi.org/10.1007/978-3-319-97220-6_6

importance to help classify patients into immune complex (IC), pauci-immune, and anti-GBM antibody-mediated RPGN. This helps guide therapy; the biopsy can also provide prognostic information, as will be discussed in subsequent sections. While in adults, especially older adults, pauci-immune RPGN is the most common type of RPGN, in children most RPGN has been seen in the setting of IC-mediated GN such as post-streptococcal GN, systemic lupus erythematosus, IgA nephropathy, and Henoch-Schonlein purpura nephritis [2, 3]; however recent data and our own personal experience raise the concern that pauci-immune RPGN may be becoming more common in children [4]. A detailed discussion of each of the IC-mediated RPGN diseases is beyond the scope of this chapter; the reader is referred to other sections of this book for additional information on some of these conditions. Suffice it to state that the outcome in children with IC-mediated RPGN is generally better when compared to those with pauci-immune RPGN and anti-GBM antibody-mediated RPGN [2]; the management of RPGN in the setting of an IC-mediated GN is driven predominantly by the underlying etiology of the GN. Based predominantly on anecdotal data, high-dose IV "pulse" corticosteroids and plasmapheresis are sometimes initiated in the context of IC-mediated RPGN, especially when the clinical course is complicated by concomitant alveolar hemorrhage [5–9].

In addition to helping classify patients with RPGN into various categories that have therapeutic implications, a renal biopsy provides additional prognostic benefit; a large multicenter pediatric study on patients with RPGN demonstrated that 50% of children with RPGN progressed to end-stage renal disease (ESRD); poor prognostic features included chronic changes on biopsy and a higher percentage of large and cellular crescents and breaks in the Bowman's capsule. Interestingly the percentage of glomeruli affected with crescent formation (beyond the 50% that was required for study entry) was not associated with a poorer prognosis [2].

In the next section, we will discuss pauci-immune RPGN and anti-GBM antibody-mediated RPGN in greater detail.

Anti-GBM Antibody-Mediated RPGN

Anti-GBM antibody-mediated RPGN, also referred to as Goodpasture's disease (GD) or Goodpasture's syndrome (GS) (when the renal disease is accompanied by alveolar hemorrhage), is exceedingly uncommon in adults (estimated incidence of 0.5–1 per million per year) and even more so in children. A review of the largest series of pediatric cases of anti-GBM antibody-mediated RPGN identified only 23 reported children with this entity as of 2012 [10]. In addition to the typical expected manifestations of RPGN outlined previously, children often present with signs of alveolar hemorrhage (cough and hemoptysis); prodromal signs and symptoms such as fever and malaise may precede the renal and pulmonary manifestations of the disease [10]. Rare clinical manifestations include central nervous system vasculitis manifesting with seizures [11, 12] and autoimmune inner ear disease with hearing loss, tinnitus, and vertigo [13]. Interestingly there may be a considerable time lag between the pulmonary and renal manifestations of the disease, and patients may sometimes have a more indolent presentation and may present with iron deficiency anemia due to ongoing slow pulmonary hemorrhage [10]. A bimodal age distribution has been described with an early peak in the young adult years and a later peak in the sixth to eighth decade of life. An inconsistent gender predilection has been reported; the pediatric series reported a female predominance [10].

Anti-GBM antibody-mediated RPGN is a prototypical autoimmune disease, with a strong HLA association [14]; 80% of patients exhibit DRB1*15 or DRB1*04 haplotypes which likely confer susceptibility to the disease while the DRB1*07 has a protective effect. These HLA associations reflect the ability of certain Class II molecules to bind and present peptides derived from an autoantigen to helper T cells. It has been hypothesized that when an insult, such as a respiratory illness [15], smoking [16], hydrocarbon exposure [17], or the use of a lymphocyte-depleting agent such as alemtuzumab [18], is experienced by a genetically susceptible individual, it leads to unmasking of a previously cryptic epitope in the non-collagenous-1 domain of the α 3 chain (α3NC1) of type IV collagen. This leads to the production of autoantibodies to this native antigen, mainly of the complement binding IgG1 and IgG3 subtypes. These autoreactive antibodies incite inflammation at sites where this antigen is expressed, namely, the alveolar and glomerular basement membranes, explaining the clinical manifestations of this disease. The diagnosis is established by serologic testing for anti-GBM antibodies which are almost universally present and by renal (or alveolar) biopsy demonstrating crescentic GN with linear IgG staining along the GBM. A substantial number of patients (20–30%) [19] with anti-GBM antibody-mediated RPGN also have coexisting ANCA positivity which may have implications for long-term outcome [20], pointing to the importance of checking for these antibodies even when the diagnosis of anti-GBM antibody-mediated RPGN has been established. Such dual-positive patients may experience recurrences, which are otherwise uncommon in anti-GBM antibody-mediated RPGN, and may possibly have a poorer prognosis, although this has not been consistently demonstrated in the literature.

Prior to the advent of immunosuppressive therapy and plasmapheresis, the mortality in patients with GD/GS was extremely high, and while newer treatment approaches have reduced this, the mortality rate remains inordinately high, especially in children, ranging from a low of 10% [10] to a high of 30% [21], stemming from complications related to alveolar hemorrhage and renal failure. Due to the limited data in children, prognostic information and therapeutic guidelines for anti-GBM antibody-mediated RPGN are derived from adult data. Poor prognostic markers for progression to ESRD include dialysis dependence at presentation and the presence of 100% crescents on renal biopsy [22]; anti-GBM antibody titers have not been consistently found to be associated with disease severity or outcome. Clinically significant recurrences are uncommon, even after renal transplantation, although histological recurrence, defined as the presence of linear IgG deposits along the GBM, is seen in about 50% of patients if transplantation is performed while circulating antibodies are present [23]. Postponing transplantation for at least 6 months after antibodies have become undetectable reduces the recurrence rate significantly and is the accepted guideline [24]. Treatment strategies are targeted at removing preformed antibodies (since there seems to be a very clear pathogenic link between the antibodies and tissue injury) and at preventing more antibodies from being formed; this is achieved via a combination of plasmapheresis and aggressive combination immunosuppressive therapy. Because of its fulminant course and high mortality, treatment must be started promptly, sometimes even before final diagnostic confirmation can be achieved. Much of our data on treatment comes from the retrospective studies from the Hammersmith Hospital which documented reasonable renal and patient survival in patients except those who were dialysis dependent at presentation or had 100% crescents on biopsy [22]. All patients in this series received plasmapheresis for 14 days (or until anti-GBM antibodies were undetectable) along with high-dose corticosteroids (initially IV pulse doses followed by tapering oral doses for a total duration of 6 months) and oral cyclophosphamide for 3 months. The additive role of plasmapheresis has been debated especially since it is not without risk, especially of infections and bleeding, the latter resulting from depletion of fibrinogen unless fresh frozen plasma is used as replacement. Whether to offer any therapy to patients who are dialysis dependent at presentation remains unclear unless they have concomitant pulmonary hemorrhage; in patients with pulmonary hemorrhage, the mortality is so high that all therapeutic measures should be offered irrespective of the severity of renal injury. Patients poorly responsive to standard therapy or in whom there is a desire to avoid oral cyclophosphamide, due to its significant toxicity, may benefit from a combination of steroids, plasmapheresis, and rituximab [25] or mycophenolate mofetil [26]; monthly IV cyclophosphamide has also been used anecdotally with good results [27]. In spite of the limited evidence base, at our center, our standard practice is to initiate therapy with high-dose IV methylprednisolone at a dose of 30 mg/kg/day (maximum of 1 g/day) for 3–5 days followed by 2 mg/kg/day (maximum 60 mg/day) of oral prednisolone, along with four weekly doses of rituximab (375 mg/m^2/dose); all children receive daily plasmapheresis until pulmonary hemorrhage (if present) resolves and then receive alternate day exchanges for a maximum total of 14 treatments. Albumin is used as the replacement fluid, unless fibrinogen levels get depleted, in which case fresh frozen plasma is used; some recommend empirically using plasma as replacement at the end of the exchanges in patients with pulmonary hemorrhage to replace coagulation factors and reduce risk of further bleeding [28]. Unlike many other autoimmune diseases, maintenance immunosuppressive therapy is not needed for patients with GD/GS; anti-GBM antibody titers should be monitored serially, although the reappearance or rise in titers does not necessarily herald a relapse and therefore should not be used as an indicator to resume or intensify therapy, in the absence of clinical signs or symptoms.

Table 6.1 outlines treatment recommendations for patients with anti-GBM antibody-mediated RPGN and for pauci-immune RPGN.

Table 6.1 Summary of treatment recommendations for patients with anti-GBM antibody-mediated and ANCA-positive pauci-immune RPGN

	Anti-GBM antibody mediated	Pauci-immune ANCA positive
Plasmapheresis	For alveolar hemorrhage: 14 treatments or until antibodies negative	For alveolar hemorrhage or severe renal disease (including dialysis dependence): 7 treatments over 14 days. If alveolar hemorrhage, daily until hemorrhage stops and then every other day (total of 7–10 treatments)
Corticosteroids	If not dialysis dependent at presentation and if <100% crescents on renal biopsy, intravenous methylprednisolone 30 mg/kg/day (maximum 1 gram) for 3–5 days, followed by oral prednisolone 2 mg/kg/day (maximum 60 mg/day) with slow taper over 6–9 months	Intravenous methylprednisolone 30 mg/kg/day (maximum 1 gram) for 3–5 days, followed by oral prednisolone 2 mg/kg/day (maximum 60 mg/day) with slow taper
Additional immunosuppression	If not dialysis dependent at presentation and if <100% crescents on renal biopsy, intravenous cyclophosphamide 500–1000 mg/m^2/dose monthly for 3 months *OR* Oral cyclophosphamide 2 mg/kg/day for 3 months *OR* Rituximab 375 mg/m^2 monthly for 4 months	*Induction therapy* Intravenous cyclophosphamide 500–1000 mg/m^2/dose monthly for 3 months with possible extension up to 6 months *OR* Oral cyclophosphamide 2 mg/kg/day for 3 months *OR* Rituximab 375 mg/m^2 monthly for 4 months *Maintenance therapy*: oral steroids + one of the following: Azathioprine (1–2 mg/kg/day) *OR* Mycophenolate *OR* Methotrexate *OR* Rituximab

Pauci-immune RPGN

As the term suggests, patients with pauci-immune RPGN have few or no IC deposits seen on renal biopsy by IF staining (<2+) and electron microscopy; the vast majority of such patients are also ANCA positive, and therefore this section will address ANCA-positive pauci-immune RPGN only. Due to the infrequent numbers of patients with ANCA-negative pauci-immune RPGN (10–20% of those with pauci-immune GN), there are no consensus guidelines on management of this entity; the general treatment approach and outcomes are very similar to those in ANCA-positive RPGN [29]. As for other types of RPGN, due to the rarity of this condition in children, most of our data is derived from adult studies with some contribution from smaller retrospective pediatric series [4, 30].

ANCA-positive GN comprises a group of conditions causing necrotizing vasculitis affecting small and medium vessels: granulomatosis with polyangiitis (GPA) previously referred to as Wegener's granulomatosis (characterized by granulomatous inflammation of the upper and lower respiratory tract along with necrotizing GN), microscopic polyangiitis (MPA) with frequent pulmonary capillaritis but absence of granulomas, and eosinophilic granulomatosis with polyangiitis (EGPA) previously referred to as Churg-Strauss syndrome, with eosinophil-rich granulomatous inflammation [31]; some patients with any of these aforementioned conditions may present with renal-limited vasculitis. Renal biopsy findings in patients with ANCA-positive RPGN have been noted to have significant prognostic value; in 2010, an international working group of renal pathologists proposed a histological classification [32]: focal (>50% normal glomeruli), crescentic (>50% cellular crescents), sclerotic (>50% sclerotic glomeruli), and mixed (any other combination). A validation study was carried out using the biopsies of 100 adult patients and confirmed the prognostic value of the classification system over a 1- and 5-year period, with patients in the focal class experiencing the best outcomes in terms of estimated GFR and renal survival followed in order by those in the crescentic, mixed, and sclerotic classes. A number of validation studies have since been published worldwide and have all confirmed the predictive value of this system, both in adults (as recently reviewed by Tanna et al.) [33] and in children [34]. In the pediatric study, the probability of having an estimated GFR of >60 ml/min/1.73 m^2 at 2 years was 100% in the focal group, 56% in the crescentic/mixed group, and 0% in the sclerotic group.

The peak age of onset for ANCA-positive RPGN is between the fifth and sixth decade of life; within the pediatric age group, most patients present during adolescence with a slight female preponderance [4, 30]. Children with MPA tend to be younger than those with GPA. The majority of children have constitutional symptoms including fever, malaise, and fatigue and present with some respiratory symptoms attributable to upper airway (in GPA) or lower airway (both in MPA and GPA) involvement such as shortness of breath, cough, hemoptysis, epistaxis, sinusitis, and nasal septal perforation [35]; many reports also document subglottic stenosis as a relatively unique pediatric presentation of GPA, compared to adults [36, 37]. Chest imaging in patients with respiratory symptoms may show signs of alveolar hemorrhage (in MPA) or pulmonary nodules (in GPA). Other extrarenal manifestations include musculoskeletal (arthritis), gastrointestinal (nausea and abdominal pain), ocular (conjunctivitis, uveitis), neurologic (such as mononeuritis and seizures), and dermatologic (palpable purpura) [35]; venous thromboembolism may also be seen [37]. EGPA is extremely rare in children and is typically associated with extrarenal symptoms; since none of the reported pediatric patients with EGPA have had renal involvement and all were ANCA negative, this entity will not be discussed any further here [38]. The severity of renal involvement in MPA and GPA varies considerably, but all patients have hematuria and proteinuria, as can be expected [30].

In addition to renal biopsy, serologic testing for ANCA is essential. By enzyme-linked immunosorbent assay (ELISA) or indirect IF (IIF), ANCA positivity has a sensitivity and specificity of 93% and 90%, respectively; in GPA the majority of children (63%) have a c-ANCA pattern on IIF and are positive for proteinase-3 (PR-3) antibodies on ELISA [39], while most children (55%) with MPA have a p-ANCA pattern on IIF and are positive for myeloperoxidase (MPO) antibodies [40]. Consensus recommendations propose testing for ANCA both by IIF and ELISA to increase sensitivity of test results. ANCA are predominantly IgG antibodies directed against the primary granules of neutrophils and monocytes and play a pathogenic role in causing tissue inflammation [41]. Hypotheses and data related to why ANCA develop in patients and how they lead to tissue injury have been comprehensively described by Bosch et al. in their review article and will therefore not be discussed in great detail [41]; suffice it to say that in the setting of an inflammatory insult, PR-3 and MPO are translocated to the cell surface of neutrophils and monocytes where they interact with ANCA and stimulate neutrophils to undergo a respiratory burst and release their primary granule contents leading to tissue inflammation and endothelial damage. Soluble MPO and PR-3 can also be released and bind to endothelial cells leading to additional cytotoxic effects when ANCA bind to them. In addition to having diagnostic value, ANCA can also be used to monitor for disease recurrence/relapse, although in the absence of clinical symptoms, reappearance or a rise in titers of ANCA should not be used to modify therapy [42].

There have been many clinical trials, and several more that are ongoing, investigating optimal treatment options for adults with ANCA-positive pauci-immune RPGN, and these have guided the treatment offered to children. The largest and longest study of plasmapheresis in ANCA-positive RPGN, the MEPEX study, included patients with a serum creatinine >500 μM/L (5.8 mg/dl) and showed that compared to high-dose IV methylprednisolone, plasmapheresis was associated with a significant reduction in progression to ESRD at 12 months (from 43% to 19%) with no difference in mortality or adverse events [43]. However, at the 4-year follow-up, there was no significant difference in outcomes, and the renal function in those who were not on maintenance dialysis was comparable, raising questions about the benefit of plasma exchange in the treatment of patients; moreover outcomes were universally very poor, highlighting the need for better therapies for patients with severe renal disease [44]. In this study, deaths from infections were more common in the plasmapheresis group. Nevertheless, plasmapheresis continues to be used and recommended for patients with severe renal disease (including those who are dialysis dependent on presentation, unless advanced chronic changes are noted on biopsy) [45]; plasmapheresis has also been recommended as adjunctive treatment for patients with diffuse alveolar hemorrhage and for those who have dual-antibody-positive RPGN [46]. Some small studies have suggested a benefit of leukocytapheresis in ANCA-positive RPGN, attributed to its ability to remove leukocytes that are responsible for mediating tissue injury [47]; larger studies are needed before this becomes a recommended treatment option. Ongoing studies are underway to clarify the precise role of plasmapheresis in the treatment of renal disease and alveolar hemorrhage in ANCA-positive RPGN and should help clarify its role in the treatment of this condition.

In addition to plasmapheresis, patients with ANCA-positive RPGN traditionally receive induction therapy followed by long-term maintenance immunosuppression.

Induction therapy had traditionally consisted of high-dose IV methylprednisolone followed by an oral prednisolone taper (as part of maintenance therapy) [46]; in addition to methylprednisolone, at least one additional immunosuppressive agent is used, most commonly cyclophosphamide. Several studies have compared the use of IV pulse and continuous oral administration of cyclophosphamide and found that the use of IV cyclophosphamide leads to equivalent remission rates but at the cost of an increased risk of relapse (pooled relative risk from four studies: 1.79, 95% CI 1.11–2.87) compared to oral cyclophosphamide [48]. Prolonging the duration of IV cyclophosphamide to 12 months has been suggested as one way to reduce the risk of relapses, although this has not been demonstrated consistently [49, 50]. Benefits of IV cyclophosphamide include lower incidence of leukopenia, infections, and gonadal toxicity due to lower cumulative drug exposure [51]. Based on these observations, many centers, including ours, preferentially use IV cyclophosphamide as opposed to oral cyclophosphamide as the induction agent of choice. Recent studies have suggested equivalent remission rates with the use of rituximab instead of cyclophosphamide as the induction agent. The RAVE trial compared four doses to IV rituximab to oral cyclophosphamide [52, 53] and demonstrated comparable remission rates at 6 and 18 months and superiority in inducing remission in patients who had relapsed and were being re-induced. The RITUXIVAS trial compared a regimen of IV cyclophosphamide (3–6 months) to a combination of four doses of IV rituximab along with two doses of IV cyclophosphamide and also demonstrated equivalence in inducing remission in newly diagnosed patients, all of whom had renal involvement [54, 55]. Combination therapy with cyclophosphamide and rituximab, compared to rituximab alone, may offer an advantage in reducing the risk of future relapses; most relapses occurred in the setting of B-cell repopulation [56]. Due to our concern about long-term gonadal toxicity in pediatric patients, especially adolescents, our institutional practice is to use rituximab as the preferred induction agent, in combination with IV methylprednisolone. There has also been some interest in using mycophenolate mofetil (MMF) as an alternative induction agent to cyclophosphamide or rituximab due to its safety profile. Data pertaining to MMF use in ANCA-positive RPGN are very limited at this point in time; two studies in Chinese patients suggest equivalent, if not better, remission rates with the use of MMF compared to IV cyclophosphamide [57, 58]. Eagerly awaited are published data from larger trials and trials enrolling a more diverse ethnic population, comparing the two agents, including the MYCYC trial (https://clinicaltrials.gov/ct2/show/NCT00414128). Unlike for anti-GBM antibody RPGN, patients with ANCA-positive RPGN who are dialysis dependent at presentation respond much better to immunosuppressive therapy, and a substantial proportion will be able to come off dialysis. The treatment approach for such patients remains the same as that for those who are not on dialysis [59]. For those who are dialysis dependent and do not recover sufficient renal function to come off dialysis by 3 months and do not have extrarenal disease, immunosuppressive therapy should be stopped [46].

Following induction therapy, about 60% of patients go into remission at 6 months, with the percentage remaining in sustained remission dropping to about 50% by

12 months, based on data from the aforementioned studies. For those who do not enter into remission, reattempts at induction with an alternative agent or additional doses of the same agent used previously are typically tried. Other strategies that are sometimes used include the addition of intravenous immunoglobulin [60] or T-cell depleting agents [61]. There are no clear consensus guidelines on how to approach the management of such patients. For those who achieve remission after induction therapy, maintenance immunosuppression is necessary to reduce relapses; this always includes oral corticosteroids at tapering doses. In addition to corticosteroids, azathioprine remains the standard maintenance immunosuppressive agent [62]. Both of these should be continued for 18–24 months until after remission is achieved. Alternatives to azathioprine include MMF at 2 g/day (although it should be used with caution and only if azathioprine is contraindicated due to the significantly higher relapse rate compared to azathioprine) [63], methotrexate at a dose of 0.3 mg per kilogram per week, progressively increased to 25 mg per week (except in patients with a GFR <60 ml/min/1.73 m^2) [46, 64], or rituximab. Rituximab has been shown in one randomized trial to be more effective than azathioprine in reducing relapses following induction with corticosteroids and IV cyclophosphamide; low-dose rituximab (500 mg/dose) was administered on days 0 and 14 after randomization and then at months 6, 12, and 18 after the first infusion [65]. A major relapse was seen in 5% of the rituximab cohort compared to 29% in the azathioprine group, at 28 months. Oral co-trimoxazole, which was previously recommended as an adjunctive therapy, has not been shown to reduce relapses significantly and therefore is not recommended for that purpose, although its use may help in reducing the risk of pneumocystis infections.

Relapses, as mentioned above, are common in patients with ANCA-positive RPGN, in spite of using recommended induction and maintenance therapies. Predictive factors for relapse have included the presence of PR-3 ANCA (as opposed to MPO ANCA), a higher PR-3 titer [66], the presence of upper or lower respiratory involvement [50], and the persistence of ANCA positivity [67], although titers in themselves have a poor positive predictive value for a relapse and therefore should not be used to drive changes in therapy. For those patients who remain dialysis dependent and are transplant candidates, transplant should be delayed until patients are in extrarenal remission for at least 12 months; ANCA titers (or their persistence) should not be used in determining optimal timing for transplantation [46].

Conclusions

In summary, RPGN is uncommon in children and adolescents, such that most treatment recommendations and outcome data are derived from adult studies. Early diagnosis and treatment at experienced centers and in a multidisciplinary team approach are essential to reduce morbidity and mortality. Serologic testing and tissue diagnoses are important since therapeutic guidelines vary based on the cause of

RPGN. Immunosuppressive therapies, with the possible use of plasmapheresis, remain the cornerstone of management. In spite of optimal therapy, many patients relapse and/or progress to ESRD and may benefit from renal transplantation; this should be planned and timed based on evidence of disease activity, both clinical and serologic.

References

1. Miller MN, Baumal R, Poucell S, Steele BT. Incidence and prognostic importance of glomerular crescents in renal diseases of childhood. Am J Nephrol. 1984;4(4):244–7.
2. A clinico-pathologic study of crescentic glomerulonephritis in 50 children. A report of the southwest pediatric nephrology study group. Kidney Int. 1985;27(2):450–8.
3. Little MA, Pusey CD. Rapidly progressive glomerulonephritis: current and evolving treatment strategies. J Nephrol. 2004;17(Suppl 8):S10–9.
4. Khalighi MA, Wang S, Henriksen KJ, Bock M, Keswani M, Chang A, et al. Pauci-immune glomerulonephritis in children: a clinicopathologic study of 21 patients. Pediatr Nephrol. 2015;30(6):953–9.
5. Rajagopala S, Parameswaran S, Ajmera JS, Ganesh RN, Katrevula A. Diffuse alveolar hemorrhage in IgA nephropathy: case series and systematic review of the literature. Int J Rheum Dis. 2017;20(1):109–21.
6. Shenoy M, Ognjanovic MV, Coulthard MG. Treating severe Henoch-Schonlein and IgA nephritis with plasmapheresis alone. Pediatr Nephrol. 2007;22(8):1167–71.
7. Mara-Koosham G, Stoltze K, Aday J, Rendon P. Pulmonary renal syndrome after streptococcal pharyngitis: a case report. J Investig Med High Impact Case Rep. 2016;4(2):1–4. 2324709616646127
8. Harada T, Ozono Y, Miyazaki M, Sasaki O, Miyazaki K, Abe K, et al. Plasmapheresis in the treatment of rapidly progressive glomerulonephritis. Ther Apher. 1997;1(4):366–9.
9. Stratta P, Canavese C, Fenoglio R, Priolo G, Grillo A, Aimo G, et al. Dual effect of methylprednsolone pulses on apoptosis of peripheral leukocytes in patients with renal diseases. Int J Immunopathol Pharmacol. 2006;19(3):647–59.
10. Bayat A, Kamperis K, Herlin T. Characteristics and outcome of Goodpasture's disease in children. Clin Rheumatol. 2012;31(12):1745–51.
11. Gittins N, Basu A, Eyre J, Gholkar A, Moghal N. Cerebral vasculitis in a teenager with Goodpasture's syndrome. Nephrol Dial Transplant. 2004;19(12):3168–71.
12. Kim JY, Ahn KJ, Jung JI, Jung SL, Kim BS, Hahn ST. Imaging findings of central nervous system vasculitis associated with Goodpasture's syndrome: a case report. Korean J Radiol. 2007;8(6):545–7.
13. Greco A, Rizzo MI, De Virgilio A, Gallo A, Fusconi M, Pagliuca G, et al. Goodpasture's syndrome: a clinical update. Autoimmun Rev. 2015;14(3):246–53.
14. Fisher M, Pusey CD, Vaughan RW, Rees AJ. Susceptibility to anti-glomerular basement membrane disease is strongly associated with HLA-DRB1 genes. Kidney Int. 1997;51(1):222–9.
15. Shah MK, Hugghins SY. Characteristics and outcomes of patients with Goodpasture's syndrome. South Med J. 2002;95(12):1411–8.
16. Donaghy M, Rees AJ. Cigarette smoking and lung haemorrhage in glomerulonephritis caused by autoantibodies to glomerular basement membrane. Lancet. 1983;2(8364):1390–3.
17. Bombassei GJ, Kaplan AA. The association between hydrocarbon exposure and anti-glomerular basement membrane antibody-mediated disease (Goodpasture's syndrome). Am J Ind Med. 1992;21(2):141–53.

18. Meyer D, Coles A, Oyuela P, Purvis A, Margolin DH. Case report of anti-glomerular basement membrane disease following alemtuzumab treatment of relapsing-remitting multiple sclerosis. Mult Scler Relat Disord. 2013;2(1):60–3.
19. Jayne DR, Marshall PD, Jones SJ, Lockwood CM. Autoantibodies to GBM and neutrophil cytoplasm in rapidly progressive glomerulonephritis. Kidney Int. 1990;37(3):965–70.
20. Srivastava A, Rao GK, Segal PE, Shah M, Geetha D. Characteristics and outcome of crescentic glomerulonephritis in patients with both antineutrophil cytoplasmic antibody and anti-glomerular basement membrane antibody. Clin Rheumatol. 2013;32(9):1317–22.
21. Poddar B, Singhal S, Azim A, Gulati S, Baronia A. Goodpasture's syndrome in children. Saudi J Kidney Dis Transpl. 2010;21(5):935–9.
22. Levy JB, Turner AN, Rees AJ, Pusey CD. Long-term outcome of anti-glomerular basement membrane antibody disease treated with plasma exchange and immunosuppression. Ann Intern Med. 2001;134(11):1033–42.
23. Kotanko P, Pusey CD, Levy JB. Recurrent glomerulonephritis following renal transplantation. Transplantation. 1997;63(8):1045–52.
24. Chapter 14: anti-glomerular basement membrane antibody glomerulonephritis. Kidney Int Suppl (2011). 2012;2(2):240–2.
25. Touzot M, Poisson J, Faguer S, Ribes D, Cohen P, Geffray L, et al. Rituximab in anti-GBM disease: a retrospective study of 8 patients. J Autoimmun. 2015;60:74–9.
26. Garcia-Canton C, Toledo A, Palomar R, Fernandez F, Lopez J, Moreno A, et al. Goodpasture's syndrome treated with mycophenolate mofetil. Nephrol Dial Transplant. 2000;15(6):920–2.
27. Bjerre A, Hogasen K, Grotta J, Scott H, Tangeraas T, Dorje C. Rescue of kidney function in a toddler with anti-GBM nephritis. Clin Kidney J. 2012;5(6):584–6.
28. Clark WF, Huang SS, Walsh MW, Farah M, Hildebrand AM, Sontrop JM. Plasmapheresis for the treatment of kidney diseases. Kidney Int. 2016;90(5):974–84.
29. Shah S, Havill J, Rahman MH, Geetha D. A historical study of American patients with anti-neutrophil cytoplasmic antibody negative pauci-immune glomerulonephritis. Clin Rheumatol. 2016;35(4):953–60.
30. Kouri AM, Andreoli SP. Clinical presentation and outcome of pediatric ANCA-associated glomerulonephritis. Pediatr Nephrol. 2017;32(3):449–55.
31. Jennette JC, Falk RJ, Bacon PA, Basu N, Cid MC, Ferrario F, et al. 2012 Revised International Chapel Hill consensus conference nomenclature of vasculitides. Arthritis Rheum. 2013;65(1):1–11.
32. Berden AE, Ferrario F, Hagen EC, Jayne DR, Jennette JC, Joh K, et al. Histopathologic classification of ANCA-associated glomerulonephritis. J Am Soc Nephrol. 2010;21(10):1628–36.
33. Tanna A, Pusey CD. The histopathological classification of ANCA-associated glomerulonephritis comes of age. J Rheumatol. 2017;44(3):265–7.
34. Noone DG, Twilt M, Hayes WN, Thorner PS, Benseler S, Laxer RM, et al. The new histopathologic classification of ANCA-associated GN and its association with renal outcomes in childhood. Clin J Am Soc Nephrol. 2014;9(10):1684–91.
35. Plumb LA, Oni L, Marks SD, Tullus K. Paediatric anti-neutrophil cytoplasmic antibody (ANCA)-associated vasculitis: an update on renal management. Pediatr Nephrol. 2018; 33(1):25–39. https://doi.org/10.1007/s00467-016-3559-2. Epub 2017 Jan 6.
36. Rottem M, Fauci AS, Hallahan CW, Kerr GS, Lebovics R, Leavitt RY, et al. Wegener granulomatosis in children and adolescents: clinical presentation and outcome. J Pediatr. 1993;122(1):26–31.
37. Akikusa JD, Schneider R, Harvey EA, Hebert D, Thorner PS, Laxer RM, et al. Clinical features and outcome of pediatric Wegener's granulomatosis. Arthritis Rheum. 2007;57(5):837–44.
38. Gendelman S, Zeft A, Spalding SJ. Childhood-onset eosinophilic granulomatosis with polyangiitis (formerly Churg-Strauss syndrome): a contemporary single-center cohort. J Rheumatol. 2013;40(6):929–35.

39. Ozen S, Pistorio A, Iusan SM, Bakkaloglu A, Herlin T, Brik R, et al. EULAR/PRINTO/PRES criteria for Henoch-Schonlein purpura, childhood polyarteritis nodosa, childhood Wegener granulomatosis and childhood Takayasu arteritis: Ankara 2008. Part II: final classification criteria. Ann Rheum Dis. 2010;69(5):798–806.
40. Cabral DA, Canter DL, Muscal E, Nanda K, Wahezi DM, Spalding SJ, et al. Comparing presenting clinical features in 48 children with microscopic polyangiitis to 183 children who have granulomatosis with polyangiitis (Wegener's): an ARChiVe cohort study. Arthritis Rheum. 2016;68(10):2514–26.
41. Bosch X, Guilabert A, Font J. Antineutrophil cytoplasmic antibodies. Lancet. 2006;368(9533):404–18.
42. Schmitt WH, van der Woude FJ. Clinical applications of antineutrophil cytoplasmic antibody testing. Curr Opin Rheumatol. 2004;16(1):9–17.
43. Jayne DR, Gaskin G, Rasmussen N, Abramowicz D, Ferrario F, Guillevin L, et al. Randomized trial of plasma exchange or high-dosage methylprednisolone as adjunctive therapy for severe renal vasculitis. J Am Soc Nephrol. 2007;18(7):2180–8.
44. Walsh M, Casian A, Flossmann O, Westman K, Hoglund P, Pusey C, et al. Long-term follow-up of patients with severe ANCA-associated vasculitis comparing plasma exchange to intravenous methylprednisolone treatment is unclear. Kidney Int. 2013;84(2):397–402.
45. de Lind van Wijngaarden RA, Hauer HA, Wolterbeek R, Jayne DR, Gaskin G, Rasmussen N, et al. Chances of renal recovery for dialysis-dependent ANCA-associated glomerulonephritis. J Am Soc Nephrol. 2007;18(7):2189–97.
46. Chapter 13: Pauci-immune focal and segmental necrotizing glomerulonephritis. Kidney Int Suppl (2011). 2012;2(2):233–9.
47. Hotta O, Ishida A, Kimura T, Taguma Y. Improvements in treatment strategies for patients with antineutrophil cytoplasmic antibody-associated rapidly progressive glomerulonephritis. Ther Apher Dial. 2006;10(5):390–5.
48. Walters G, Willis NS, Craig JC. Interventions for renal vasculitis in adults. Cochrane Database Syst Rev. 2015;(9):CD003232.
49. Guillevin L, Cohen P, Mahr A, Arene JP, Mouthon L, Puechal X, et al. Treatment of polyarteritis nodosa and microscopic polyangiitis with poor prognosis factors: a prospective trial comparing glucocorticoids and six or twelve cyclophosphamide pulses in sixty-five patients. Arthritis Rheum. 2003;49(1):93–100.
50. Hogan SL, Falk RJ, Chin H, Cai J, Jennette CE, Jennette JC, et al. Predictors of relapse and treatment resistance in antineutrophil cytoplasmic antibody-associated small-vessel vasculitis. Ann Intern Med. 2005;143(9):621–31.
51. Haubitz M, Schellong S, Gobel U, Schurek HJ, Schaumann D, Koch KM, et al. Intravenous pulse administration of cyclophosphamide versus daily oral treatment in patients with antineutrophil cytoplasmic antibody-associated vasculitis and renal involvement: a prospective, randomized study. Arthritis Rheum. 1998;41(10):1835–44.
52. Stone JH, Merkel PA, Spiera R, Seo P, Langford CA, Hoffman GS, et al. Rituximab versus cyclophosphamide for ANCA-associated vasculitis. N Engl J Med. 2010;363(3):221–32.
53. Specks U, Merkel PA, Seo P, Spiera R, Langford CA, Hoffman GS, et al. Efficacy of remission-induction regimens for ANCA-associated vasculitis. N Engl J Med. 2013;369(5):417–27.
54. Jones RB, Tervaert JW, Hauser T, Luqmani R, Morgan MD, Peh CA, et al. Rituximab versus cyclophosphamide in ANCA-associated renal vasculitis. N Engl J Med. 2010;363(3):211–20.
55. Jones RB, Furuta S, Tervaert JW, Hauser T, Luqmani R, Morgan MD, et al. Rituximab versus cyclophosphamide in ANCA-associated renal vasculitis: 2-year results of a randomised trial. Ann Rheum Dis. 2015;74(6):1178–82.
56. McGregor JG, Hogan SL, Kotzen ES, Poulton CJ, Hu Y, Negrete-Lopez R, et al. Rituximab as an immunosuppressant in antineutrophil cytoplasmic antibody-associated vasculitis. Nephrol Dial Transplant. 2015;30(Suppl 1):i123–31.

57. Han F, Liu G, Zhang X, Li X, He Q, He X, et al. Effects of mycophenolate mofetil combined with corticosteroids for induction therapy of microscopic polyangiitis. Am J Nephrol. 2011;33(2):185–92.
58. Hu W, Liu C, Xie H, Chen H, Liu Z, Li L. Mycophenolate mofetil versus cyclophosphamide for inducing remission of ANCA vasculitis with moderate renal involvement. Nephrol Dial Transplant. 2008;23(4):1307–12.
59. Pepper RJ, Chanouzas D, Tarzi R, Little MA, Casian A, Walsh M, et al. Intravenous cyclophosphamide and plasmapheresis in dialysis-dependent ANCA-associated vasculitis. Clin J Am Soc Nephrol. 2013;8(2):219–24.
60. Jayne DR, Chapel H, Adu D, Misbah S, O'Donoghue D, Scott D, et al. Intravenous immunoglobulin for ANCA-associated systemic vasculitis with persistent disease activity. QJM. 2000;93(7):433–9.
61. Lockwood CM, Thiru S, Stewart S, Hale G, Isaacs J, Wraight P, et al. Treatment of refractory Wegener's granulomatosis with humanized monoclonal antibodies. QJM. 1996;89(12):903–12.
62. Jayne D, Rasmussen N, Andrassy K, Bacon P, Tervaert JW, Dadoniene J, et al. A randomized trial of maintenance therapy for vasculitis associated with antineutrophil cytoplasmic autoantibodies. N Engl J Med. 2003;349(1):36–44.
63. Hiemstra TF, Walsh M, Mahr A, Savage CO, de Groot K, Harper L, et al. Mycophenolate mofetil vs azathioprine for remission maintenance in antineutrophil cytoplasmic antibody-associated vasculitis: a randomized controlled trial. JAMA. 2010;304(21):2381–8.
64. Pagnoux C, Mahr A, Hamidou MA, Boffa JJ, Ruivard M, Ducroix JP, et al. Azathioprine or methotrexate maintenance for ANCA-associated vasculitis. N Engl J Med. 2008;359(26):2790–803.
65. Guillevin L, Pagnoux C, Karras A, Khouatra C, Aumaitre O, Cohen P, et al. Rituximab versus azathioprine for maintenance in ANCA-associated vasculitis. N Engl J Med. 2014;371(19):1771–80.
66. Westman KW, Bygren PG, Olsson H, Ranstam J, Wieslander J. Relapse rate, renal survival, and cancer morbidity in patients with Wegener's granulomatosis or microscopic polyangiitis with renal involvement. J Am Soc Nephrol. 1998;9(5):842–52.
67. Kyndt X, Reumaux D, Bridoux F, Tribout B, Bataille P, Hachulla E, et al. Serial measurements of antineutrophil cytoplasmic autoantibodies in patients with systemic vasculitis. Am J Med. 1999;106(5):527–33.

Chapter 7
IgA Nephropathy

Aris Oates

Abbreviations

ESRD	End-stage renal disease
GWAS	Genome-wide association studies
IgAN	Immunoglobulin A nephropathy
KDIGO	Kidney disease improving global outcomes

Introduction

Immunoglobulin A nephropathy (IgAN) is a lifelong disease, primarily characterized clinically by persistent microscopic hematuria with and without macroscopic hematuria, proteinuria, or hypertension, and carries a risk of progression to renal failure. It is the most common cause of glomerulonephritis worldwide. In this chapter we review the worldwide epidemiology of the disease in adolescents and children to explore the pathologic and histologic defining features. Consensus diagnosis and treatment options will be reviewed and discussed. It is now established as a slowly progressive disease with variable course, and close follow-up with optimized supportive care is recommended in patients without severe disease to help improve renal survival. Although the initial presentation of many patients may have contributed to the belief that this was a benign entity, we now know that IgAN is a major cause of end-stage renal disease (ESRD). Investigations into the optimal subset of patients to benefit from immunosuppressive therapy and new treatment targets are ongoing.

A. Oates
University of California, San Francisco, CA, USA
e-mail: Aris.Oates@ucsf.edu

M. N. Haddad et al. (eds.), *Adolescents with Chronic Kidney Disease*,
https://doi.org/10.1007/978-3-319-97220-6_7

Case

A previously healthy 13-year-old Mongolian male presented to an acute care clinic with a 2-day history of painless red urine. Parents reported no medications or allergies but that he had been sick with rhinorrhea, cough, and congestion for several days prior to presentation. Urinalysis sent from clinic revealed 3+ protein and 250 RBC/HPF. He had no hypertension, rash, or edema on physical exam, and he was referred to nephrology clinic where he was seen 1 week later. In clinic, he noted this has been happening for 1–2 years; this was the fourth episode he could remember of grossly bloody urine. The episodes were always associated with an upper respiratory infection. This episode was typical in that his urine color became clear again after 1–2 days, and he has otherwise been well. He had no history of urinary tract infections or kidney stones. There is no known family history of renal disease. Blood pressure was not elevated and physical exam was normal. Lab tests were notable for normal kidney function (eGFR >120 ml/min/1.73 m^2), normal complement levels, negative antinuclear antibody, a urinalysis with microscopy showing 10–20 RBC/HPF with no protein (urine protein/creatinine ratio 0.12 mg/mg creatinine), and no hypercalciuria (urine calcium/creatinine ratio 0.1 mg/mg creatinine).

Clinical Presentation

Originally reported by Jean Berger in 1968 [1] and formerly recognized by the eponymic name of Berger's disease, the report highlighted the occurrence of macroscopic hematuria with a concurrent episode of pharyngitis and persistent microscopic hematuria. Although it was initially described as having an almost benign disease course, over the subsequent decades, longitudinal studies showed that patients are at risk for progression to ESRD.

Symptoms present over a broad-spectrum ranging from incidental findings of microscopic and macroscopic hematuria to hypertension, proteinuria, and rapidly progressive glomerulonephritis. Screening methods of the population being studied can alter the presenting symptoms greatly. Some studies reported isolated macroscopic hematuria and/or asymptomatic proteinuria as the most common presentation (60–80% of patients). Presentation with isolated microscopic hematuria is more common in cohorts with extensive urine screening. The incidence of macroscopic hematuria is lower in adults than in children [2]. Episodes of macroscopic hematuria often are triggered by upper respiratory tract infections or less commonly with other gastrointestinal or sinus infections and often recur with subsequent similar infections. The intervals between and subsequent number of recurrences typically vary by patient. Although the majority of pediatric patients present with either no proteinuria or sub-nephrotic range proteinuria, normal renal function, and normal blood pressure, there is a smaller subset of patients that present with either acute nephritic syndrome, nephrotic syndrome, or with renal failure.

Given the indolent course and unknown rate of progression with gradual evolution of mesangial hypercellularity into glomerulosclerosis, many studies have attempted to understand factors that portend a poor prognosis. In adults, poor prognostic indicators include older age at time of diagnosis, absence of macroscopic hematuria, persistent proteinuria, persistent hypertension, high degree of crescents and glomerular sclerosis, and reduced renal function at time of diagnosis [2, 3]. Children, in general, are thought to have better clinical course [4, 5] especially for those with minimal proteinuria (<0.5 g/day/1.73 m^2) at the time of diagnosis [6]. A retrospective analysis of 385 Japanese children showed that those with minimal proteinuria at diagnosis had improved renal survival free from chronic kidney disease stages III–V compared to those with proteinuria, 100% vs. 78.7%, respectively [6].

Although several studies found a negative association between macroscopic hematuria and long-term renal prognosis, these generally did not hold up with multivariate analysis [7] or in the pediatric population [8]. Hypertension and renal function impairment at presentation can be reversible in children and are not seen as good predictive markers [2]. Heavy proteinuria (≥1 g/day/m^2) is the strongest predictor of poor outcomes in children [9] and the degree of proteinuria can correlate with the severity of glomerular lesions [2]. Other poor prognostic indicators in children include the number of glomeruli displaying crescents, sclerosis, and adhesions; diffuse mesangial proliferation; and moderate to severe tubulointerstitial changes [9].

Several long-term follow-up studies have demonstrated the increasing risk of progression to ESRD from 5 to 15% after 5 years to as high as 10–50% 20 years after diagnosis [10, 11]. Importantly, some patients do not progress and simply maintain their clinical condition, while some can also achieve spontaneous remission. Renal survival is improved in patients who were diagnosed as children versus adults [4, 5], although the actual improvement may be overstated [4, 12] and may be related to thresholds for biopsy and/or age at diagnosis. When comparing younger children and adolescent patients, those patients diagnosed prior to 16 years of age had more favorable outcomes than those diagnosed after age 16 [5]. It is worth noting that the improved pediatric outcomes are not always accounted for by difference in chronic changes or histologic activity seen on biopsy.

Epidemiology

Although the prevalence can vary based on geography, IgAN is the most frequently occurring primary glomerulonephritis worldwide [3, 13, 14]. In adolescents and children, the prevalence of IgAN varies greatly based on screening, referral patterns, and biopsy criteria; rates should also be regarded with some degree of caution given the potential subclinical nature of the disease. In pediatrics, IgAN is likely the most common type of glomerulonephritis [8, 15]; this is particularly evident from studies in Asia where standardized, large-scale screenings of school-age children are more routine [2, 8].

Worldwide, the incidence of IgAN in pediatric patients ranges from 0.5 to 5 per 100,000 per year [14], with considerable variation based on ethnic and geographic makeup of the populations being studied. Populations in Asia, Australia, and Europe have reported the highest prevalence [16]. In Japan the incidence was reported as high as 4.5–9.9 cases per 100,000 per year for children [17, 18], while in Italy [19] and Venezuela [20], the incidence rate was 0.31 and 0.03 cases per 100,000 per year for children, respectively [13].

Most studies have reported a male predominance ranging from 1.5 to 2.3:1 over female patients although the ratio has been noted to vary based on the geographic region of the study [3, 8]. While the first presentation of symptoms can occur in patients as young as 2 years of age, the mean age of presentation is during the first to third decades of life [3, 8, 21].

In the United States, the incidence of IgAN in Kentucky was reported to be higher in adolescents aged 10–19 years, 1.02 cases per 100,000 per year, compared to younger children aged 1–9 years, 0.56 per 100,000 per year [22]. In a study from Tennessee, the incidence of IgAN for Black and White children was similar at 0.57 and 0.3 cases per 100,000 per year, respectively [23]. The socioeconomic makeup of the population has also been shown to influence incidence, as those adults living in socioeconomically deprived postal codes had a higher incidence of IgAN [24].

Diagnosis

The definitive diagnosis of IgAN requires a renal biopsy. While other markers such as an elevated serum IgA levels, in particular serum galactose-deficient IgA1, can be suggestive for disease, the diagnosis is definitively made by histopathologic analysis of renal tissue with immunohistochemical or immunofluorescent staining for IgA dominant deposits. Skin biopsies have been shown to be of low yield and of nonspecific utility [25]. Although clinical practice can vary by region, in patients with IgAN who have isolated hematuria and no clinical or laboratory signs of more progressive disease (e.g., proteinuria, hypertension, elevated creatinine), close long-term observation for these signs prior to a biopsy could be considered [6, 26].

Patients with other systemic illnesses can have similar pathological features seen in the glomeruli. These are thought to be distinct diseases, simply sharing a common pathological result, such as alcoholic liver disease, portal systemic shunts, celiac disease, dermatitis herpetiformis, IgA monoclonal gammopathy, mycosis fungoides, mucin-secreting and other cancers, leprosy, pulmonary hemosiderosis, ankylosing spondylitis, other rheumatologic diseases, cyclical neutropenia [27], and Henoch-Schönlein purpura nephritis [14, 28].

Pathophysiology and Histology

The defining feature of IgAN seen on biopsy is a predominance of IgA mesangial deposits diffusely found throughout all glomeruli and points to IgAN being an immune complex-mediated disease process [2, 3]. IgAN is thought to be centered around abnormalities in IgA, autoimmune responses to abnormal IgA, and/or aberrant, excessive IgA production. The kidney manifests an expression of these abnormalities [29], with multiple "hits" predisposing to or exacerbating the injury through genetic and/or environmental modifiers and factors [14, 30]. After mesangial deposition occurs, the associated complement cascade and immune activation lead to mesangial cell damage and ongoing glomerulosclerosis.

IgA, after IgG, is the second most common immunoglobulin and exists in two subclasses, IgA1 and IgA2. The vast majority of IgA in serum, 90% [29], is monomeric and produced by lymphocytes and plasma cells, whereas polymeric IgA is produced by enteric and respiratory tract lymphocytes and plasma cells. In 50–70% of adult patients with IgAN, serum levels of both monomeric and polymeric forms of IgA are increased (the ratio of dimer/monomer was also increased), along with varied increases in several autoantibodies such as IgA rheumatoid factor, antinuclear protein IgA antibodies, and anticollagen IgA antibodies [2, 31]. In contrast, only 8–16% of pediatric IgAN patients have elevated serum IgA levels [2].

How elevated serum IgA levels are linked to IgAN is not completely understood. Elevated serum IgA level may lead to stimulation of lymphocytes and is exacerbated by some defective clearance of IgA [30], although the causative infectious or allergic [15] stimulating antigens have yet to be conclusively detected [2]. In vitro studies have demonstrated peripheral blood lymphocytes in patients with IgAN produce more IgA than controls [32], and there is increased helper T-lymphocyte function and secretion of IgA in IgAN patients [33]. The majority of IgA deposits in the mesangium are IgA1 subclass, like 90% of serum IgA, and are polymeric [30, 34]. The lack of galactose in the hinge region of serum IgA with truncated O-linked glycan in IgAN patients has drawn attention to this terminal galactose on circulating IgA1 as a possible cause for mesangial deposition. Numerous studies show that under-glycosylation of IgA1 contributes to self-aggregation of IgA and mesangial accumulation [35, 36]. Some studies have also pointed to the potential for disease-specific markers from a glycan-specific IgG antibody in IgAN patients [37] and complex formation with IgG autoantibodies. Although to date no binding sites or receptor for IgA in the mesangium have been found, binding may be associated and exacerbated not with a structural change but mediated via altered anion charge [34].

IgA deposits can be found in isolation or along with variable mesangial deposits of IgG, IgM, C3, C4, C4d, mannose-binding lectin, and/or C5b-C9. Classically, C1q is usually not present [14]. Light microscopy findings are variable, ranging from mesangial hypercellularity and mesangial enlargement/expansion to crescentic disease. The degree of tubulointerstitial damage corresponds to the degree of glomerular injury. Several studies have shown that the progression of mild histologic lesions to severe lesions appears to be rare [4, 38]. Crescentic lesions occur in an estimated 18% of adult IgAN patients [39]. In one case series of five patients with rapidly progressive crescentic IgAN, 41% of these patients were less than 16 years of age [40].

Electron microscopy highlights electron dense deposits in the mesangium and para-mesangium that can extend into the subendothelial and/or subepithelial regions [14]. The basement membrane can also frequently appear lysed in pediatric biopsies [28]. Epithelial foot process is usually preserved, although diffuse podocyte foot process effacement can be seen in presentation with nephrotic syndrome.

In addition to IgA binding to the mesangium and triggering cytokines (such as IL-6 and TNF-alpha) and complement (alternative and lectin pathways) activation [14, 30], other immune cells are likely involved in the response. Glomerular infiltration by macrophages and T cells correlates with the degree of proteinuria in IgAN, and in adults this histological finding also correlates with renal function [21]. Activation of mesangial cell mitogens, such as PDGF-B and IL-1 from macrophage invasion, has been shown to induce mesangial cell proliferation in mouse models. Glomerular endothelial and mesangial cell injury is caused by macrophage interaction and release of cytokines (such as IL-1 and TNF-alpha). Macrophages have also been shown to induce expression of alpha-smooth muscle actin, which is a feature of the proliferation of mesangial cells and associated with progression of disease [21, 41].

Histologic differences seen between pediatric and adult patients with IgAN are notable. Pediatric patients have more minimal histologic lesions on biopsy than adults, 24% vs. 14%, respectively, as well as have less advanced chronic lesions, 3% vs. 17% [4]. Arterial or arteriolar sclerosis is less common in pediatric biopsies compared to adults. The most prominent and common biopsy finding in early-stage pediatric IgAN is hypercellularity of the glomeruli with mild matrix expansion which corresponds with the degree of proteinuria. By contrast, with early-stage adult IgAN, there is more marked matrix expansion rather than hypercellularity; there is little correlation seen between adult mesangial proliferation and proteinuria. Crescents were more frequently seen in pediatric biopsies [42], and there were also differences in the crescentic composition. Forty-one percent of pediatric versus 16% of adult biopsies were entirely cellular crescents and 59% of pediatric versus 84% of adult biopsies had some degree of fibrous organization. Adult biopsy samples also had a higher deposition of fibrinogen, while pediatric biopsy samples had more staining for glomerular IgM and C3c [21]. Several other studies have shown increased tubular atrophy, segmental glomerulosclerosis, and higher grade of glomerular pathology in adult biopsies [5]. While the mechanistic cause and clinical correlation for the different histological appearances is not entirely clear, worse renal survival does correlate with more interstitial fibrosis and higher histologic grade [4]. This may explain improved survival seen in IgAN patients diagnosed as children versus adults.

Classification

In 2009, the Oxford Classification of IgAN aimed to identify reproducible, pathologic features of biopsy results. Four categories were identified: mesangial hypercellularity (M), endocapillary hypercellularity (E), segmental glomerulosclerosis (S), and tubular atrophy/interstitial fibrosis (T). A resulting MEST score was assigned based on each category and used to predict renal outcome, independent of clinical assessments at the time of the biopsy (Table 7.1). Notably absent from the original scoring system is a designation for crescents; given the low prevalence in the study biopsy specimens, they were not included in the original classification [43]. The score was further modified, as MEST-C, to include crescents [44] (See Figs. 7.1, 7.2, and 7.3). This classification and scoring schema has been validated in both pediatric and adult populations [42, 44], as well as different patient cohorts with various presentations and therapies [45]. Prior classification systems used for IgAN have included the Memphis [46] and Haas [47] schemas.

The MEST score can be used in clinical practice as well. Barbour et al. reported that combining the MEST score with clinical data at the time of biopsy significantly

Table 7.1 Oxford classification of IgAN with definitions and scoring (MEST with C score)

Biopsy pathologic feature and definition	Assigned score
M – Mesangial hypercellularity: percentage of the glomeruli have >3 cells in a mesangial area Or Mean score of all glomeruli: <4 mesangial cells/mesangial area = 0 4–5 mesangial cells/mesangial area = 1 6–7 mesangial cells/mesangial area = 2 ≥8 mesangial cells/mesangial area = 3	M0: ≤50% of the glomeruli have >3 cells in a mesangial area M1: >50% of the glomeruli have >3 cells in a mesangial area Or M0: mean score ≤0.5 M1: mean score >0.5
E – Endocapillary hypercellularity: any amount of the tuft involved in sclerosis, but not involving the whole tuft or the presence of an adhesion	E0: Absent E1: Present
S – Segmental glomerulosclerosis: hypercellularity due to increased number of cells within glomerular capillary lumina causing narrowing of the lumina or podocytopathic features	S0: Absent S1: Present
T – Tubular atrophy/interstitial fibrosis: percentage of cortical area involved by the tubular atrophy or interstitial fibrosis, whichever is greater	T0: 0–25% T1: 26–50% T2: >50%
C – Cellular/fibrocellular crescents: frequency of cellular and/or fibrocellular crescents	C0: Absent C1: Present in at least one glomerulus, but <25% C2: Present ≥25% of glomeruli

Optimal yield of glomeruli needed for scoring ≥8

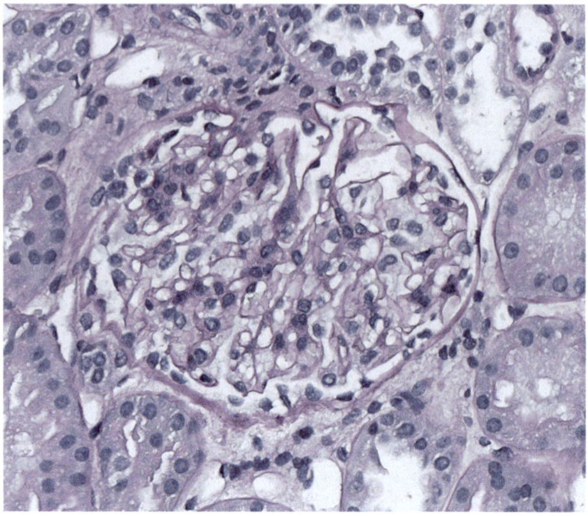

Fig. 7.1 An 11 years old M with IgA nephropathy noting minimal glomerular changes on light microscopy. H&E stain; 400 × magnification

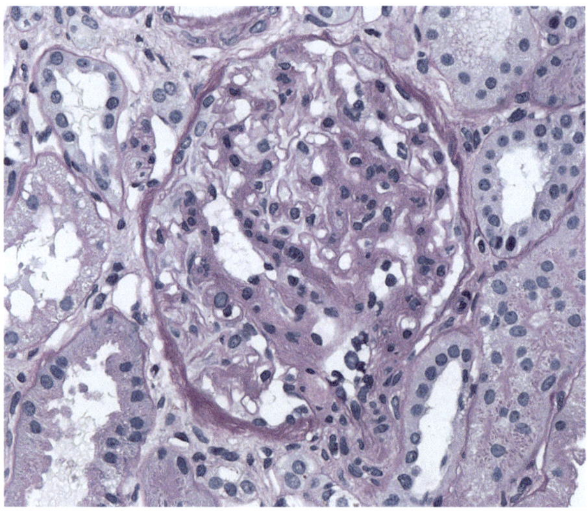

Fig. 7.2 A 14 years old M with IgA nephropathy noting mesangial proliferative changes. H&E stain; 400 × magnification

improves the clinical outcome prediction models for risk of a 50% decline in renal function or end-stage renal disease (ESRD) [48]. It has been proposed that the MEST score would also be a useful marker for comparing follow-up biopsies with IgAN to gauge treatment response [44]. Multiple studies have shown variable strengths of associations between MEST components and renal outcome [49], although there are fewer studies showing such correlation in children. One study of 98 Chinese children with IgAN showed the T score (tubular atrophy and interstitial fibrosis) was the only pathologic feature independently associated with renal

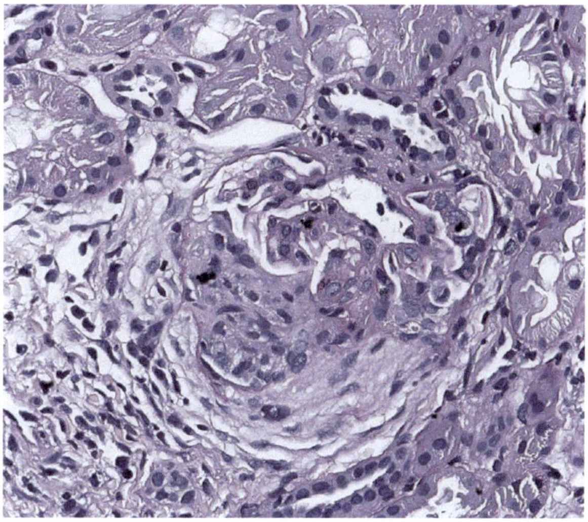

Fig. 7.3 A 15 years old F with IgA nephropathy noting fibrocellular crescent. H&E stain; 400 × magnification

outcomes [50], and a Japanese study of 250 children and adolescents only noted a correlation between the presence of crescents and renal outcomes [51]. Several other studies have failed to show any association [44], although it is unclear if these results were due to limited number of pediatric patients. The timing of the renal biopsy in children and the acute versus chronic changes seen may be possible explanations for these differences [51]. In a study of 196 adult patients, Yoon et al. reported that the M1 (mesangial hypercellularity) feature was significantly associated with the development of persistent proteinuria as well as predicted the progression of kidney disease in patients with IgAN. Importantly, while steroid therapy was shown to reduce proteinuria in patients with M1 scores, steroid use was not able to improve kidney function in these select patients. The authors argue that a M1 score could be an early predictor of adverse outcomes and could guide the clinical decision-making process regarding the initiation of immunosuppressive therapy in IgAN patients [49]. Within the European validation study of the Oxford Classification of IgAN (VALIGA) cohort, the authors studied a subset of 262 pediatric patients and young adults less than 23 years of age and found that the M1 score was associated with proteinuria and progression of disease [52]. Patients with a M0 score were at higher risk for progression as well if proteinuria at presentation was greater than or equal to 0.4 g/day/1.73 m^2 and eGFR was less than 90 ml/min/1.73 m^2. However, in a subgroup analysis of 174 children less than 18 years of age, the M, S, and T scores failed to have any predictive value. The authors did report that in children less than 16 years of age who at presentation had a score of M0 and well-preserved renal function (eGFR >90 ml/min/1.73 m^2) did exhibit a higher probability of proteinuria remission during follow-up and treatment with immunosuppressive therapy.

Treatment

The long and variable course of IgAN can present a therapeutic dilemma as it is crucial to differentiate those at high risk of disease progression to ESRD from those who have a milder disease and can be observed or managed with less toxic or less invasive interventions. Many advocate that the severity of glomerular changes seen on biopsy, the degree of renal function impairment, and the degree of proteinuria are key markers for identifying potential candidates for more aggressive treatment options. It is important to note that these surrogate outcome markers, such as doubling of serum creatinine and reduction in urinary protein excretion, have not been fully validated in children as markers for disease progression to ESRD [53].

Treatment options fall in the category of supportive, immune prophylaxis, immune suppression, and immune modulation. The 2012 Kidney Disease Improving Global Outcomes (KDIGO) Clinical Practice Guideline for Glomerulonephritis recommended primary treatment long term with an ACE inhibitor or angiotensin receptor blocker when the degree of proteinuria exceeds 1 g/day, with titration of the drug as needed (Grade 1B recommendation). No other Grade 1 recommendations were proposed by KDIGO, although there were several other consensus recommendations. In children specifically, expert opinion suggests a proteinuria goal of less than 0.5 g/day per $1.73m^2$. A 6-month course of steroid therapy was recommended for patients with an eGFR greater than 50 ml/min/1.73 m^2 and proteinuria persistently greater than 1 g/day after 3–6 months of optimized supportive care. In crescentic disease (>50% of glomeruli on renal biopsy), steroids and cyclophosphamide are suggested [54].

Supportive Therapy

Supportive therapies attempt to control proteinuria to reduce long-term tubular and glomerular damage. The mainstay of treatment is with ACE inhibition; several studies have shown that ACE inhibitors decrease the degree of proteinuria by 21–61% in IgAN patients [55]. As with other proteinuric diseases, ACE inhibitors work by reducing glomerular capillary hypertension, improve permeability characteristics of the glomerular basement membrane, and improve long-term renal function [56–59]. Moreover, in addition to reducing proteinuria, ACE inhibitors may delay disease progression through limiting intrarenal angiotensin II hyperreactivity, as studies have shown a potential role of renin-angiotensin in the progression of IgAN [2, 34, 55]. This must be balanced with the nephrotoxicity of ACE inhibitors as well as the prolonged disease course of IgAN.

Angiotensin receptor blockers (ARBs) have been compared to ACE inhibitors and have equivalent effects on proteinuria and likely have similar long-term benefits [60, 61]. Small studies in adults and pediatrics have shown some potential benefit to the combination of ACE inhibitors and ARBs in reducing proteinuria in IgAN patients, although the effect of this on long-term renal function is unclear [62, 63]. Certainly, other large studies in different adult patient populations have shown that combination therapy increases the risks of serious adverse events without benefit to renal disease, mortality, or cardiovascular disease [64, 65]. Combination therapy should be used with caution in IgAN patients.

Adequate control of blood pressure is recommended [53, 54]. Multiple antihypertensive medications may be needed to achieve blood pressure goals: adults <130 mmHg [54] and children <90th percentile, adjusted for age, height, and sex [67, 68]. The ESCAPE trial in children with CKD showed that more intensive blood pressure control, lowering blood pressure to less than the 50th percentile, could delay the progression of renal disease [69]. Additional supportive measures may also help blood pressure control including regular physical activity and exercise [66], maintaining a healthy weight, smoking cessation, dietary sodium restriction, restrictions on analgesic use, and diuretics. The importance of optimizing supportive therapy was demonstrated in the STOP-IgAN trial where a third of study participants had a response to supportive therapy alone and did not require immunosuppressive therapy [70].

Immune Prophylaxis

Because recurrent gross hematuria in IgAN may recur with upper respiratory infections, tonsillectomy has been evaluated as a prophylactic measure. The tonsils receive direct exogenous antigen stimulation from the oral and sinus cavities, and they include both local and systemic immune responses to these stimuli. Kawasaki et al. compared the effect of tonsillectomy plus prednisolone, warfarin, and dipyridamole versus prednisolone, warfarin, dipyridamole, and mizorbine for treatment of diffuse IgAN disease in Japanese children. Diffuse disease was defined as moderate or severe mesangial proliferation in at least 80% of sampled glomeruli. They reported no significant difference between the two groups related to urine protein excretion or serum creatinine and noted both treatments were effective in reducing proteinuria. There were a greater number of acute exacerbations of IgAN in the non-tonsillectomy group; however, the significance of this on short- and long-term outcomes, including progression of disease, is unclear [71]. Two recent meta-analyses found that tonsillectomy used as stand-alone or adjunct therapy has the potential to induce remission and lower rates of ESRD in adult and pediatric patients with IgAN [72, 73]. Recent data has focused on finding select patients, such as those outlined by Suzuki et al. with high expression of TLR9 [74] that may benefit the most from this treatment option.

It has been proposed that omega-3 fatty acids could be used to treat IgAN based on the premise that they can limit the production and/or action of cytokines from the initial immune response to renal injury [75]. While some initial trials were able to show benefit in terms of proteinuria and risk of ESRD [54], subsequent studies have been conflicting [76]. A meta-analysis of five randomized control trials comprising

233 patients showed that while omega-3 fatty acids reduced proteinuria, there was no observed preservation of renal function in patients with IgAN [77]. One possible explanation for the varied results is the observed dose-dependent effect of omega-3 fatty acids on plasma phospholipid eicosapentaenoic acid (EPA) and docosahexaenoic acid (DHA) levels and the resulting effect seen on proteinuria [78]. Given the relative low risk for harm, many experts including the KDIGO recommendations have advocated that omega-3 fatty acid therapy could still be offered to patients with IgAN. It may be particularly useful in patients with >1 g/day of proteinuria despite optimized supportive therapies [54].

Other therapies such as vitamin E, antiplatelet agents, anticoagulant agents, statins, and phenytoin have limited and inconsistent evidence to demonstrate efficacy in the treatment of IgAN [76].

Immune Suppression and Immune Modulation

Steroids have been shown to reduce proteinuria and preserve renal function in adult patients with IgAN [79–81]. Ten-year renal survival in patients with 1–3.5 g/day of proteinuria was 97% in patients receiving steroids versus 53% in those receiving supportive therapy alone [82]. A subset of IgAN patients with nephrotic range proteinuria may benefit more from steroids than other IgAN patients. Although uncommon, IgAN patients with histological features similar to minimal change disease respond similarly to those with minimal change nephrotic syndrome disease alone, and this is a clear indication for steroids [83, 84].

Vecchio et al. published an extensive review of randomized controlled trials of immunosuppressive medication for adults and children with IgAN. In 6 studies comprising 341 patients, steroids lowered the risk of progression to ESRD, doubling of serum creatinine, and urinary protein excretion. In 4 studies with 138 patients, steroids preserved glomerular filtration rate when compared to controls with a mean difference of 17.8 ml/min/1.73 m^2. In 2 studies with 160 patients, steroids combined with renin-angiotensin system inhibitors improved the risk of progression to ERSD, relative risk of RR 0.16. In 1 study with 38 patients, the addition of steroids lowered proteinuria more than renin-angiotensin system inhibitors use alone with a mean difference of −0.20 g/day [80]. Immunosuppressive therapy with steroids does not come without potential harms and increases the risk of adverse events such as severe infections and impaired glucose tolerance [70, 81].

Less data is available for other immunosuppressive regimes. In 1 study with 78 patients, azathioprine combined with steroids and dipyridamole improved remission of proteinuria, RR 1.24, compared to steroids alone, although the effect on other outcomes was unclear. In 1 study with 40 patients, mycophenolate mofetil combined with renin-angiotensin system inhibitors was shown to reduce the risk of progression to ESRD and lower urinary protein excretion. Other immunosuppressive agents such as cyclosporine and leflunomide showed inconclusive results due to insufficient data. Of note, Vecchio et al. argued the risks of bias in many of these studies was high given the inherent selective reporting bias and smaller sample sizes [80].

Cyclophosphamide may be of potential use especially in cases of proliferative lesions with severe renal involvement histologically [54, 85]. In 1 randomized control trial of 38 IgAN patients from the United Kingdom, cyclophosphamide and prednisolone followed by azathioprine for maintenance improved 5-year renal survival, 72% versus 5% in the control group without any immunosuppression [86].

Investigations with other therapies such as rituximab, plasma exchange, and calcineurin inhibitors have, to date, not yielded promising results regarding preservation of long-term renal function [8, 87–89]. Given the potential role that activation of C3 and generation of C5b-9 complex plays in the development of IgAN, some authors have proposed using eculizumab, a monoclonal antibody and terminal complement inhibitor [90], although there is little available data on outcomes.

Immunosuppressant therapy is used more widely in children with IgAN than in adults [42]. Studies of immunosuppression specifically for pediatric patients are also more limited, despite the fact that steroids have been reported to lower urinary protein excretion and preserve renal function [91]. Yoshikawa et al. investigated the use of prednisone, azathioprine, heparin-warfarin, and dipyridamole in a nonrandomized controlled trial of Japanese children with newly diagnosed IgAN and diffuse mesangial proliferation on biopsy [92]. They compared a group of 40 children receiving prednisolone, azathioprine, heparin-warfarin, and dipyridamole to a group of 38 children receiving only heparin-warfarin and dipyridamole. Of note, few patients were treated with ACE inhibitors in this study. Over a 2-year follow-up period, the treatment group had a reduction in urinary protein excretion and serum IgA concentrations. On repeat biopsy, the treatment group had less mesangial IgA deposition and fewer sclerosed glomeruli. A follow-up study by Kamei et al. demonstrated that the treatment group receiving the 2-year combination therapy of prednisolone, azathioprine, heparin-warfarin, and dipyridamole demonstrated a better 10-year renal survival, 97.1% vs. 84.8% compared to the control group receiving heparin-warfarin and dipyridamole only [93].

Yoshikawa et al. also investigated the use of prednisone alone versus combination therapy with prednisolone, azathioprine, warfarin, and dipyridamole in 80 children with newly diagnosed IgAN and diffuse mesangial proliferation on biopsy. After 2 years, those in the prednisone alone group had an increased number of sclerotic glomeruli, while those in the combination therapy group had no change. Again the follow-up was only 2 years. The other endpoints such as a reduction in urinary protein excretion, hematuria, serum IgA concentrations, and renal function were the same in both groups [94].

Given the mixed results that immunosuppressive therapy has on proteinuria reduction and long-term renal function preservation, many have continued to question the exact pathogenesis of IgAN. Some have proposed that the effects of steroid treatment may be through direct steroid action on the glomerulus to change the filtration rate instead of immune system modulation. More investigation in this area is needed.

Genetics

The strongest evidence for a genetic component to IgAN is seen in observational reports of familial aggregations of IgAN in affected sibling-sibling and parent-child pairs from a variety of different ethnic backgrounds [2, 10]. It is presumed that the genetic architecture of IgAN is more complex than a classic Mendelian inheritance. An environmental exposure triggering an underlying genetic susceptibility to disease has been the proposed model for the IgAN phenotype seen in humans [95].

Several genome-wide association studies (GWAS) have attempted to identify genomic signals associated with IgAN. Gharavi et al. studied 24 families from Italy and 6 from the United States and identified a potential locus at 6q22–23 which they named IGAN1 [96]. However, no known genes identified in this locus have been associated with disease manifestations, nor was this locus identified when studying a Japanese family with IgAN [95]. A GWAS from the UK Glomerulonephritis DNA Bank showed a reported strong association on chromosome 6p and with HLA region, particularly HLA-DQ in this European population [97]. Other GWAS have found associations with the loci on major histocompatibility complex Class I (HLA-B12, Bw35, B37) and Class II (HLA-DR1, DR4), complement factor H, complement factor H-related proteins 1 and 3, and cytokines related to mucosal immunity and inflammation [2, 98, 99]. These linkage studies have continued to identify loci thought to predispose to IgAN; however, the percentage of conferred, overall disease risk remains small. Genes underlying the pathogenesis of IgAN have yet to be identified [30].

Experimental models show that blockage of the renin-aldosterone system and, in particular, the intrarenal axis is successful in slowing the progression of IgAN [100]. Thus polymorphisms of the angiotensinogen gene and the angiotensin II type 1 receptor have been extensively studied with respect to the D allele (and DD genotype) [101]. However, to date, no identified polymorphism has been found to be associated with disease susceptibility or progression in IgAN patients [10, 55].

Several murine models of spontaneously developing IgAN have provided insight into the genetic components of the disease. Murine models have investigated and found separate, genetic loci that have a synergistic effect on IgA serum levels as well as other combinations of independent loci having a separate synergistic effect on potential glomerular deposition of IgA [95]. The ddY mouse, first isolated for the development of mammary gland tumors, was noted to have spontaneous development of IgAN. Research on this phenotype has yielded clues to the immunologic and, in particular, the gut-associated lymphoreticular tissue role in the serum levels of IgA and the deposition of IgA in the glomerulus. Uteroglobin-deficient mouse models have shown a possible role of uteroglobin in the prevention of glomerular deposition of IgA [10]. More investigation of these mice models could help provide understanding of the genetic links, pathogenesis, and potential treatment targets.

Transplant

Recurrent IgAN disease based on histopathologic examination can occur in 30–60% of patients after renal transplant [102, 103]. There does not appear to be a difference in recurrence rate among different ethnic groups [103]. However, of those patients with recurrence, it is more difficult to parse out allograft dysfunction and loss secondary to disease recurrence versus from other causes such as chronic rejection. One study estimated recurrence of IgAN was responsible for 2–16% of graft loss [104, 105] with a mean time from transplant to ESRD of 63 months [106]. However, the 10-year patient and graft survivals are the same for IgAN as for other renal diseases requiring transplantation [107]. Therefore, there remains a debate whether recurrent disease plays a clinically significant role on long-term graft survival.

Without protocol biopsies, recurrent disease is primarily detected after the appearance of microscopic hematuria, proteinuria, or both [107]. Graft dysfunction due to disease recurrence is rare before 3-years posttransplant, and recurrent disease likely follows a similar progressive course to the original IgAN clinical course [105]. Although forecasting recurrent disease progression in the transplanted organ based on the original disease progression may prove challenging as the patient milieu has been altered with multiple immunosuppressive medications associated with the transplantation. While some studies have highlighted young age of recipient, serum creatinine at 6-months posttransplant, proteinuria (≥1 g/day) at 6-months posttransplant, previous graft loss from recurrent disease, and recipient male sex as predictors of graft dysfunction, the predictive effect of these factors has been inconsistent across studies. By and large, in multiple studies, the major predictor of graft dysfunction from recurrent disease is time posttransplantation [106–109]. In those with recurrent IgAN after renal transplant, high-grade proteinuria, hypertension, and glomerulosclerosis involving at least 30% of the biopsy were predictive factors for graft failure [106, 109].

Induction regimens for renal transplantation using antithymocyte globulin have been shown to reduce the rate of IgAN disease recurrence. In a retrospective study of 116 transplant patients with IgAN, the disease recurrence rate at 10 years was 9% versus 41% in those with and without antithymocyte globulin used for induction, respectively [110]. Those on cyclosporine or mycophenolate mofetil for renal transplant maintenance immunosuppression had similar rates of disease recurrence and graft loss from disease recurrence, although more studies are needed [104, 106, 111]. Decreased donor and living donor transplant recipients also did not have different graft survival rates for IgAN [108, 109, 112], although there is some conflicting evidence regarding the graft survival of living-related and living-unrelated transplants [103, 112]. However, if a living-related donor is being considered, even minor urinary abnormalities should be thoroughly investigated before proceeding due to the increased risk of progression to ESRD in familial IgAN [109].

Treatment options for disease recurrence mimic those for IgAN in native kidneys. Options range from supportive measures such as reducing proteinuria and controlling high blood pressures to additional immunosuppressive regimes. Short pulses of high-dose steroids with a taper to prior transplant maintenance doses and/ or cyclophosphamide can be considered. If additional immunosuppression is indicated for disease recurrence, consideration should be given to the total burden of immunosuppression. Patients should be monitored closely for cytomegalovirus infection and prophylaxis for *Pneumocystis jirovecii* have been strongly advocated [106]. Some Japanese studies have shown that treatment with tonsillectomy in patients with recurrent disease after transplant can decrease the degree of proteinuria and improve histological features on biopsy, although this has not been investigated in other populations [106, 113].

Summary

IgAN, once thought to be a benign entity in adults and children, is a common cause of glomerulonephritis worldwide and a major cause of ESRD. Established as a slowly progressive disease with variable course, close follow-up and optimized supportive care are recommended in patients without severe disease to help improve renal survival. Investigations into the optimal subset of patients to benefit from more aggressive immunosuppressive therapy and new treatment options are ongoing.

Acknowledgments The authors wish to thank Dr. Zoltan Laszik for the pathology images in Figs. 7.1, 7.2, and 7.3.

References

1. Berger J. IgA glomerular deposits in renal disease. Transplant Proc. 1969;1(4):939–44.
2. Yoshikawa N, Tanaka R, Iijima K. Pathophysiology and treatment of IgA nephropathy in children. Pediatr Nephrol. 2001;16(5):446–57.
3. D'Amico G. The commonest glomerulonephritis in the world: IgA nephropathy. Q J Med. 1987;64(245):709–27.
4. Haas M, Rahman MH, Cohn RA, Fathallah-Shaykh S, Ansari A, Bartosh SM. IgA nephropathy in children and adults: comparison of histologic features and clinical outcomes. Nephrol Dial Transplant. 2008;23(8):2537–45.
5. Ronkainen J, Ala-Houhala M, Autio-Harmainen H, Jahnukainen T, Koskimies O, Merenmies J, et al. Long-term outcome 19 years after childhood IgA nephritis: a retrospective cohort study. Pediatr Nephrol. 2006;21(9):1266–73.
6. Higa A, Shima Y, Hama T, Sato M, Mukaiyama H, Togawa H, et al. Long-term outcome of childhood IgA nephropathy with minimal proteinuria. Pediatr Nephrol. 2015;30(12):2121–7.
7. Moreno JA, Martín-Cleary C, Gutiérrez E, Rubio-Navarro A, Ortiz A, Praga M, et al. Haematuria: the forgotten CKD factor? Nephrol Dial Transplant. 2012;27(1):28–34.
8. Delos Santos NM, Wyatt RJ. Pediatric IgA nephropathies: clinical aspects and therapeutic approaches. Semin Nephrol. 2004;24(3):269–86.
9. Yoshikawa N, Ito H, Nakamura H. Prognostic indicators in childhood IgA nephropathy. Nephron. 1992;60(1):60–7.

10. Hsu SI, Ramirez SB, Winn MP, Bonventre JV, Owen WF. Evidence for genetic factors in the development and progression of IgA nephropathy. Kidney Int. 2000;57(5):1818–35.
11. Schena FP. A retrospective analysis of the natural history of primary IgA nephropathy worldwide. Am J Med. 1990;89(2):209–15.
12. Wyatt RJ, Kritchevsky SB, Woodford SY, Miller PM, Roy S 3rd, Holland NH, et al. IgA nephropathy: long-term prognosis for pediatric patients. J Pediatr. 1995;127(6):913–9.
13. McGrogan A, Franssen CFM, de Vries CS. The incidence of primary glomerulonephritis worldwide: a systematic review of the literature. Nephrol Dial Transplant. 2011;26(2):414–30.
14. Wyatt RJ, Julian BA. IgA nephropathy. N Engl J Med. 2013;368(25):2402–14.
15. Hogg RJ. Idiopathic immunoglobulin A nephropathy in children and adolescents. Pediatr Nephrol. 2010;25(5):823–9.
16. Donadio JV, Grande JP. IgA nephropathy. N Engl J Med. 2002;347(10):738–48.
17. Shibano T, Takagi N, Maekawa K, Mae H, Hattori M, Takeshima Y, et al. Epidemiological survey and clinical investigation of pediatric IgA nephropathy. Clin Exp Nephrol. 2016;20(1):111–7.
18. Utsunomiya Y, Koda T, Kado T, Okada S, Hayashi A, Kanzaki S, et al. Incidence of pediatric IgA nephropathy. Pediatr Nephrol. 2003;18(6):511–5.
19. Coppo R, Gianoglio B, Porcellini MG, Maringhini S. Frequency of renal diseases and clinical indications for renal biopsy in children (report of the Italian National Registry of Renal Biopsies in Children). Group of Renal Immunopathology of the Italian Society of Pediatric Nephrology and Group of Renal Immunopathology of the Italian Society of Nephrology. Nephrol Dial Transplant. 1998;13(2):293–7.
20. Orta-Sibu N, Lopez M, Moriyon JC, Chavez JB. Renal diseases in children in Venezuela, South America. Pediatr Nephrol. 2002;17(7):566–9.
21. Ikezumi Y, Suzuki T, Imai N, Ueno M, Narita I, Kawachi H, et al. Histological differences in new-onset IgA nephropathy between children and adults. Nephrol Dial Transplant. 2006;21(12):3466–74.
22. Wyatt RJ, Julian BA, Baehler RW, Stafford CC, McMorrow RG, Ferguson T, et al. Epidemiology of IgA nephropathy in central and eastern Kentucky for the period 1975 through 1994. Central Kentucky Region of the Southeastern United States IgA Nephropathy DATABANK Project. J Am Soc Nephrol. 1998;9(5):853–8.
23. Sehic AM, Gaber LW, Roy S 3rd, Miller PM, Kritchevsky SB, Wyatt RJ. Increased recognition of IgA nephropathy in African-American children. Pediatr Nephrol. 1997;11(4):435–7.
24. McQuarrie EP, Mackinnon B, McNeice V, Fox JG, Geddes CC. The incidence of biopsy-proven IgA nephropathy is associated with multiple socioeconomic deprivation. Kidney Int. 2014;85(1):198–203.
25. Hasbargen JA, Copley JB. Utility of skin biopsy in the diagnosis of IgA nephropathy. Am J Kidney Dis. 1985;6(2):100–2.
26. Hoshino Y, Kaga T, Abe Y, Endo M, Wakai S, Tsuchiya K, et al. Renal biopsy findings and clinical indicators of patients with hematuria without overt proteinuria. Clin Exp Nephrol. 2015;19(5):918–24.
27. Clarkson AR, Woodroffe AJ, Aarons I, Hiki Y, Hale G. IgA nephropathy. Annu Rev Med. 1987;38:157–68.
28. Yoshikawa N, Yoshiara S, Yoshiya K, Matsuo T, Okada S. Lysis of the glomerular basement membrane in children with IgA nephropathy and Henoch-Shönlein nephritis. J Pathol. 1986;150(2):119–26.
29. Lai KN. Pathogenic IgA in IgA nephropathy: still the blind men and the elephant? Kidney Int. 2006;69(7):1102–3.
30. Barratt J, Feehally J, Smith AC. Pathogenesis of IgA nephropathy. Semin Nephrol. 2004;24(3):197–217.
31. Hiki Y, Saitoh M, Kobayashi Y. Serum IgA class anti-IgA antibody in IgA nephropathy. Nephron. 1991;59(4):552–60.

32. Iijima K, Yoshikawa N, Shiozawa S, Matsuyama S, Kobayashi K, Yoshiya K, et al. Immune abnormalities and clinical course in childhood IgA nephropathy. Nephron. 1990;56(3):255–60.
33. Kameda A, Yoshikawa N, Shiozawa S, Doi K, Nakamura H. Lymphocyte subpopulations and function in childhood IgA nephropathy. Nephron. 1991;59(4):546–51.
34. Lai KN, Leung JCK. Pathogenic role of the IgA molecule in IgA nephropathy. Nephrology. 2002;7:S86–91.
35. Novak J, Vu HL, Novak L, Julian BA, Mestecky J, Tomana M. Interactions of human mesangial cells with IgA and IgA-containing immune complexes. Kidney Int. 2002;62(2):465–75.
36. Sano T, Hiki Y, Kokubo T, Iwase H, Shigematsu H, Kobayashi Y. Enzymatically deglycosylated human IgA1 molecules accumulate and induce inflammatory cell reaction in rat glomeruli. Nephrol Dial Transplant. 2002;17(1):50–6.
37. Suzuki H, Fan R, Zhang Z, Brown R, Hall S, Julian BA, et al. Aberrantly glycosylated IgA1 in IgA nephropathy patients is recognized by IgG antibodies with restricted heterogeneity. J Clin Invest. 2009;119(6):1668–77.
38. Lee HS, Lee MS, Lee SM, Lee SY, Lee ES, Lee EY, et al. Histological grading of IgA nephropathy predicting renal outcome: revisiting H. S. Lee's glomerular grading system. Nephrol Dial Transplant. 2005;20(2):342–8.
39. Lee MJ, Kim SJ, Oh HJ, Ko KI, Koo HM, Kim CH, et al. Clinical implication of crescentic lesions in immunoglobulin A nephropathy. Nephrol Dial Transplant. 2014;29(2):356–64.
40. Abuelo JG, Esparza AR, Matarese RA, Endreny RG, Carvalho JS, Allegra SR. Crescentic IgA nephropathy. Medicine. 1984;63(6):396–406.
41. Utsunomiya Y, Kawamura T, Abe A, Imai H, Hirano K, Maruyama N, et al. Significance of mesangial expression of alpha-smooth muscle actin in the progression of IgA nephropathy. Am J Kidney Dis. 1999;34(5):902–10.
42. Working Group of the International IgA Nephropathy Network and the Renal Pathology Society, Coppo R, Troyanov S, Camilla R, Hogg RJ, Cattran DC, et al. The Oxford IgA nephropathy clinicopathological classification is valid for children as well as adults. Kidney Int. 2010;77(10):921–7.
43. Working Group of the International IgA Nephropathy Network and the Renal Pathology Society, Cattran DC, Coppo R, Cook HT, Feehally J, Roberts ISD, et al. The Oxford classification of IgA nephropathy: rationale, clinicopathological correlations, and classification. Kidney Int. 2009;76(5):534–45.
44. Trimarchi H, Barratt J, Cattran DC, Cook HT, Coppo R, Haas M, et al. Oxford classification of IgA nephropathy 2016: an update from the IgA nephropathy classification working group. Kidney Int. 2017;91(5):1014–21.
45. Coppo R, Troyanov S, Bellur S, Cattran D, Cook HT, Feehally J, et al. Validation of the Oxford classification of IgA nephropathy in cohorts with different presentations and treatments. Kidney Int. 2014;86(4):828–36.
46. Wyatt RJ, Emancipator SN, Kon V, Waldo FB, Donadio J, Grande JP, et al. IgA nephropathy databank: development of a system for management of renal biopsy acquired data. Am J Kidney Dis. 1997;29(6):817–28.
47. Haas M. Histologic subclassification of IgA nephropathy: a clinicopathologic study of 244 cases. Am J Kidney Dis. 1997;29(6):829–42.
48. Barbour SJ, Espino-Hernandez G, Reich HN, Coppo R, Roberts ISD, Feehally J, et al. The MEST score provides earlier risk prediction in IgA nephropathy. Kidney Int [Internet]. 2015; https://doi.org/10.1038/ki.2015.322.
49. Yoon C-Y, Chang TI, Kang EW, Lim BJ, Kie JH, Kee YK, et al. Clinical usefulness of the Oxford classification in determining immunosuppressive treatment in IgA nephropathy. Ann Med. 2017;49(3):217–29.
50. Le W, Zeng C-H, Liu Z, Liu D, Yang Q, Lin R-X, et al. Validation of the Oxford classification of IgA nephropathy for pediatric patients from China. BMC Nephrol. 2012;13:158.
51. Shima Y, Nakanishi K, Hama T, Sato M, Mukaiyama H, Togawa H, et al. Biopsy timing and Oxford classification variables in childhood/adolescent IgA nephropathy. Pediatr Nephrol. 2015;30(2):293–9.

52. Coppo R, Lofaro D, Camilla RR, Bellur S, Cattran D, Cook HT, et al. Risk factors for progression in children and young adults with IgA nephropathy: an analysis of 261 cases from the VALIGA European cohort. Pediatr Nephrol. 2017;32(1):139–50.
53. Lau KK, Butani L. Treatment of pediatric IgA nephropathy. Hong Kong J Nephrol. 2007;9(2):70–6.
54. Chapter 10: immunoglobulin A nephropathy. Kidney Int Suppl. 2012;2(2):209–17.
55. Dillon JJ. Angiotensin-converting enzyme inhibitors and angiotensin receptor blockers for IgA nephropathy. Semin Nephrol. 2004;24(3):218–24.
56. Abbate M, Zoja C, Corna D, Capitanio M, Bertani T, Remuzzi G. In progressive nephropathies, overload of tubular cells with filtered proteins translates glomerular permeability dysfunction into cellular signals of interstitial inflammation. J Am Soc Nephrol. 1998;9(7):1213–24.
57. Jafar TH, Schmid CH, Landa M, Giatras I, Toto R, Remuzzi G, et al. Angiotensin-converting enzyme inhibitors and progression of nondiabetic renal disease. A meta-analysis of patient-level data. Ann Intern Med. 2001;135(2):73–87.
58. Jafar TH, Stark PC, Schmid CH, Strandgaard S, Kamper A-L, Maschio G, et al. The effect of angiotensin-converting-enzyme inhibitors on progression of advanced polycystic kidney disease. Kidney Int. 2005;67(1):265–71.
59. Kanno Y, Okada H, Yamaji Y, Nakazato Y, Suzuki H. Angiotensin-converting-enzyme inhibitors slow renal decline in IgA nephropathy, independent of tubulointerstitial fibrosis at presentation. QJM. 2005;98(3):199–203.
60. Doggrell SA. ACE inhibitors and AT-1-receptor antagonists COOPERATE in non-diabetic renal disease. Expert Opin Pharmacother. 2003;4(7):1185–8.
61. Nakao N, Yoshimura A, Morita H, Takada M, Kayano T, Ideura T. Combination treatment of angiotensin-II receptor blocker and angiotensin-converting-enzyme inhibitor in non-diabetic renal disease (COOPERATE): a randomised controlled trial. Lancet. 2003;361(9352):117–24.
62. Chow K-M, Szeto C-C, Kwan BC-H, Leung C-B, Chung K-Y, Li PK-T. Dual therapy with ACE inhibitors and angiotensin II receptor blockers in proteinuric IgA nephropathy patients. Hong Kong J Nephrol. 2007;9(2):89–93.
63. Yang Y, Ohta K, Shimizu M, Nakai A, Kasahara Y, Yachie A, et al. Treatment with low-dose angiotensin-converting enzyme inhibitor (ACEI) plus angiotensin II receptor blocker (ARB) in pediatric patients with IgA nephropathy. Clin Nephrol. 2005;64(1):35–40.
64. Fried LF, Emanuele N, Zhang JH, Brophy M, Conner TA, Duckworth W, et al. Combined angiotensin inhibition for the treatment of diabetic nephropathy. N Engl J Med. 2013;369(20):1892–903.
65. ONTARGET Investigators, Yusuf S, Teo KK, Pogue J, Dyal L, Copland I, et al. Telmisartan, ramipril, or both in patients at high risk for vascular events. N Engl J Med. 2008;358(15):1547–59.
66. Fuiano G, Mancuso D, Cianfrone P, Comi N, Mazza G, Marino F, et al. Can young adult patients with proteinuric IgA nephropathy perform physical exercise? Am J Kidney Dis. 2004;44(2):257–63.
67. Hadtstein C, Schaefer F. Hypertension in children with chronic kidney disease: pathophysiology and management. Pediatr Nephrol. 2008;23(3):363–71.
68. National High Blood Pressure Education Program Working Group on High Blood Pressure in Children and Adolescents. The fourth report on the diagnosis, evaluation, and treatment of high blood pressure in children and adolescents. Pediatrics. 2004;114(2 Suppl 4th Report):555–76.
69. ESCAPE Trial Group, Wühl E, Trivelli A, Picca S, Litwin M, Peco-Antic A, et al. Strict blood-pressure control and progression of renal failure in children. N Engl J Med. 2009;361(17):1639–50.
70. Rauen T, Eitner F, Fitzner C, Sommerer C, Zeier M, Otte B, et al. Intensive supportive care plus immunosuppression in IgA nephropathy. N Engl J Med. 2015;373(23):2225–36.
71. Kawasaki Y, Takano K, Suyama K, Isome M, Suzuki H, Sakuma H, et al. Efficacy of tonsillectomy pulse therapy versus multiple-drug therapy for IgA nephropathy. Pediatr Nephrol. 2006;21(11):1701–6.

72. Duan J, Liu D, Duan G, Liu Z. Long-term efficacy of tonsillectomy as a treatment in patients with IgA nephropathy: a meta-analysis. Int Urol Nephrol. 2017;49(1):103–12.
73. Liu L-L, Wang L-N, Jiang Y, Yao L, Dong L-P, Li Z-L, et al. Tonsillectomy for IgA nephropathy: a meta-analysis. Am J Kidney Dis. 2015;65(1):80–7.
74. Sato D, Suzuki Y, Kano T, Suzuki H, Matsuoka J, Yokoi H, et al. Tonsillar TLR9 expression and efficacy of tonsillectomy with steroid pulse therapy in IgA nephropathy patients. Nephrol Dial Transplant. 2012;27(3):1090–7.
75. Donadio JV Jr, Bergstralh EJ, Offord KP, Spencer DC, Holley KE. A controlled trial of fish oil in IgA nephropathy. Mayo Nephrology Collaborative Group. N Engl J Med. 1994;331(18):1194–9.
76. Reid S, Cawthon PM, Craig JC, Samuels JA, Molony DA, Strippoli GF. Non-immunosuppressive treatment for IgA nephropathy. Cochrane Database Syst Rev. 2011;16(3):CD003962.
77. Chou H-H, Chiou Y-Y, Hung P-H, Chiang P-C, Wang S-T. Omega-3 fatty acids ameliorate proteinuria but not renal function in IgA nephropathy: a meta-analysis of randomized controlled trials. Nephron Clin Pract. 2012;121(1–2):c30–5.
78. Hogg RJ, Fitzgibbons L, Atkins C, Nardelli N, Bay RC, North American IgA Nephropathy Study Group. Efficacy of omega-3 fatty acids in children and adults with IgA nephropathy is dosage- and size-dependent. Clin J Am Soc Nephrol. 2006;1(6):1167–72.
79. Pozzi C, Bolasco PG, Fogazzi GB, Andrulli S, Altieri P, Ponticelli C, et al. Corticosteroids in IgA nephropathy: a randomised controlled trial. Lancet. 1999;353(9156):883–7.
80. Vecchio M, Bonerba B, Palmer SC, Craig JC, Ruospo M, Samuels JA, et al. Immunosuppressive agents for treating IgA nephropathy. Cochrane Database Syst Rev. 2015;(8):CD003965.
81. Lv J, Xu D, Perkovic V, Ma X, Johnson DW, Woodward M, et al. Corticosteroid therapy in IgA nephropathy. J Am Soc Nephrol. 2012;23(6):1108–16.
82. Pozzi C, Andrulli S, Del Vecchio L, Melis P, Fogazzi GB, Altieri P, et al. Corticosteroid effectiveness in IgA nephropathy: long-term results of a randomized, controlled trial. J Am Soc Nephrol. 2004;15(1):157–63.
83. Clive DM, Galvanek EG, Silva FG. Mesangial immunoglobulin A deposits in minimal change nephrotic syndrome: a report of an older patient and review of the literature. Am J Nephrol. 1990;10(1):31–6.
84. Gipson DS, Massengill SF, Yao L, Nagaraj S, Smoyer WE, Mahan JD, et al. Management of childhood onset nephrotic syndrome. Pediatrics. 2009;124(2):747–57.
85. Tumlin JA, Lohavichan V, Hennigar R. Crescentic, proliferative IgA nephropathy: clinical and histological response to methylprednisolone and intravenous cyclophosphamide. Nephrol Dial Transplant. 2003;18(7):1321–9.
86. Ballardie FW, Roberts ISD. Controlled prospective trial of prednisolone and cytotoxics in progressive IgA nephropathy. J Am Soc Nephrol. 2002;13(1):142–8.
87. Xie X, Lv J, Shi S, Zhu L, Liu L, Chen M, et al. Plasma exchange as an adjunctive therapy for crescentic IgA nephropathy. Am J Nephrol. 2016;44(2):141–9.
88. Lafayette RA, Canetta PA, Rovin BH, Appel GB, Novak J, Nath KA, et al. A randomized, controlled trial of rituximab in IgA nephropathy with proteinuria and renal dysfunction. J Am Soc Nephrol. 2017;28(4):1306–13.
89. Peng W, Tang Y, Jiang Z, Li Z, Mi X, Qin W. The effect of calcineurin inhibitors in the treatment of IgA nephropathy: a systematic review and meta-analysis (PRISMA). Medicine. 2016;95(35):e4731.
90. Ring T, Pedersen BB, Salkus G, Goodship THJ. Use of eculizumab in crescentic IgA nephropathy: proof of principle and conundrum? Clin Kidney J. 2015;8(5):489–91.
91. Waldo FB, Wyatt RJ, Kelly DR, Herrera GA, Benfield MR, Kohaut EC. Treatment of IgA nephropathy in children: efficacy of alternate-day oral prednisone. Pediatr Nephrol. 1993;7(5):529–32.

92. Yoshikawa N, Ito H, Sakai T, Takekoshi Y, Honda M, Awazu M, et al. A controlled trial of combined therapy for newly diagnosed severe childhood IgA nephropathy. The Japanese Pediatric IgA Nephropathy Treatment Study Group. J Am Soc Nephrol. 1999;10(1):101–9.
93. Kamei K, Nakanishi K, Ito S, Saito M, Sako M, Ishikura K, et al. Long-term results of a randomized controlled trial in childhood IgA nephropathy. Clin J Am Soc Nephrol. 2011;6(6):1301–7.
94. Yoshikawa N, Honda M, Iijima K, Awazu M, Hattori S, Nakanishi K, et al. Steroid treatment for severe childhood IgA nephropathy: a randomized, controlled trial. Clin J Am Soc Nephrol. 2006;1(3):511–7.
95. Hsu SI-H. Racial and genetic factors in IgA nephropathy. Semin Nephrol. 2008;28(1):48–57.
96. Gharavi AG, Yan Y, Scolari F, Schena FP, Frasca GM, Ghiggeri GM, et al. IgA nephropathy, the most common cause of glomerulonephritis, is linked to 6q22–23. Nat Genet. 2000;26(3):354–7.
97. Feehally J, Farrall M, Boland A, Gale DP, Gut I, Heath S, et al. HLA has strongest association with IgA nephropathy in genome-wide analysis. J Am Soc Nephrol. 2010;21(10):1791–7.
98. Gharavi AG, Kiryluk K, Choi M, Li Y, Hou P, Xie J, et al. Genome-wide association study identifies susceptibility loci for IgA nephropathy. Nat Genet. 2011;43(4):321–7.
99. Yu X-Q, Li M, Zhang H, Low H-Q, Wei X, Wang J-Q, et al. A genome-wide association study in Han Chinese identifies multiple susceptibility loci for IgA nephropathy. Nat Genet. 2011;44(2):178–82.
100. Lai KN, Chan LYY, Tang SCW, Tsang AWL, Li FFK, Lam MF, et al. Mesangial expression of angiotensin II receptor in IgA nephropathy and its regulation by polymeric IgA1. Kidney Int. 2004;66(4):1403–16.
101. Perna A, Ruggenenti P, Testa A, Spoto B, Benini R, Misefari V, et al. ACE genotype and ACE inhibitors induced renoprotection in chronic proteinuric nephropathies1. Kidney Int. 2000;57(1):274–81.
102. Odum J, Peh CA, Clarkson AR, Bannister KM, Seymour AE, Gillis D, et al. Recurrent mesangial IgA nephritis following renal transplantation. Nephrol Dial Transplant. 1994;9(3):309–12.
103. Wang AY, Lai FM, Yu AW, Lam PK, Chow KM, Choi PC, et al. Recurrent IgA nephropathy in renal transplant allografts. Am J Kidney Dis. 2001;38(3):588–96.
104. Chandrakantan A, Ratanapanichkich P, Said M, Barker CV, Julian BA. Recurrent IgA nephropathy after renal transplantation despite immunosuppressive regimens with mycophenolate mofetil. Nephrol Dial Transplant. 2005;20(6):1214–21.
105. Namba Y, Oka K, Moriyama T, Ichimaru N, Kyo M, Kokado Y, et al. Risk factors for graft loss in patients with recurrent IGA nephropathy after renal transplantation. Transplant Proc. 2004;36(5):1314–6.
106. Lionaki S, Panagiotellis K, Melexopoulou C, Boletis JN. The clinical course of IgA nephropathy after kidney transplantation and its management. Transplant Rev [Internet]. 2017; https://doi.org/10.1016/j.trre.2017.01.005.
107. Ponticelli C, Traversi L, Feliciani A, Cesana BM, Banfi G, Tarantino A. Kidney transplantation in patients with IgA mesangial glomerulonephritis. Kidney Int. 2001;60(5):1948–54.
108. Freese P, Svalander C, Nordén G, Nyberg G. Clinical risk factors for recurrence of IgA nephropathy. Clin Transpl. 1999;13(4):313–7.
109. Floege J. Recurrent IgA nephropathy after renal transplantation. Semin Nephrol. 2004;24(3):287–91.
110. Berthoux F, El Deeb S, Mariat C, Diconne E, Laurent B, Thibaudin L. Antithymocyte globulin (ATG) induction therapy and disease recurrence in renal transplant recipients with primary IgA nephropathy. Transplantation. 2008;85(10):1505–7.

111. Kessler M, Hiesse C, Hestin D, Mayeux D, Boubenider K, Charpentier B. Recurrence of immunoglobulin A nephropathy after renal transplantation in the cyclosporine era. Am J Kidney Dis. 1996;28(1):99–104.
112. Han SS, Huh W, Park SK, Ahn C, Han JS, Kim S, et al. Impact of recurrent disease and chronic allograft nephropathy on the long-term allograft outcome in patients with IgA nephropathy. Transpl Int. 2010;23(2):169–75.
113. Hotta K, Fukasawa Y, Akimoto M, Tanabe T, Sasaki H, Fukuzawa N, et al. Tonsillectomy ameliorates histological damage of recurrent immunoglobulin A nephropathy after kidney transplantation. Nephrology. 2013;18(12):808–12.

Chapter 8
Focal and Segmental Glomerulosclerosis (FSGS)

Stephanie Nguyen and Kuang-Yu Jen

Introduction

Focal segmental glomerulosclerosis (FSGS) is a clinicopathologic syndrome that can be classified as primary or secondary based on an identifiable underlying etiology. FSGS typically presents with nephrotic syndrome, which is defined as edema, proteinuria, and hypoalbuminemia. The form of nephrotic syndrome can be further classified based on response to treatment (Table 8.1): steroid-sensitive, frequently relapsing, steroid-dependent, or steroid-resistant nephrotic syndrome. Younger children and those who respond to steroid treatment typically do not have a renal biopsy indicated as most will have minimal change disease (MCD). Therefore, adolescents who more frequently have relapsing, steroid-dependent, or steroid-resistant nephrotic syndrome are more likely to have a renal biopsy, in which case FSGS may be diagnosed. FSGS generally features progressive glomerular scarring leading to decline of renal function and end-stage renal disease (ESRD), though with a variable clinical course depending on the underlying etiology and response to therapy.

S. Nguyen (✉)
Department of Pediatrics, UC Davis Children's Hospital, Sacramento, CA, USA
e-mail: stanguyen@ucdavis.edu

K.-Y. Jen
Department of Pathology and Laboratory Medicine, UC Davis School of Medicine, Sacramento, CA, USA
e-mail: kyjen@ucdavis.edu

M. N. Haddad et al. (eds.), *Adolescents with Chronic Kidney Disease*,
https://doi.org/10.1007/978-3-319-97220-6_8

Table 8.1 Definitions

Complete remission	Urine protein-to-creatinine ratio <20 mg/g (<20 mg/mmol) or <1+ protein on urine dipstick for three consecutive days
Partial remission	Reduction of proteinuria 50% and urine protein-to-creatinine ratio between 200 and 2000 mg/g (20–200 mg/mmol)
Steroid resistance	Failure to achieve complete remission after 8 weeks of corticosteroid therapy
Relapse	Urine protein-to-creatinine ratio ≥2,000 mg/g or ≥300 mg/dl or 1+ protein on urine dipstick
Frequent relapse	≥2 relapses within 6 months or ≥4 relapses within 12 months
Steroid dependence	Relapse while on corticosteroid therapy or within 2 weeks of stopping corticosteroid therapy

Epidemiology

In the United States, FSGS is the third most common cause of ESRD in adolescents, representing 9% of adolescents presenting for renal replacement therapy [1]. However, those with ESRD are only a fraction of true prevalence or incidence of FSGS, as not all children with nephrotic syndrome receive a kidney biopsy. The International Study of Kidney Disease in Children (ISKD) study of 561 children who received a renal biopsy at initial presentation of nephrotic syndrome found 8.6% had FSGS [2]. As steroid response was the most important factor predicting MCD, subsequent practices changed, and renal biopsy was selectively performed for steroid-resistant nephrotic syndrome (SRNS) or when there were clinical suspicions indicating a lesion other than MCD [3]. While estimates of pediatric nephrotic syndrome have remained stable, the proportion of those with FSGS has increased twofold [4, 5]. The increased incidence of FSGS was mainly seen in the group of children greater than 8 years old. Similarly, the proportion of adults with nephrotic syndrome and FSGS has increased two- to threefold, [6, 7], and in adults the incidence of FSGS has increased 11-fold between 1980 and 2000 [8].

Age appears to play an important role in the diagnosis of FSGS. In the ISKD study, children greater than 6 years presenting with nephrotic syndrome were more likely to have histology other than MCD, such as FSGS or membranoproliferative glomerulonephritis (MPGN). A later retrospective study of children 1–18 years old found that at initial presentation, those with steroid-resistant nephrotic syndrome were older (mean age 11.5 years old versus 4.6 years old) compared to those with steroid-sensitive nephrotic syndrome [9]. The subsequent renal biopsies for those with SRNS found 75% had FSGS. Similarly, in another group of adolescents, age 12–18 years old, without known proteinuric systemic disease, 55% had FSGS on renal biopsy on initial presentation with nephrotic syndrome [10].

Race also appears to play an important role in the diagnosis of FSGS. African-American children with nephrotic syndrome are more likely to present with steroid-resistant nephrotic syndrome [9] and are more likely to have FSGS than MCD on renal biopsy [10]. The reported increased incidence of FSGS in children appears to have been across all races [5].

Presenting Features

Proteinuria is a defining characteristic of FSGS. Approximately 75–90% of children and 50–60% of adults with FSGS present with nephrotic syndrome at presentation [11]. Nephrotic syndrome is defined as urine protein excretion (urine protein-to-creatinine ratio ≥2000 mg/g or ≥300 mg/dL on urine dipstick), hypoalbuminemia (serum albumin ≤2.5 g/dL), and edema [12]. Nephrotic syndrome may be accompanied by hypercholesterolemia and hypertriglyceridemia, which usually improves as proteinuria improves [13]. However, in particular the secondary nongenetic forms of FSGS can present with sub-nephrotic-range proteinuria. Compared to primary FSGS, adaptive forms of FSGS are more likely to have normal serum albumin levels even with nephrotic-range proteinuria.

Hypertension and hematuria are more likely to present with nephrotic syndrome in FSGS compared to MCD [2]. Hypertension is also more prevalent in adolescents presenting with steroid-resistant nephrotic syndrome [14]. In one case control study of children with FSGS compared to biopsy-proven MCD, those with FSGS were more likely to have hypertension (40% versus 15%), hematuria (80% versus 47%), or nephritis defined as the combination of hypertension, hematuria, and elevated serum creatinine (22% versus 2%) [15]. Though this may overestimate the prevalence as these same factors were an indication for a kidney biopsy.

Etiology

FSGS is a histological lesion resulting from the cumulative loss or damage to the glomerular filtration barrier which normally prevents proteinuria. Multiple pathways lead to this histologic diagnosis [16]. Primary or idiopathic form of FSGS has no specific known cause, though may be mediated by circulating permeability factors, for which multiple candidates are still being investigated. Secondary causes of FSGS include genetic mutations, injury due to infections or drugs, and maladaptive response to loss of renal mass (Table 8.2).

There are rapidly accumulating identified genetic mutations leading to steroid-resistant nephrotic syndrome or FSGS, now being referred to as podocytopathies, glomerular diseases in which proteinuria is due to damaged or dysfunctional podocytes. Podocytes are terminally differentiated cells that are integral to the glomerular filtration barrier. Podocyte injury leads to effacement of the podocyte foot processes which correlates with proteinuria. Change in podocyte shape requires rearrangement of actin cytoskeleton, a process that may be reversible with

Table 8.2 Etiologies of FSGS

Primary (idiopathic) FSGS
Secondary FSGS
Genetic mutations (see Table 8.3)
Viruses: HIV, Parvovirus B19
Medications: heroin, interferon therapy, lithium, pamidronate/alendronate, anabolic steroids
Adaptive structural-functional responses, e.g., glomerular hypertrophy or hyperfiltration
Reduced kidney mass: oligomeganephronia, unilateral kidney agenesis, kidney dysplasia, reflux nephropathy, chronic allograft nephropathy, advanced kidney disease with reduced nephron function, very low birth weight
Initially normal kidney mass: diabetes mellitus, hypertension, obesity, cyanotic congenital heart disease, sick cell anemia, thrombotic microangiopathy

glucocorticoid therapy but becomes irreversible and progressive in FSGS. Podocyte damage through detachment, apoptosis, or necrosis plays an important step in glomerulosclerosis. To date, there are more than 30 mutations that have been identified as causing monogenic forms of steroid-resistant nephrotic syndrome (Table 8.3) [17]. Genetic mutations are most likely to be found in infants, young children, syndromic patients, or those with family history of nephrotic syndrome. Genetic mutations can be identified in 84.8–100% of infants presenting in the first 3 months of life and 44.1–57% of children with infantile-onset nephrotic syndrome [18, 19]. Mutation detection rate of 50–67% was found for those with familial cases, defined as families with two or more affected children, one affected member of a consanguineous family, or family members affected in multiple generations [19, 20]. Mutations in the following genes can be present as isolated nephrotic syndrome or as part of a syndrome phenotype: WT-1 with Wilms tumor, Denys-Drash syndrome, or Frasier syndrome [21]; LAMB2 with Pierson syndrome; MYH9 with Epstein-Fechtner syndrome; INF2 with Charcot-Marie-Tooth disease; and LMX1B with nail-patella syndrome.

Adolescents with steroid-resistant nephrotic syndrome and without a family history have much lower mutation detection rates of 10–10.8% [19, 22]. However, identification of genetic mutations has important clinical implications. Most of the currently identified mutations are not steroid-sensitive or do not respond to cyclosporine which allows patients to stop treatments with potentially little benefit. In one cohort of children with SRNS, response rate to cyclosporine was much lower in the genetic disease group (5% complete remission and 12% partial remission) versus the nongenetic group (60% complete remission and 18% partial remission) [23]. However, especially in genetic mutations with WT1, NPHS2, or PLCE1 mutations, there are small numbers of patients that have had a partial or complete remission after cyclosporine [24–26]. Genetic mutations with autosomal dominant inheritance also have implications for living related donors who should be screened for the disease causing mutation as they may be yet to develop clinical signs or symptoms of nephrotic syndrome.

Table 8.3 Genetic mutations detected in steroid-resistant nephrotic syndrome presenting before 25 years of age

Gene	Protein	Inheritance
NPHS2	Podocin	AR
NPHS1	Nephrin	AR
WT1	Wilms tumor suppressor gene 1	AD
PLCE1	Phospholipase C, epsilon 1	AR
LAMB2	Laminin, β2	AR
SMARCAL1	SW1/SNF-related, matrix-associated, actin-dependent regulator of chromatin, subfamily a-like1	AR
INF2	Inverted formin 2	AD
TRPC6	Transient receptor potential cation channel 6	AD
COQ6	Coenzyme Q6 mono-oxygenase	AR
ITGA3	Integrin, alpha 3	AR
MYO1E	Myosin IE	AR
CUBN	Cubilin	AR
COQ2	Coenzyme Q2 4-hydroxybenzoate polyprenyltransferase	AR
LMX1B	LIM homeobox transcription factor 1, beta	AD
ADCK4	AarF doman containing kinase 4	AR
DGKE1	Diacylglycerol kinase, epsilon	AR
PDSS2	Prenyl (decaprenyl) diphosphate synthase, subunit 2	AR
ARHGAP24	Rho GTPase-activating protein 24	AD
ARHGDIA	Rho GDP diassociation inhibitor (GD1) alpha	AR
CFH	Complement factor H	AR
ITBG4	Integrin, beta 4	AR

AD autosomal dominant, *AR* autosomal recessive
Modified from Sadowski et al. [20]

Pathology

The typical histologic manifestation of FSGS is just as the name states; glomerular scars (glomerulosclerosis) are present involving only a portion of the glomerulus (segmental) and involving only some of the glomeruli (focal) in the biopsy. Hence, the characteristic lesions of FSGS may be missed if a limited number of glomeruli are sampled in a biopsy. As the disease progresses, segmental lesions evolve to become global glomerulosclerosis, and in advanced stages the more specific morphologic finding of segmental sclerosis may no longer be present in the biopsy. Instead, completely nonspecific diffuse and global glomerulosclerosis may be all that remains, and the diagnosis of FSGS cannot be made.

Podocyte injury is the common downstream effect for the diverse etiologies of FSGS, which results in foot process effacement seen on electron microscopy and the histologic manifestation of segmental glomerulosclerosis on light microscopy.

There are numerous secondary causes for FSGS including genetic mutations, viral infections, drugs or medications, and maladaptive response to glomerular hyperfiltration/hypertension, which all need to be distinguished from primary FSGS. Given that the morphologic changes of FSGS lack specificity and do not reliably distinguish between primary and secondary forms of the disease, diagnosis of FSGS on kidney biopsy can be problematic. Additionally, glomerular injury unrelated to FSGS can result in lesions that mimic segmental glomerulosclerosis seen in FSGS, such as segmental glomerular scars from chronic or sclerosing glomerulonephritides. As in all cases of renal pathology, detailed patient history and clinical data can be quite helpful to confidently secure the diagnosis.

Light Microscopic Findings

Although the "classic" sclerotic lesions of FSGS are characterized by segmental increase in extracellular matrix with associated obliteration of the glomerular capillary lumens, several histologic variants of FSGS have been described in numerous publications [27]. A concerted effort was made in 2000 by an international group of renal pathologists to histologically subclassify these variants. The resulting Columbia Classification for FSGS was published in 2004 and has become the most widely accepted categorization for the histologic variants of FSGS [28]. This system is solely based on glomerular light microscopic alterations and includes five mutually exclusive variants: collapsing, tip, cellular, perihilar, and not otherwise specified (NOS). The variants can be applied to both primary and secondary forms of FSGS. The following sections discuss the specifics of these variants with some additional remarks about distinctive tubulointerstitial findings that are not part of the Columbia Classification.

FSGS Not Otherwise Specified

This form of FSGS is essentially categorization based on exclusion of the other four variants discussed below and is the most common variant. Histologically, it shows the "classic" features of FSGS characterized by discrete segmental solidification of the glomerular tuft with increased extracellular matrix that causes obliteration of the glomerular capillary lumens [28]. Hyalinosis, foam cell entrapment, and adhesions are not required but commonly observed findings within segments of sclerosis (Fig. 8.1a–d). Prominent palisading podocytes overlying the segmental lesions can be seen and has been termed podocyte "capping." The unaffected segments of glomeruli are essentially normal if there is not another underlying glomerular disease. The juxtamedullary glomeruli appear to be preferentially affected by segmental sclerosis, and thus sampling of the corticomedullary junction is helpful to detect early FSGS. Having just one segmental lesion on biopsy is enough for the diagnosis

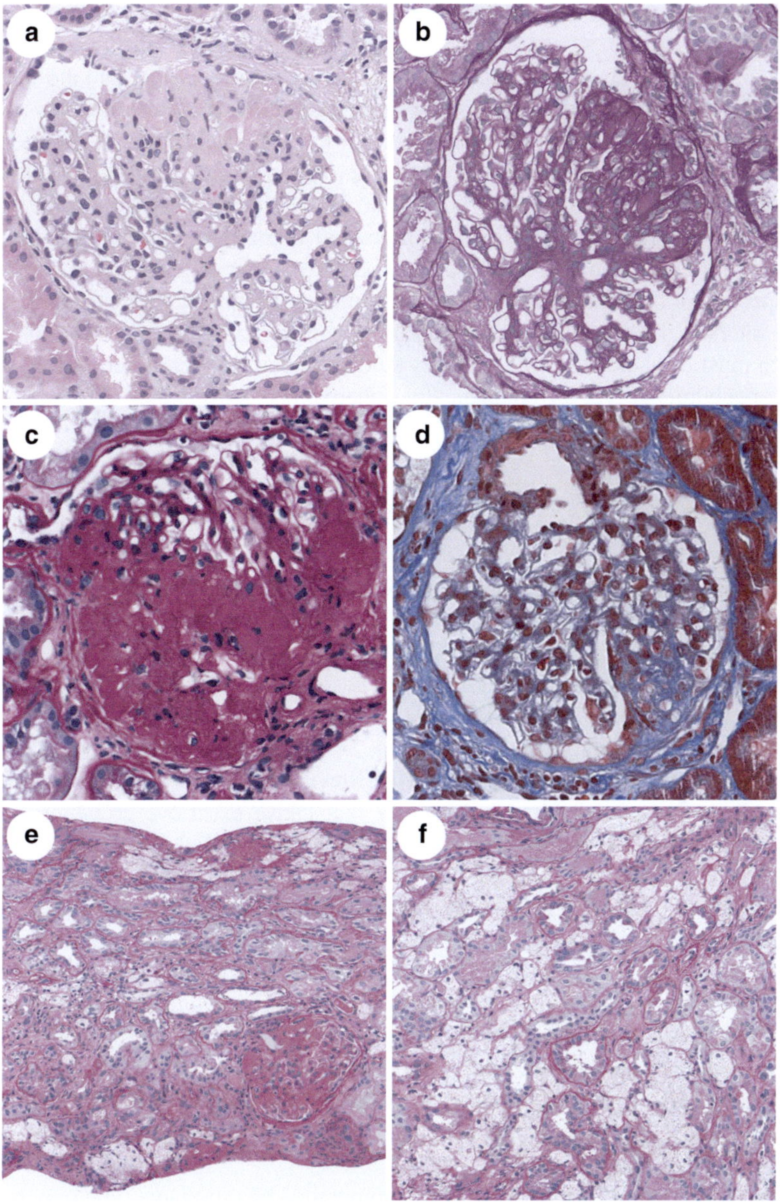

Fig. 8.1 Light microscopy findings of FSGS (NOS). (**a**) H&E stain of a glomerulus showing segmental sclerosis and hyalinosis with adhesion of the sclerotic segment to the adjacent Bowman capsule. The segmental lesion is peripheral and shows no distinctive features of the other variants of FSGS (original magnification 400×). (**b**, **c**) PAS stain helps highlight hyalinosis, wrinkling of the glomerular basement membrane, and matrix accumulation within the segments of sclerosis (original magnification 400×). (**d**) Segmental sclerosis with adhesion appears blue on Masson trichrome (original magnification 400×). (**e**, **f**) Interstitial foam cells are present in association with FSGS (NOS) and appear quite prominent in some areas (PAS; original magnification (**a**) 100× and (**b**) 200×)

of FSGS and would eliminate minimal change disease from the differential diagnosis.

Interstitial fibrosis and tubular atrophy often accompany FSGS, and the severity typically approximates the degree of overall glomerulosclerosis. Protein resorption droplets and lipid vacuoles may be present in the proximal tubules as is often the case for glomerular diseases with heavy proteinuria and nephrotic syndrome. Evidence of acute tubular injury is variable but can be prominent in some cases. Scattered individual or collections of interstitial foam cells may be present but is nonspecific and can occur in any patient with long-standing nephrotic syndrome irrespective of the cause (Fig. 8.1e, f). The finding of segmental glomerulosclerosis with interstitial foam cells is common in hereditary nephritis (Alport syndrome), which must be excluded using ancillary studies such as immunofluorescence staining for subunits of type IV collagen alpha chain and electron microscopy.

Collapsing Variant

The collapsing variant of FSGS is characterized by at least one glomerulus showing segmental or global collapse of the glomerular tuft with associated overlying podocyte hypertrophy and hyperplasia [28]. Collapse of the glomerular tuft appears implosive with wrinkling of the glomerular basement membranes that causes obliteration of the capillary lumens; however, these lesions show no increase in extracellular matrix or intracapillary cells (Fig. 8.2a). Instead, prominent extracapillary hypercellularity is commonly present in the Bowman space with podocytes exhibiting striking hypertrophy and hyperplasia that cause excessive crowding of the Bowman space. Such extracapillary lesions often mimic cellular crescents although the podocytes are plump and lack the spindled shape and pericellular matrix that is typical of true crescents [29]. Fibrin within the Bowman space and breakage of the glomerular basement membrane should be absent since such features indicate the presence of an associated necrotizing lesion and would argue in favor for a crescentic/necrotizing process. Protein resorption droplets may be quite conspicuous within the podocytes. Adhesions and hyalinosis are not usually seen in collapsing lesions. As defined, the collapsing variant trumps all other variants. Thus, having a single glomerulus with collapsing features qualifies the biopsy as collapsing variant of FSGS, irrespective of whether there are other types of segmental lesions in the biopsy.

The collapsing variant is frequently accompanied by prominent tubulointerstitial injury that appears out of proportion to the degree of glomerulosclerosis. Acute tubular injury is typically obvious and may be accompanied by swollen tubular epithelial cells containing abundant protein resorption droplets and lipid vacuoles (Fig. 8.2b). Scattered tubular microcysts consisting of ectatic tubules with proteinaceous casts are common (Fig. 8.2c). Significant interstitial fibrosis and tubular atrophy are usually present. Not surprisingly, the collapsing variant demonstrates more rapid progression and worse renal outcome than the other variants [30].

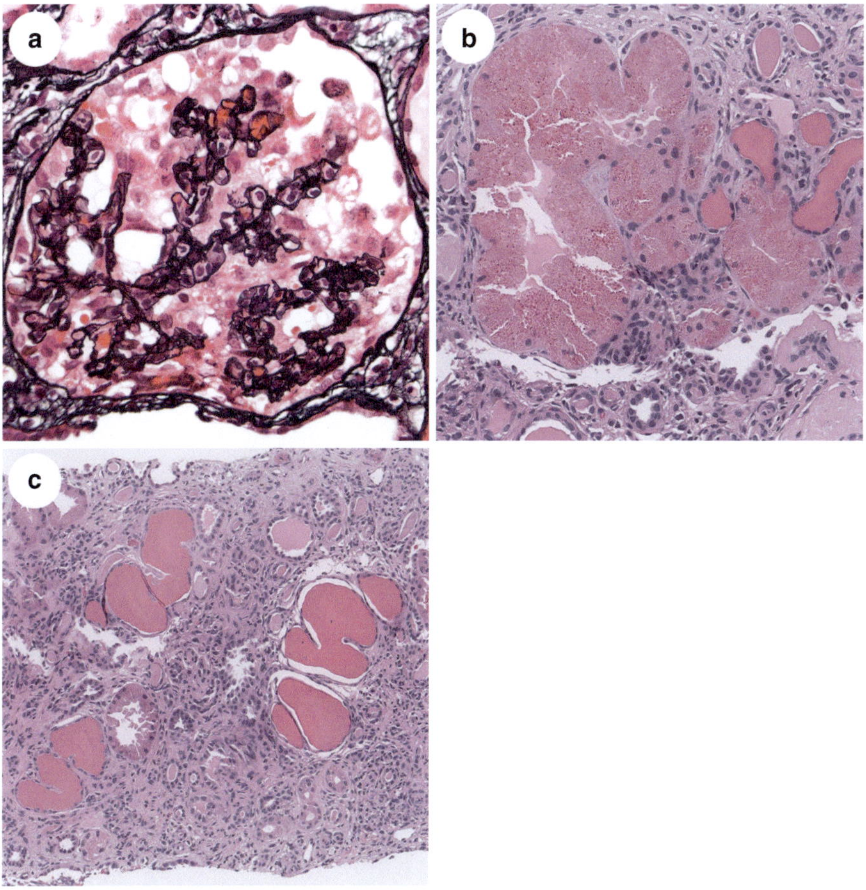

Fig. 8.2 Light microscopy findings of FSGS collapsing variant. (**a**) Glomerulus with podocyte hyperplasia/hypertrophy and associated collapse of the glomerular tuft. (Courtesy of Dr. Xin Jin Zhou, Texas A&M University (JMS; original magnification 400×)). Collapsing variant often shows associated tubulointerstitial changes including (**b**) hypertrophic proximal tubules with abundant intracytoplasmic protein resorption droplets and (**c**) tubular microcysts characterized by luminal dilatation, tubular epithelial cell flattening, and large hyaline casts (PAS; original magnification (**b**) 200× and (**c**) 100×)

Tip Variant

The tip variant of FSGS is characterized by the presence of at least one segmental lesion involving the tip domain of the glomerulus, with the tip domain defined as the outer 25% of the glomerular tuft next to the origin of the proximal tubule [28]. In identifying a definitive tip lesion, the tubular pole is involved by an adhesion between the tuft and Bowman capsule or is involved by confluence of podocytes with the parietal or tubular epithelial cells at the tubular lumen or neck. The affected segment may show endocapillary hypercellularity (often with foam cells), hyalinosis, and/or sclerosis and will frequently demonstrate associated overlying podocyte hypertrophy/hyperplasia (Fig. 8.3). Herniation of the tip lesion into the lumen of the proximal tubule is apparent in some cases. Aside from genuine tip lesions, glomeruli exhibiting segmental sclerosis or segmental endocapillary hypercellularity at the

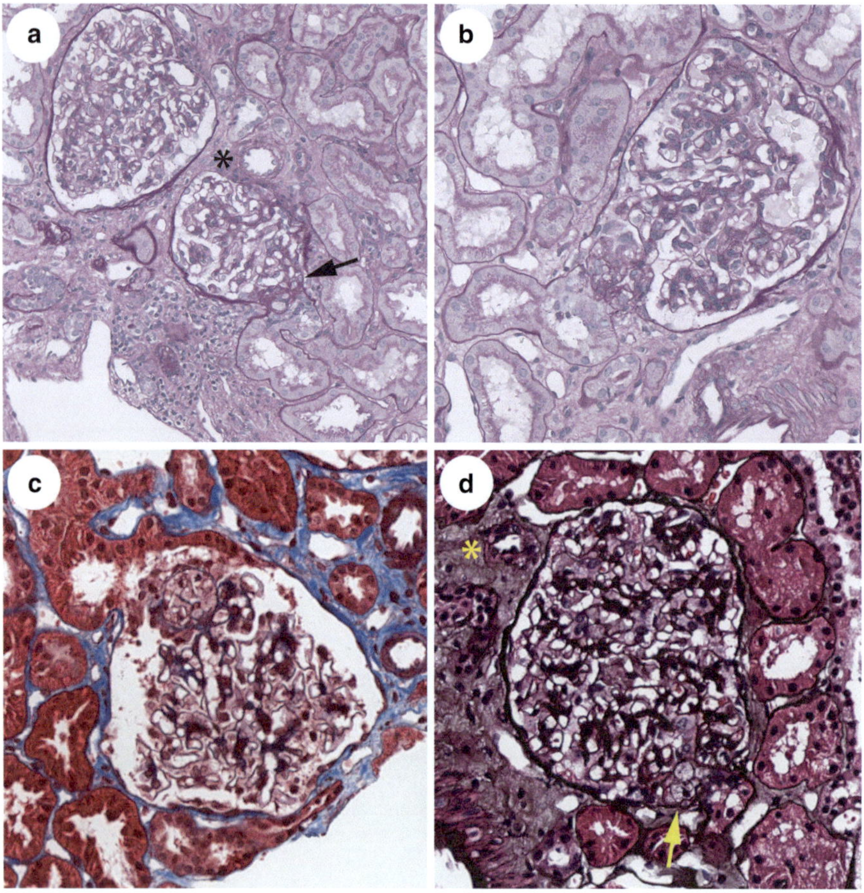

Fig. 8.3 Light microscopy findings of FSGS tip variant. (**a**) Glomerulus with sclerotic tip lesion and adhesion at the origin of the proximal tubule (arrow). An arteriole (*) at the vascular pole is noted at the opposite end of the glomerulus. The other glomerulus appears normal (PAS; original magnification 200×). (**b**) Sclerotic tip lesion and adhesion at the origin of the proximal tubule (PAS; original magnification 400×). (**c**) Intracapillary foam cells with prominent overlying podocytes are localized to the tip domain. Sclerosis is not apparent in this example of a tip lesion (Masson trichrome; original magnification 400×). (**d**) Intracapillary foam cells (arrow) are present adjacent to the partially viewed origin of the proximal tubule. An arteriole (*) is noted at the opposite end of the glomerulus, further supporting the tip domain as the location of the segmental lesion (JMS; original magnification 400×)

periphery or in an uncertain location within the glomerulus may be present in cases of the tip variant [31]. However, exclusion of the collapsing variant is mandatory and any segmental lesion that can be confidently localized to the perihilar region precludes the diagnosis of the tip variant. Tip lesions can be seen in the setting of other glomerular diseases such as membranous glomerulonephritis, IgA nephropathy, and diabetic glomerulosclerosis, among others [32]. Thus, the tip variant of FSGS should only be applied when these other forms of glomerular diseases are excluded. Overall, the tip lesion variant has the least amount of tubulointerstitial injury and chronicity when compared to the other forms of FSGS, which correlates to its better outcome [30].

Cellular Variant

In diagnosing the cellular variant of FSGS, the collapsing and tip variants must be excluded. The cellular variant is defined by the presence of at least one glomerulus with segmental endocapillary hypercellularity that occludes the capillary lumens and affects at least 25% of the tuft [28]. Any segment may be affected in this variant, although if the segmental lesions are exclusively confined to the tip domain or affect the tip domain and the peripheral segments without the presence of perihilar lesions, then by definition it is classified as the tip variant. Endocapillary hypercellularity of the cellular variant typically consists of foam cells, macrophages, and endothelial cells with variable involvement by lymphocytes, neutrophils, and other leukocytes (Fig. 8.4a, b). The intracapillary cells often fill and distend the glomerular capillaries. Some of these cells may undergo apoptosis and display pyknotic nuclei and karyorrhectic nuclear debris. Hypertrophic and hyperplastic podocytes frequently overlie the segmental lesions. This constellation of findings can present a diagnostic challenge since they greatly mimic features seen in focal and segmental proliferative glomerulonephritides, such as lupus nephritis, IgA nephropathy, or pauci-immune glomerulonephritis to name a few [29]. The lack of true necrotizing lesions on light microscopy, the absence of immune deposits by immunofluorescence and electron microscopy, and the presence of extensive severe foot process effacement help support the diagnosis of cellular variant of FSGS.

Perihilar Variant

Exclusion of the collapsing, tip, and cellular variants is mandatory for the diagnosis of the perihilar variant of FSGS. If these other variants are excluded, then a biopsy can qualify as the perihilar variant if at least one glomerulus shows perihilar hyalinosis and more than 50% of the glomeruli affected by segmental lesions demonstrate perihilar sclerosis and/or hyalinosis (Fig. 8.4c, d) [28]. This variant is often

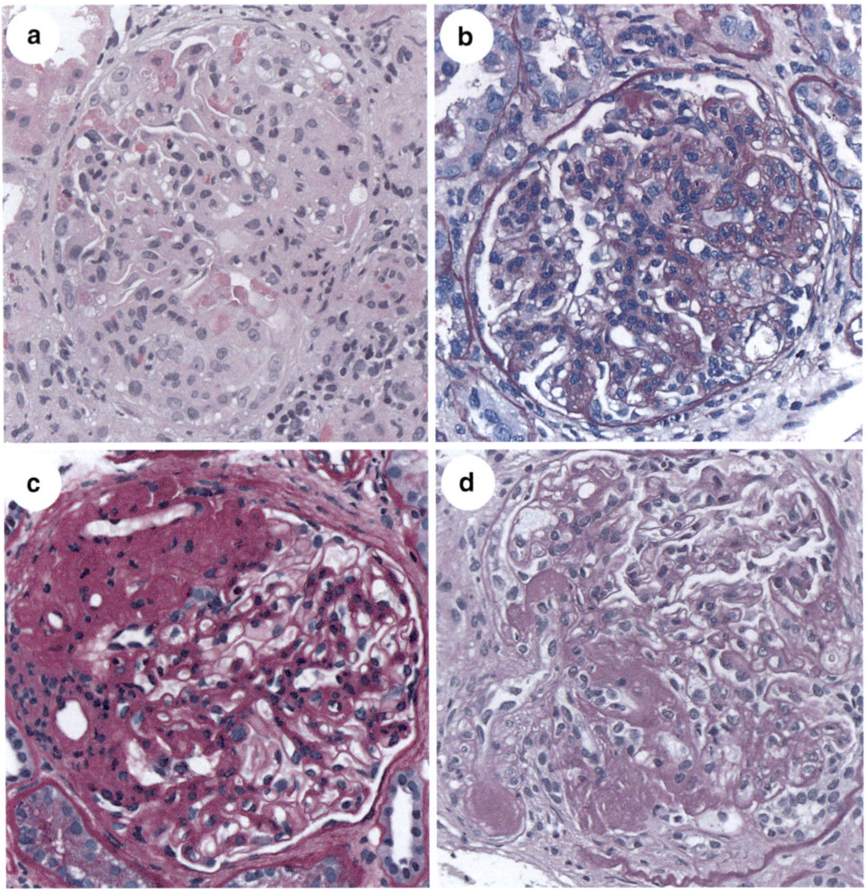

Fig. 8.4 Light microscopy findings of FSGS cellular variant and FSGS perihilar variant. (**a**) Glomerulus showing segmental endocapillary hypercellularity with presence of foam cells (near 12 o'clock). Prominent podocytes are present with intracytoplasmic protein resorption droplets (H&E; original magnification (400×). (**b**) Glomerulus with segmental endocapillary hypercellularity with foam cells and overlying hypertrophic podocytes. (Courtesy of Dr. Xin Jin Zhou, Texas A&M University (PAS; original magnification 400×)). (**c**, **d**) Glomeruli exhibiting perihilar sclerosis and hyalinosis (PAS; original magnification 400×)

associated with secondary forms of FSGS caused by maladaptive response to glomerular hyperfiltration/hypertension, thus associated glomerulomegaly is commonly encountered. By definition, perihilar hyalinosis is present and may extend into the hilar arterioles. The segmental lesions may show typical findings of segmental sclerosis including entrapped foam cells, adhesions, and prominent podocytes.

Immunofluorescence Findings

Since FSGS is not an immune complex-mediated or complement-driven glomerular disease, the immunofluorescence findings should show no convincing evidence of immune deposits. Instead, IgM and C3 staining can frequently be seen corresponding to the segmental glomerular scars and areas of hyalinosis. In some cases, less intense IgM staining may be present in non-sclerotic mesangial areas. Given that patients with FSGS often will have a high degree of proteinuria, protein resorption droplets may be present in some podocytes and proximal tubules. These intracytoplasmic protein resorption droplets typically stain for albumin and some immunoglobulins, especially IgG and IgA. This type of staining within podocytes must be distinguished from bona fide immune deposits within the glomerular tuft. Correlation with light and electron microscopic findings is often helpful to make this distinction. The immunofluorescence findings are similar for all morphologic variants of FSGS and do not serve to distinguish between the variants.

Electron Microscopic Findings

As with nearly all glomerular diseases that result in substantial proteinuria, diffuse foot process effacement is typical of FSGS. Evaluation of foot process effacement should be performed on non-sclerotic segments of the glomerulus since podocytes overlying sclerotic lesions will commonly exhibit complete foot process effacement. Although not always the case, the degree of foot process effacement roughly correlates to the severity of the proteinuria.

Ultrastructurally, areas of segmental sclerosis demonstrate solidification with marked narrowing or loss of the capillary lumens caused by prominent wrinkling of the glomerular basement membrane and matrix accumulation. Often these areas contain intramembranous hyalin, which may mimic electron-dense immune deposits. However, hyalin usually has a waxier appearance and will be largely localized to areas of sclerosis. If substantial electron-dense deposits are seen in non-sclerotic portions of the glomerulus, then an immune complex-mediated process is likely present, and the diagnosis of FSGS should be reconsidered. Intracapillary foam cells may be present and are identified by the presence of numerous intracytoplasmic electron-lucent vacuoles. Podocyte detachment from the glomerular basement membrane may occur and will often show multiple layers of intervening new basement membrane material.

Similar to immunofluorescence findings, electron microscopic features do not distinguish between FSGS variants as the Columbia Classification is solely based on glomerular histologic findings. However, specific ultrastructural findings may point to some secondary causes of FSGS. For example, a case of collapsing variant of FSGS with tubuloreticular inclusions within endothelial cells on electron microscopy would be highly suspicious for HIV-associated nephropathy and should be correlated to clinical data to support this diagnosis.

Treatment

Treatment may vary according to the underlying etiology of FSGS. However, almost all forms of FSGS may benefit from renin-angiotensin system (RAS) blockade. One observational study found that angiotensin-converting enzyme inhibitor (ACEI) and angiotensin receptor blocker (ARB) use was associated with increased likelihood of remission and predictive of renal survival in children [33]. There are two randomized clinical trials that showed proteinuria reduction in children with steroid-resistant nephrotic syndrome [34, 35]. Low- and high-dose enalapril (0.2–0.6 mg/kg daily) reduce proteinuria for those with SRNS by 33–52% [34].

The mainstay of treatment in nephrotic syndrome is steroid therapy with oral prednisone 2 mg/kg or 60 mg/m^2 per day with maximum dose 60 mg per day for 4–6 weeks tapered to 1.5 mg/kg or 40 mg/m^2 every other day for an additional 4–6 weeks [36]. Response to steroid therapy determines subsequent treatment, indications for a diagnostic kidney biopsy, and prognosis. 12.4–21.9% of children are resistant to steroid therapy at initial presentation [3, 37]. Additional immunosuppressant therapies are used to treat those with steroid-dependent, frequently relapsing, and steroid-resistant nephrotic syndrome or those intolerant of steroid therapy.

There are published guidelines for the treatment of nephrotic syndrome based on the evidence and consensus among experts in the field [38, 39]. For idiopathic forms of FSGS, FSGS can be initially steroid-sensitive later to become frequently relapsing, steroid-dependent, or steroid-resistant. While the majority of genetic forms of FSGS will not respond to therapy, there are some mutations that have at least a partial response to calcineurin inhibitor therapy, and current guidelines still recommend at least a 6-month trial of therapy.

Steroid-Dependent/Frequently Relapsing Nephrotic Syndrome

For those with steroid-dependent or frequently relapsing nephrotic syndrome, a steroid-sparing agent is prescribed to avoid steroid-related adverse effects. Meta-analysis by the Cochrane group and the KDIGO practice guidelines has summarized the randomized clinical trials of steroid-sparing agents [38, 40].

Alkylating agents such as cyclophosphamide or chlorambucil reduced the risk of relapse at 6–12 months and 12–24 months compared to prednisone alone. Oral cyclophosphamide at a dose of 2 mg/kg per day given for 8–12 weeks for a maximum cumulative dose of 168 mg/kg is started after remission is achieved with corticosteroid. Oral cyclophosphamide reduced the risk of relapse by half compared to corticosteroids alone, risk ratio 0.44–0.47 [38, 40]. Chlorambucil 0.1–0.2 mg/kg per day given for 8 weeks, for a maximum cumulative dose of 11.2 mg/kg, also reduced the risk of relapse by approximately 80%, risk ratio 0.13–019 [38, 40]. There is no evidence a second course of alkylating agents improved the relapse rate. Both alkylating agents are associated with leukopenia, thrombocytopenia, and infections.

Alternatively, intravenous cyclophosphamide given monthly for 6 months had fewer relapses compared to oral cyclophosphamide at 6 months but was similar to oral cyclophosphamide at 24 months. The infection rate was lower in the intravenous group but had similarly rates of other side effects: bone marrow suppression, hair loss, nausea, and vomiting.

Concern for gonadal toxicity is the primary reason for hesitation in use of cyclophosphamide in adolescents. Females with sustained amenorrhea may have premature ovarian failure, characterized by elevated gonadotropins and low levels of estradiol. Observational studies in postpubertal females with systemic lupus erythematosus (SLE) found that the risk of amenorrhea was related to both cumulative dose of cyclophosphamide and age at time of exposure [41–43]. For females less than 30 years old, the risk of sustained amenorrhea was 10–14% versus 50–60% for those over 40 years old [41, 42]. The risk of sustained amenorrhea for those less than 25 years and who received a cumulative dose of cyclophosphamide of 10 g or less was negligible though the overall number of study participants was small ($n = 37$) [41, 42]. Few studies in girls with nephrotic syndrome report gonadal toxicity with alkylating agents [44].

In males with nephrotic syndrome, the risk of azoospermia was also associated with the cumulative dose or duration of exposure to cyclophosphamide, especially with cumulative doses over 300 mg/kg [43, 44]. Treatment before onset of puberty entails less risk of azoospermia. Observational studies in males with nephrotic syndrome or malignancies found the recovery of azoospermia often occurred after the end of therapy but could take up to 3 years or longer. Recovery occurred in 80% of males who received cumulative doses of cyclophosphamide less than 7.5 g/m^2 but was less than 10% for those who received cumulative doses greater than 7.5 g/m^2.

Calcineurin inhibitors (CNIs), cyclosporine or tacrolimus, are recommended as steroid-sparing agents in frequently relapsing or steroid-dependent nephrotic syndrome. Cyclosporine is given at a starting dose 4–5 mg/kg/day in two divided doses or tacrolimus 0.1 mg/kg/day in two divided doses. Earlier clinical trials aimed for 10–14 h cyclosporine trough levels of 50–150 ng/mL or 200–600 ng/mL, though lower levels 60–80 ng/mL appear to be effective to maintain remission [45–47]. Cyclosporine was as effective as cyclophosphamide or chlorambucil at reducing the relapse rate, but the effect was not sustained after cyclosporine was stopped [46, 47]. The suggested minimum duration of therapy is 1 year though some have recommend use for less than 2 years due to the risk of renal damage [48, 49]. Creatinine levels were significantly higher, and hirsutism and gum hypertrophy were more common with cyclosporine compared to alkylating agents. Tacrolimus use is often preferred over cyclosporine due to the negative cosmetic side effects of cyclosporine (hypertrichosis, gum hyperplasia) though there are no randomized controlled trials comparing cyclosporine and tacrolimus in steroid-dependent or frequently relapsing nephrotic syndrome. Both CNIs have side effects that include hypertension, acute kidney injury, and renal interstitial fibrosis.

For those with serious adverse effects from prior alkylating agent therapy or CNIs or who continue to have steroid-dependent or frequently relapsing nephrotic syndrome despite corticosteroid-sparing agents, the addition of rituximab, a chimeric anti-CD 20 monoclonal antibody, can decrease the relapse rate and reduce prednisone and CNI treatment. Children with steroid-dependent nephrotic syndrome given one dose of rituximab 375 mg/m^2 intravenously had a median relapse-free survival of 18 months while being taken off corticosteroids [50].

Children with steroid- and CNI-dependent nephrotic syndrome given one to two doses of rituximab 375 mg/m^2 intravenously had a lower relapse rate at 3 months compared to CNIs and prednisone alone, 48.1% versus 18.5% [51]. Prednisone and CNIs were tapered 1 month after rituximab. At 3 months, 77.8% was off prednisone and 62.9% were off CNIs in the rituximab group versus 7.4% and 3.7% in the control group. Relapse-free rate for rituximab was 50% and 25% at 6 and 12 months, respectively. Children with steroid- and CNI-dependent nephrotic syndrome given four weekly infusions of rituximab 375 mg/m^2 (maximum 500 mg) had a median relapse-free survival of 267 days versus 101 days compared to placebo and had decreased steroid usage, prednisolone 8.37 mg/m^2 per day versus 21 mg/m^2 per day, compared to placebo [52]. The reported adverse effects of rituximab included bronchospasm, hypotension, fever, skin rash, and joint pain. More serious adverse reactions reported include *Pneumocystis jiroveci* pneumonia [53, 54], and rare but sometimes fatal cases of pulmonary fibrosis have been associated with rituximab administration given for nephrotic syndrome [55–57].

Steroid-Resistant Nephrotic Syndrome

As many as 12.4–21.9% of children are resistant to steroid therapy at initial presentation [3, 37]. A kidney biopsy is indicated for children with SRNS to help guide therapy. Children with SRNS are more likely to have FSGS but may have minimal change disease (MCD), mesangial proliferative glomerulonephritis, or other histopathologic diagnoses. Those who do not achieve a partial or complete remission are at risk for progression to ESRD.

Current KDIGO Glomerulonephritis 2012 guidelines recommend a calcineurin inhibitor as the initial therapy combined with corticosteroids for children with SRNS [39]. Treatment with CNIs is recommended to continue for a minimum of 6 months and then stopped if a partial or complete remission is not achieved. One observational case series of 20 children with SRNS and FSGS had a complete remission rate of 30% with a cyclosporine trough level 100–200 ng/mL [58]. In a meta-analysis of three randomized clinical trials of 49 children with SRNS, cyclosporine achieved complete remission in 31% and partial remission in 38% of patients within 6 months of therapy versus none in the control arms [39, 59]. The goal cyclosporine trough level varied widely between the randomized clinical trials from 100 to 250 ng/ml [60], <200 ng/ml [61], 250 to 600 ng/ml [62], and 300 to 500 ng/ml [63]. Complete and partial remission rates were higher with higher cyclosporine levels.

One randomized controlled trial comparing tacrolimus to cyclosporine in children with SRNS had similar remission rates overall 85.7% versus 80% at 6 months and 85.7% versus 75% at 12 months when compared to cyclosporine [64]. Tacrolimus complete and partial remission rates at 6 months were 42.8% and 42.8%, respectively, compared to cyclosporine 50% and 30%, respectively. Median time to complete or partial remission was similar at 8 and 12 weeks for tacrolimus and cyclosporine, respectively. Relapse rate was lower in tacrolimus compared cyclosporine. The trough levels for tacrolimus were adjusted for goal 5–8 ng/ml and for cyclosporine 100–150 ng/ml. After 12 months of therapy, the estimated glomerular filtration rate (eGFR) was lower compared to start of therapy in both groups but did not differ between tacrolimus and cyclosporine. Reversible nephrotoxicity and hypertension occurred similarly in both groups. Cosmetic side effects of hypertrichosis and gum hypertrophy were much more commonly seen in the cyclosporine-treated group, 95% and 60%, respectively, versus in the tacrolimus treated group, 0% and 4.7%. Diarrhea was much more commonly seen in the tacrolimus treated group, 28.6% versus 5%, in the cyclosporine treated group.

In a randomized controlled trial of children with SRNS, tacrolimus had higher complete or partial remission rates compared to monthly intravenous cyclophosphamide, 82.5% versus 45.8% [65]. Tacrolimus had a higher sustained remission at 12 months 73.1% versus 42.9% compared to intravenous cyclophosphamide. There was no significant difference in eGFR at 12 months between the two treatment groups. Serious infections were higher in the cyclophosphamide treated group, 16 events in 8 patients including 1 death.

For those with steroid- and CNI-resistant nephrotic syndrome, the KDIGO guidelines suggest mycophenolate mofetil, high-dose corticosteroids, or a combination of both immunosuppressant therapies though the quality level of evidence was low. There is no randomized controlled trial of an effective therapy for steroid- and CNI-resistant nephrotic syndrome at this time. In one open-label randomized controlled trial of 31 children with steroid- and CNI-resistant nephrotic syndrome, two doses of rituximab as an add-on therapy did not significantly reduce proteinuria or improve remission rates [66]. Multiple potential therapies for multidrug-resistant nephrotic syndrome are currently underway: ofatumumab, a humanized anti-CD20 monoclonal antibody which is currently FDA approved for multidrug-resistant chronic lymphocytic leukemia (NCT02394106) [67–69]; abatacept (CTLA4-Ig), a recombinant fusion protein that modifies T-cell activation which is currently FDA approved for rheumatoid arthritis (NCT02592798) [70]; and low-density lipoprotein apheresis (LDL-A) which was originally developed for severe dyslipidemias but approved by the FDA for humanitarian device use in children with FSGS (NCT02235857) [71, 72].

Prognosis

Multiple factors are associated with renal survival in children and adolescents with FSGS. Renal survival appears inversely related to proteinuria. In a FSGS disease registry of 78 children and adolescents, there was a 90% decreased risk of ESRD for those with a complete remission compared to those with no remission [33]. The 3-year renal survival rate was 100% for those in complete remission, 92% for those in partial remission, and 47% if no remission. Another observational study in Brazilian children reported a 10-year renal survival of 95% for steroid-responsive versus 54% for steroid-nonresponsive FSGS [73].

Those with a genetic form of FSGS also have a reported higher rate of progression to ESRD. Similarly, they were also less like to achieve a complete or partial remission after cyclosporine therapy. The complete and partial remission rate were 3% and 16%, respectively, in those with genetic FSGS as compared to 55% and 13%, respectively, in nongenetic forms [23].

The histologic subclassification of FSGS variants is also important in the prognosis in children. The collapsing variant of FSGS not only presents initially with lower renal function but also progresses faster [74]. Collapsing variant of FSGS also initially present with higher measures of chronic injury as indicated by degree interstitial fibrosis, tubular atrophy, arteriosclerosis, and glomerular sclerosis. Those with collapsing lesions are also less likely to be steroid responsive or achieve remission of proteinuria [74–76].

Transplant

The majority of FSGS diagnosed in renal transplant recipients represent recurrence of primary FSGS with a smaller number of de novo cases. Proteinuria is the first sign of disease recurrence and can develop sometimes within hours after surgery. Overall the risk of FSGS recurrence for adolescents has reported to be between, 5.8% and 24%, from large registries like United Network of Organ Sharing (UNOS) and North American Pediatric Renal Trials and Collaborative Studies (NAPTRCS) [77–79]. In addition, those with an idiopathic FSGS have a higher risk of posttransplant recurrence compared to those with a genetic form of FSGS, 28.5% versus 4.5% [80].

Adolescents with FSGS face worse posttransplant outcomes than adolescents with other diagnoses. Acute tubular necrosis (ATN) requiring dialysis during the 1st week posttransplantation was nearly twice as high in adolescents with FSGS compared to other adolescents in both living and decreased donor recipients [81]. The most significant risk for graft failure was due to disease recurrence which accounted for 15.2% of graft failures in adolescents with FSGS compared to 3.2% of graft failure for adolescences with other diagnoses [81]. Adolescents with FSGS also have worse outcomes for graft survival compared to younger children with FSGS.

Race appears to be an important factor as Black children with FSGS face worse outcome after renal transplant with a higher risk of graft failure, acute rejection, and delayed graft function compared to other races [82]. However, there was no difference in patient mortality or FSGS recurrence. In fact, others have reported a higher risk of recurrence in White children compared to all other races, 19% versus 12% [79].

References

1. Ferris ME, Gipson DS, Kimmel PL, Eggers PW. Trends in treatment and outcomes of survival of adolescents initiating end-stage renal disease care in the United States of America. Pediatr Nephrol. 2006;21(7):1020–6.
2. Nephrotic syndrome in children: prediction of histopathology from clinical and laboratory characteristics at time of diagnosis. A report of the International Study of Kidney Disease in Children. Kidney Int. 1978;13(2):159–65.
3. The primary nephrotic syndrome in children. Identification of patients with minimal change nephrotic syndrome from initial response to prednisone. A report of the International Study of Kidney Disease in Children. J Pediatr 1981;98(4):561–4.
4. Borges FF, Shiraichi L, da Silva MPH, Nishimoto EI, Nogueira PCK. Is focal segmental glomerulosclerosis increasing in patients with nephrotic syndrome? Pediatr Nephrol. 2007;22(9):1309–13.
5. Bonilla-Felix M, Parra C, Dajani T, Ferris M, Swinford RD, Portman RJ, et al. Changing patterns in the histopathology of idiopathic nephrotic syndrome in children. Kidney Int. 1999;55(5):1885–90.
6. Braden GL, Mulhern JG, O'Shea MH, Nash SV, Ucci AA Jr, Germain MJ. Changing incidence of glomerular diseases in adults. Am J Kidney Dis. 2000;35(5):878–83.
7. Haas M, Spargo BH, Coventry S. Increasing incidence of focal-segmental glomerulosclerosis among adult nephropathies: a 20-year renal biopsy study. Am J Kidney Dis. 1995;26(5):740–50.
8. Kitiyakara C, Eggers P, Kopp JB. Twenty-one-year trend in ESRD due to focal segmental glomerulosclerosis in the United States. Am J Kidney Dis. 2004;44(5):815–25.
9. Kim JS, Bellew CA, Silverstein DM, Aviles DH, Boineau FG, Vehaskari VM. High incidence of initial and late steroid resistance in childhood nephrotic syndrome. Kidney Int. 2005;68(3):1275–81.
10. Baqi N, Singh A, Balachandra S, Ahmad H, Nicastri A, Kytinski S, et al. The paucity of minimal change disease in adolescents with primary nephrotic syndrome. Pediatr Nephrol. 1998;12(2):105–7.
11. Bose B, Cattran D, Toronto Glomerulonephritis R. Glomerular diseases: FSGS. Clin J Am Soc Nephrol. 2014;9(3):626–32.
12. Chapter 3: steroid-sensitive nephrotic syndrome in children. Kidney Int Suppl. 2(2):163–71.
13. Querfeld U. Should hyperlipidemia in children with the nephrotic syndrome be treated? Pediatr Nephrol. 1999;13(1):77–84.
14. Trautmann A, Bodria M, Ozaltin F, Gheisari A, Melk A, Azocar M, et al. Spectrum of steroid-resistant and congenital nephrotic syndrome in children: the PodoNet registry cohort. Clin J Am Soc Nephrol. 2015;10(4):592–600.
15. Alshami A, Roshan A, Catapang M, Jöbsis JJ, Kwok T, Polderman N, et al. Indications for kidney biopsy in idiopathic childhood nephrotic syndrome. Pediatr Nephrol. 2017;32:1–9.
16. Fogo AB. Causes and pathogenesis of focal segmental glomerulosclerosis. Nat Rev Nephrol. 2015;11(2):76–87.

17. Lovric S, Ashraf S, Tan W, Hildebrandt F. Genetic testing in steroid-resistant nephrotic syndrome: when and how? Nephrol Dial Transplant. 2016;31(11):1802–13.
18. Hinkes BG, Mucha B, Vlangos CN, Gbadegesin R, Liu J, Hasselbacher K, et al. Nephrotic syndrome in the first year of life: two thirds of cases are caused by mutations in 4 genes (NPHS1, NPHS2, WT1, and LAMB2). Pediatrics. 2007;119(4):e907–19.
19. Santín S, Bullich G, Tazón-Vega B, García-Maset R, Giménez I, Silva I, et al. Clinical utility of genetic testing in children and adults with steroid-resistant nephrotic syndrome. Clin J Am Soc Nephrol. 2011;6(5):1139–48.
20. Sadowski CE, Lovric S, Ashraf S, Pabst WL, Gee HY, Kohl S, et al. A single-gene cause in 29.5% of cases of steroid-resistant nephrotic syndrome. J Am Soc Nephrol. 2015;26(6):1279–89.
21. Stefanidis CJ, Querfeld U. The podocyte as a target: cyclosporin A in the management of the nephrotic syndrome caused by WT1 mutations. Eur J Pediatr. 2011;170(11):1377–83.
22. Lipska BS, Iatropoulos P, Maranta R, Caridi G, Ozaltin F, Anarat A, et al. Genetic screening in adolescents with steroid-resistant nephrotic syndrome. Kidney Int. 2013;84(1):206–13.
23. Büscher AK, Beck BB, Melk A, Hoefele J, Kranz B, Bamborschke D, et al. Rapid response to cyclosporin a and favorable renal outcome in nongenetic versus genetic steroid–resistant nephrotic syndrome. Clin J Am Soc Nephrol. 2016;11(2):245–53.
24. Ruf RG, Lichtenberger A, Karle SM, Haas JP, Anacleto FE, Schultheiss M, et al. Patients with mutations in NPHS2 (podocin) do not respond to standard steroid treatment of nephrotic syndrome. J Am Soc Nephrol. 2004;15(3):722–32.
25. Klaassen I, Ozgoren B, Sadowski CE, Moller K, van Husen M, Lehnhardt A, et al. Response to cyclosporine in steroid-resistant nephrotic syndrome: discontinuation is possible. Pediatr Nephrol. 2015;30(9):1477–83.
26. Hinkes B, Wiggins RC, Gbadegesin R, Vlangos CN, Seelow D, Nurnberg G, et al. Positional cloning uncovers mutations in PLCE1 responsible for a nephrotic syndrome variant that may be reversible. Nat Genet. 2006;38(12):1397–405.
27. Jennette JC, Olson JL, Silva FG, D'Agati VD. Heptinstall's pathology of the kidney. 7th ed. Philadelphia: Wolters Kluwer Health/Lippincott Williams & Wilkins; 2015. 2 volumes p
28. D'Agati VD, Fogo AB, Bruijn JA, Jennette JC. Pathologic classification of focal segmental glomerulosclerosis: a working proposal. Am J Kidney Dis. 2004;43(2):368–82.
29. D'Agati VD, Jennette JC, Silva FG, American Registry of Pathology., Armed Forces Institute of Pathology (U.S.). Non-neoplastic kidney diseases. Washington, DC: American Registry of Pathology in collaboration with the Armed Forces Institute of Pathology; 2005. p. xvii. 721 p. p
30. D'Agati VD, Alster JM, Jennette JC, Thomas DB, Pullman J, Savino DA, et al. Association of histologic variants in FSGS clinical trial with presenting features and outcomes. Clin J Am Soc Nephrol. 2013;8(3):399–406.
31. Stokes MB, Markowitz GS, Lin J, Valeri AM, D'Agati VD. Glomerular tip lesion: a distinct entity within the minimal change disease/focal segmental glomerulosclerosis spectrum. Kidney Int. 2004;65(5):1690–702.
32. Howie AJ. Changes at the glomerular tip: a feature of membranous nephropathy and other disorders associated with proteinuria. J Pathol. 1986;150(1):13–20.
33. Gipson DS, Chin H, Presler TP, Jennette C, Ferris ME, Massengill S, et al. Differential risk of remission and ESRD in childhood FSGS. Pediatr Nephrol. 2006;21(3):344–9.
34. Bagga A, Mudigoudar BD, Hari P, Vasudev V. Enalapril dosage in steroid-resistant nephrotic syndrome. Pediatr Nephrol. 2004;19(1):45–50.
35. Yi Z, Li Z, Wu XC, He QN, Dang XQ, He XJ. Effect of fosinopril in children with steroid-resistant idiopathic nephrotic syndrome. Pediatr Nephrol. 2006;21(7):967–72.
36. Gipson DS, Massengill SF, Yao L, Nagaraj S, Smoyer WE, Mahan JD, et al. Management of childhood onset nephrotic syndrome. Pediatrics. 2009;124(2):747–57.
37. McKinney PA, Feltbower RG, Brocklebank JT, Fitzpatrick MM. Time trends and ethnic patterns of childhood nephrotic syndrome in Yorkshire, UK. Pediatr Nephrol. 2001;16(12):1040–4.
38. Lombel RM, Gipson DS, Hodson EM. Treatment of steroid-sensitive nephrotic syndrome: new guidelines from KDIGO. Pediatr Nephrol. 2013;28(3):415–26.

39. Lombel RM, Hodson EM, Gipson DS. Treatment of steroid-resistant nephrotic syndrome in children: new guidelines from KDIGO. Pediatr Nephrol. 2013;28(3):409–14.
40. Pravitsitthikul N, Willis N, Hodson EM, Craig JC. Non-corticosteroid immunosuppressive medications for steroidsensitive nephrotic syndrome in children. Cochrane Database Syst Rev. 2013;(10):CD002290. https://doi.org/10.1002/14651858.CD002290.pub4. Pages 1–121.
41. Chiu Mok C, Sing Lau C, Woon Sing Wong R. Risk factors for ovarian failure in patients with systemic lupus erythematosus receiving cyclophosphamide therapy. Arthritis Rheumatism. 1998;41(5):831–7.
42. Ioannidis JPA, Katsifis GE, Tzioufas AG, Moutsopoulos HM. Predictors of sustained amenorrhea from pulsed intravenous cyclophosphamide in premenopausal women with systemic lupus erythematosus. J Rheumatol. 2002;29(10):2129–35.
43. Wetzels JFM. Cyclophosphamide-induced gonadal toxicity: a treatment dilemma in patients with lupus nephritis? Neth J Med. 2004;62(10):347–52.
44. Latta K, von Schnakenburg C, Ehrich JHH. A meta-analysis of cytotoxic treatment for frequently relapsing nephrotic syndrome in children. Pediatr Nephrol. 2001;16(3):271–82.
45. Ishikura K, Ikeda M, Hattori S, Yoshikawa N, Sasaki S, Iijima K, et al. Effective and safe treatment with cyclosporine in nephrotic children: a prospective, randomized multicenter trial. Kidney Int. 2008;73(10):1167–73.
46. Niaudet P. Comparison of cyclosporin and chlorambucil in the treatment of steroid-dependent idiopathic nephrotic syndrome: a multicentre randomized controlled trial. The French Society of Paediatric Nephrology. Pediatr Nephrol. 1992;6(1):1–3.
47. Ponticelli C, Edefonti A, Ghio L, Rizzoni G, Rinaldi S, Gusmano R, et al. Cyclosporin versus cyclophosphamide for patients with steroid-dependent and frequently relapsing idiopathic nephrotic syndrome: a multicentre randomized controlled trial. Nephrol Dial Transplant. 1993;8(12):1326–32.
48. Iijima K, Hamahira K, Tanaka R, Kobayashi A, Nozu K, Nakamura H, et al. Risk factors for cyclosporine-induced tubulointerstitial lesions in children with minimal change nephrotic syndrome. Kidney Int. 2002;61(5):1801–5.
49. Myers BD, Sibley R, Newton L, Tomlanovich SJ, Boshkos C, Stinson E, et al. The long-term course of cyclosporine-associated chronic nephropathy. Kidney Int. 1988;33(2):590–600.
50. Ravani P, Rossi R, Bonanni A, Quinn RR, Sica F, Bodria M, et al. Rituximab in children with steroid-dependent nephrotic syndrome: a multicenter, open-label, noninferiority, randomized controlled trial. J Am Soc Nephrol. 2015;26(9):2259–66.
51. Ravani P, Magnasco A, Edefonti A, Murer L, Rossi R, Ghio L, et al. Short-term effects of rituximab in children with steroid- and calcineurin-dependent nephrotic syndrome: a randomized controlled trial. Clin J Am Soc Nephrol. 2011;6(6):1308–15.
52. Iijima K, Sako M, Nozu K, Mori R, Tuchida N, Kamei K, et al. Rituximab for childhood-onset, complicated, frequently relapsing nephrotic syndrome or steroid-dependent nephrotic syndrome: a multicentre, double-blind, randomised, placebo-controlled trial. Lancet. 2014;384(9950):1273–81.
53. Guigonis V, Dallocchio A, Baudouin V, Dehennault M, Hachon-Le Camus C, Afanetti M, et al. Rituximab treatment for severe steroid- or cyclosporine-dependent nephrotic syndrome: a multicentric series of 22 cases. Pediatr Nephrol. 2008;23(8):1269.
54. Ravani P, Bonanni A, Rossi R, Caridi G, Ghiggeri GM. Anti-CD20 antibodies for idiopathic nephrotic syndrome in children. Clin J Am Soc Nephrol. 2016;11(4):710–20.
55. Chaumais M-C, Garnier A, Chalard F, Peuchmaur M, Dauger S, Jacqz-Agrain E, et al. Fatal pulmonary fibrosis after rituximab administration. Pediatr Nephrol. 2009;24(9):1753–5.
56. Grenda R, Jarmużek W, Rubik J, Migdał M, Pronicki M. Fatal rituximab-associated lung injury syndrome in a patient treated with rituximab for recurrence of post-transplant nephrotic syndrome. Pediatr Transplant. 2015;19(5):E115–E20.
57. Bitzan M, Anselmo M, Carpineta L. Rituximab (B-cell depleting antibody) associated lung injury (RALI): a pediatric case and systematic review of the literature. Pediatr Pulmonol. 2009;44(9):922–34.

58. Niaudet P. Treatment of childhood steroid-resistant idiopathic nephrosis with a combination of cyclosporine and prednisone. French Society of Pediatric Nephrology. J Pediatr. 1994;125(6 Pt 1):981–6.
59. Hahn D, Hodson EM, Willis NS, Craig JC. Interventions for preventing and treating kidney disease in Henoch-Schönlein Purpura (HSP). Cochrane Database Syst Rev. 2015;(8):CD005128. https://doi.org/10.1002/14651858.CD005128.pub3. Pages 1–78.
60. Gipson DS, Trachtman H, Kaskel FJ, Greene TH, Radeva MK, Gassman JJ, et al. Clinical trial of focal segmental glomerulosclerosis in children and young adults. Kidney Int. 2011;80(8):868–78.
61. Garin EH, Orak JK, Hiott KL, Sutherland SE. Cyclosporine therapy for steroid-resistant nephrotic syndrome. A controlled study. Am J Dis Child. 1988;142(9):985–8.
62. Ponticelli C, Rizzoni G, Edefonti A, Altieri P, Rivolta E, Rinaldi S, et al. A randomized trial of cyclosporine in steroid-resistant idiopathic nephrotic syndrome. Kidney Int. 1993;43(6):1377–84.
63. Lieberman KV, Tejani A. A randomized double-blind placebo-controlled trial of cyclosporine in steroid-resistant idiopathic focal segmental glomerulosclerosis in children. J Am Soc Nephrol. 1996;7(1):56–63.
64. Choudhry S, Bagga A, Hari P, Sharma S, Kalaivani M, Dinda A. Efficacy and safety of tacrolimus versus cyclosporine in children with steroid-resistant nephrotic syndrome: a randomized controlled trial. Am J Kidney Dis. 2009;53(5):760–9.
65. Gulati A, Sinha A, Gupta A, Kanitkar M, Sreenivas V, Sharma J, et al. Treatment with tacrolimus and prednisolone is preferable to intravenous cyclophosphamide as the initial therapy for children with steroid-resistant nephrotic syndrome. Kidney Int. 2012;82(10):1130–5.
66. Magnasco A, Ravani P, Edefonti A, Murer L, Ghio L, Belingheri M, et al. Rituximab in children with resistant idiopathic nephrotic syndrome. J Am Soc Nephrol. 2012;23(6):1117–24.
67. Basu B. Ofatumumab for rituximab-resistant nephrotic syndrome. N Engl J Med. 2014;370(13):1268–70.
68. Bonanni A, Rossi R, Murtas C, Ghiggeri GM. Low-dose of atumumab for rituximab-resistant nephrotic syndrome. BMJ Case Rep. 2015:Published online 16 Sep 2015, https://doi.org/10.1136/bcr-2015-210208.
69. Wang CS, Liverman RS, Garro R, George RP, Glumova A, Karp A, et al. Ofatumumab for the treatment of childhood nephrotic syndrome. Pediatr Nephrol. 2017;32(5):835–41.
70. Yu CC, Fornoni A, Weins A, Hakroush S, Maiguel D, Sageshima J, et al. Abatacept in B7-1-positive proteinuric kidney disease. N Engl J Med. 2013;369(25):2416–23.
71. Hattori M, Chikamoto H, Akioka Y, Nakakura H, Ogino D, Matsunaga A, et al. A combined low-density lipoprotein apheresis and prednisone therapy for steroid-resistant primary focal segmental glomerulosclerosis in children. Am J Kidney Dis. 2003;42(6):1121–30.
72. Moriarty PM. Lipoprotein apheresis: present and future uses. Curr Opin Lipidol. 2015;26(6):544–52.
73. Abrantes MM, Cardoso LS, Lima EM, Penido Silva JM, Diniz JS, Bambirra EA, et al. Predictive factors of chronic kidney disease in primary focal segmental glomerulosclerosis. Pediatr Nephrol. 2006;21(7):1003–12.
74. Silverstein DM, Craver R. Presenting features and short-term outcome according to pathologic variant in childhood primary focal segmental glomerulosclerosis. Clin J Am Soc Nephrol. 2007;2(4):700–7.
75. Schwartz MM, Evans J, Bain R, Korbet SM. Focal segmental glomerulosclerosis: prognostic implications of the cellular lesion. J Am Soc Nephrol. 1999;10(9):1900–7.
76. Singh HK, Baldree LA, McKenney DW, Hogan SL, Jennette JC. Idiopathic collapsing glomerulopathy in children. Pediatr Nephrol. 2000;14(2):132–7.
77. Huang K, Ferris ME, Andreoni KA, Gipson DS. The differential effect of race among pediatric kidney transplant recipients with focal segmental glomerulosclerosis. Am J Kidney Dis. 2004;43(6):1082–90.

78. Tejani A, Stablein DH. Recurrence of focal segmental glomerulosclerosis posttransplantation: a special report of the North American Pediatric Renal Transplant Cooperative Study. J Am Soc Nephrol. 1992;2(12 Suppl):S258–63.
79. Nehus EJ, Goebel JW, Succop PS, Abraham EC. Focal segmental glomerulosclerosis in children: multivariate analysis indicates that donor type does not alter recurrence risk. Transplantation. 2013;96(6):550–4.
80. Trautmann A, Bodria M, Ozaltin F, Gheisari A, Melk A, Azocar M, et al. Spectrum of steroid-resistant and congenital nephrotic syndrome in children: the PodoNet Registry Cohort. Clin J Am Soc Nephrol. 2015;10(4):592–600.
81. Baum MA, Ho M, Stablein D, Alexander SR, North American Pediatric Renal Transplant Cooperative S. Outcome of renal transplantation in adolescents with focal segmental glomerulosclerosis. Pediatr Transplant. 2002;6(6):488–92.
82. Guan I, Singer P, Frank R, Chorny N, Infante L, Sethna CB. Role of race in kidney transplant outcomes in children with focal segmental glomerulosclerosis. Pediatr Transplant. 2016;20(6):790–7.

Chapter 9
Lupus Nephritis

Kartik Pillutla and Kuang-Yu Jen

Introduction

Systemic lupus erythematosus (SLE) is an autoimmune disease with a relapsing and remitting course that affects multiple systems in the body. Young females of child-bearing age, including adolescents, are the most commonly affected. Lupus nephritis, an immune complex-mediated glomerulonephritis, is a common manifestation in juvenile-onset SLE. Adolescent patients are confronted with a disease that carries a significant risk of complications such as infertility, end-stage renal disease (ESRD), and cardiovascular mortality. Cosmetic side effects from medications such as Cushingoid facies, weight gain, and stretch marks pose significant challenges for adolescents and their peer relationships [1].

Pathogenesis

Though the pathogenesis of lupus and lupus nephritis has not been fully elucidated, SLE is characterized by the loss of immune tolerance to nuclear autoantigens [2]. This results in autovaccination, the formation of antinuclear antibodies, and activation of autoreactive lymphocytes [2]. Upon stimulation from an infective, environmental, or hormonal trigger, there is expansion of autoreactive immune cells which

K. Pillutla (✉)
Department of Pediatrics, Dell Medical School, University of Texas at Austin,
Dell Children's Medical Center of Central Texas, Pediatric Nephrology, Austin, TX, USA
e-mail: kpillutla@seton.org

K.-Y. Jen
Department of Pathology and Laboratory Medicine, UC Davis School of Medicine,
Sacramento, CA, USA

M. N. Haddad et al. (eds.), *Adolescents with Chronic Kidney Disease*,
https://doi.org/10.1007/978-3-319-97220-6_9

results in organ injury. Lupus nephritis is characterized by the formation of immune complexes that can deposit in the mesangial, subendothelial, and/or subepithelial areas of the glomerulus. Immune complex deposition activates complement, Toll-like receptors, and other inflammatory mediators that lead to renal injury [3]. Individuals may possess genetic variants that predispose them to renal injury from lupus nephritis such as the APOL1 nephropathy risk allele in African-Americans [2].

Epidemiology

Though SLE is a disease that predominantly affects women of reproductive age, 10–20% cases of SLE are diagnosed in children [4]. Similar to adults, the disease is found more commonly among females, though juvenile-onset SLE has a higher proportion of affected males versus adult-onset SLE. Non-White populations including Black, Hispanic, and Asian are disproportionally affected [5]. Juveniles are generally diagnosed during adolescence [4]. The disease course of juvenile-onset SLE is often more severe compared to adult-onset lupus [1, 4, 6]. Hematologic and neurologic manifestations are more common among patients diagnosed with juvenile-onset SLE [4].

Renal involvement and damage is more common among patients with juvenile-onset SLE with up to 80% affected [6–8]. Manifestations can range from mild hematuria and proteinuria to nephrotic syndrome and significant acute and chronic renal injury. The presence of renal disease in SLE has been demonstrated to be a significant predictor of morbidity and outcome including a 10–20% risk of ESRD 10 years after the initial diagnosis [1, 6]. Black and Hispanic adolescents have an increased risk of developing severe renal disease [9, 10]. Although morbidity and mortality remain significant, the advent of immunosuppressive therapies has improved lupus nephritis survival over time. Prior to the introduction of corticosteroid therapy, 5-year patient survival was 17% for patients with lupus nephritis. With the introduction of cyclophosphamide-based regimens, 5-year patient survival improved to 80% [11]. The 5-year patient survival rate is currently 90–95% [12].

Presentation

In addition to the extrarenal manifestations commonly seen in SLE including fatigue, arthritis, serositis, and cerebritis, the presentation of lupus nephritis can vary from asymptomatic microscopic hematuria or proteinuria to rapidly progressive glomerulonephritis. Lupus nephritis is classified based on renal biopsy according to the International Society of Nephrology and Renal Pathology Society (ISN/RPS) 2003 guidelines as outlined in Table 9.1 [19]. Patients with milder forms of lupus nephritis (class I and class II) are often asymptomatic, with renal manifestations such as hematuria and proteinuria only detected on laboratory testing [13]. Patients with more severe forms of lupus nephritis (class III and class IV) may have

Table 9.1 The International Society of Nephrology/Renal Pathology Society (ISN/RPS) classification of lupus nephritis (2003) with associated clinical findings [19]

Lupus nephritis class	Pathological findings	Clinical findings
Class I: minimal mesangial lupus nephritis	LM: normal glomeruli IF/EM: mesangial immune deposits	Hematuria, mild proteinuria
Class II: mesangial proliferative lupus nephritis	LM: mesangial proliferation with mesangial matrix expansion IF/EM: mesangial immune deposits	Hematuria, mild proteinuria
Class III: focal lupus nephritis	LM: active or chronic segmental or global glomerulonephritis involving <50% of glomeruli IF/EM: predominately subendothelial and mesangial immune deposits	Hematuria, proteinuria, hypertension
Class IV: diffuse lupus nephritis	LM: active or chronic segmental or global glomerulonephritis involving ≥50% of glomeruli IF/EM: predominately subendothelial and mesangial immune deposits	Hematuria, severe proteinuria (often nephrotic range), hypertension, acute kidney injury
Class V: membranous lupus nephritis	LM: thickening of glomerular capillary walls often with "spikes" and "holes" on silver stain IF/EM: subepithelial and intramembranous immune deposits	Nephrotic syndrome
Class VI: Advanced sclerosis lupus nephritis	≥90% glomeruli sclerosed without residual activity	Advanced CKD/ESRD

LM light microscopy, *IF* immunofluorescence, *EM* electron microscopy

gross hematuria, nephrotic range proteinuria, edema, hypertension, or a rapidly progressive glomerulonephritis. Studies have demonstrated that class III and class IV are the most common forms of lupus nephritis in the pediatric population [1, 14, 15].

Class V membranous lupus nephritis is a relatively less common form of lupus nephritis among pediatric patients. Among pediatric patients with lupus nephritis, the prevalence of class V disease can range from 9% to 30% [16]. Nephrotic syndrome may be the patient's initial symptom with no extrarenal manifestations when the diagnosis is made [16].

Diagnosis

Clinical and Laboratory Findings

Patients are diagnosed with SLE based on the American College of Rheumatology criteria and revised by the Systemic Lupus International Collaborating Clinics (SLICC) in 2012 (Table 9.2). The diagnosis of lupus nephritis should be considered in the presence of proteinuria greater than 500 mg/day or spot protein/creatinine

Table 9.2 Diagnostic criteria for systemic lupus erythematosus. Diagnosis is made with four positive criteria including one clinical and one immunological criteria or renal biopsy positive for lupus nephritis with elevated ANA or anti-dsDNA [17]

Clinical criteria	Immunological criteria
Acute cutaneous lupus	Elevated ANA
Chronic cutaneous lupus	Elevated anti-dsDNA
Oral or nasal ulcers	Elevated anti-Sm
Non-scarring alopecia	Elevated antiphospholipid Ab
Synovitis	Low complement
Serositis	Positive direct coombs
Renal involvement	
Neurological involvement	
Hemolytic anemia	
Leukopenia	
Thrombocytopenia	

ratio greater than 0.5, active sediment including cellular casts, hematuria, or an abnormal creatinine that cannot be explained by other causes [17]. Patients are diagnosed with lupus nephritis if they have a renal biopsy consistent with lupus nephritis and a positive ANA or anti-dsDNA, or they fulfill four diagnostic criteria, including one immunological and one clinical criteria [18].

Renal Biopsy

A renal biopsy to diagnose and classify lupus nephritis is strongly recommended if there is a presence of proteinuria greater than 1 g in a 24 h urine collection or spot urine protein/creatinine ratio, proteinuria more than 500 mg/day with hematuria or cellular casts, or an abnormal creatinine [17]. The renal biopsy specimens are analyzed with light, immunofluorescence (IF), and electron microscopy (EM). Classification based on the ISN/RPS 2003 guidelines is determined by glomerular features only and mainly relies on light microscopic findings [19]. However, it should be noted that in a minority of lupus patients with renal disease, pathologic lesions may be confined to the tubulointerstitium and/or vessels, without glomerular involvement.

For accurate diagnosis and classification, it is recommended that the biopsy sample contains at least ten glomeruli for light microscopic examination as lupus nephritis often has focal involvement in the kidney [20]. Each glomerulus is evaluated for active and chronic lesions (Table 9.3). If such lesions are absent and the glomeruli demonstrate mesangial immune deposits by IF and EM, then the diagnosis of class I lupus nephritis is rendered if the light microscopy shows no glomerular abnormalities. However, if the glomeruli exhibit mesangial hypercellularity, then class II lupus nephritis is the appropriate diagnosis (Fig. 9.1a). A simple way to view these milder forms of lupus nephritis is that they express pathologic changes that are confined to the mesangium, without involvement of the peripheral glomerular capillary loops. In contrast, the more severe forms of lupus nephritis demonstrate

Table 9.3 Active and chronic glomerular lesions of the International Society of Nephrology/Renal Pathology Society (ISN/RPS) classification of lupus nephritis (2003)

Active lesions	Chronic lesions
Endocapillary hypercellularity with or without leukocyte infiltration and with substantial luminal reduction	Glomerulosclerosis, segmental or global
Karyorrhexis	Fibrous adhesions
Fibrinoid necrosis	Fibrous crescents
Rupture of glomerular basement membrane	
Crescents, cellular or fibrocellular	
Subendothelial deposits identifiable by light microscopy (wire loops)	
Intraluminal immune aggregates (hyaline thrombi)	

Adapted from Weening et al. [19]

evidence of renal injury that has spread beyond the mesangium to involve the glomerular capillary loops and Bowman space. When any active or chronic glomerular lesion is present, then the biopsy supports class III lupus nephritis if there is focal (<50%) glomerular involvement and class IV lupus nephritis if there is diffuse (≥50%) glomerular involvement (Fig. 9.1b–d).

On biopsy, class V membranous lupus nephritis is characterized by subepithelial (and often mesangial) immune deposits. The typical features seen on light microscopy described as "holes" and "spikes" on Jones methenamine silver stain for primary/idiopathic membranous nephropathy are often observed in membranous lupus nephritis as well (Fig. 9.1d). Importantly, if active or chronic glomerular lesions are superimposed on membranous lupus nephritis, then concurrent class III or class IV disease should be reported. However, class V lupus nephritis cannot occur simultaneously with class I or class II disease since the mesangial findings of class I and class II lupus nephritis are encompassed within the spectrum of what is seen in class V membranous lupus nephritis.

Patients with the advanced sclerosing lupus nephritis of class VI disease have no active glomerular disease but instead show widespread global glomerulosclerosis (≥90%) associated with previous class III, IV, or V disease [19]. This class essentially represents ESRD due to lupus nephritis.

In addition to the classification of lupus nephritis, the renal biopsy is also examined for degree of activity and chronicity, with the NIH activity and chronicity index being the most widely used [19]. The activity index represents the degree of inflammatory injury to the kidney, while the chronicity index represents the degree of irreversible damage that the kidney has sustained [21]. Typically, abundant immune deposits are present in lupus nephritis, which are easily detected on IF and EM. IgG staining is invariably positive and usually strongest in intensity (Fig. 9.2a). Frequently, IF reveals positive staining for all immunoglobulins and complement components that are routinely tested, including IgG, IgA, IgM, C3, and C1q. The term "full-house" positivity is applied to describe such IF findings and is highly characteristic of lupus nephritis.

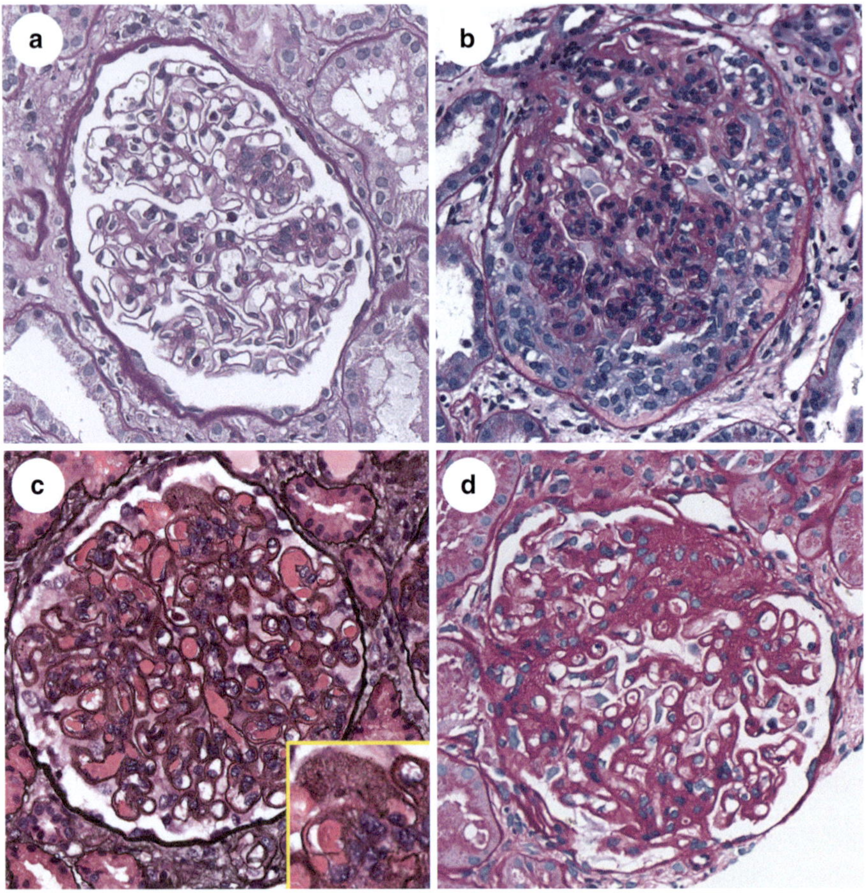

Fig. 9.1 Light microscopy findings of lupus nephritis. Common histologic findings in various classes of lupus nephritis are shown. (**a**) Glomerulus with segmental mesangial widening and mesangial hypercellularity in class II mesangial proliferative lupus nephritis (periodic acid-Schiff). Note the absence of active and chronic lesions. (**b**) Glomerulus showing global endocapillary proliferation and crescent formation from a case of class IV diffuse lupus nephritis (periodic acid-Schiff). (**c**) Glomerulus from a case with both class IV diffuse lupus nephritis and class V membranous lupus nephritis. Note the extensive wire loops (subendothelial deposits) and hyaline thrombi (intraluminal immune aggregates) of class IV disease. Tangential sections of the glomerular basement membrane appear mottled (best seen at 12 o'clock in inset), indicative of subepithelial deposits of class V disease (methenamine silver). (**d**) Glomerulus with chronic lesions represented by segmental scar and fibrous adhesions (periodic acid-Schiff)

On EM, the corresponding immune deposits may be mesangial, subendothelial, and/or subepithelial in location and typically correlates to the class of disease (Fig. 9.2b). For class I and class II lupus nephritis, the deposits are essentially confined to the mesangium, while class III and class IV disease will show subendothelial deposits. Widespread subepithelial deposits indicate a component of membranous lupus nephritis (class V). The immune deposits often show a variegated appear-

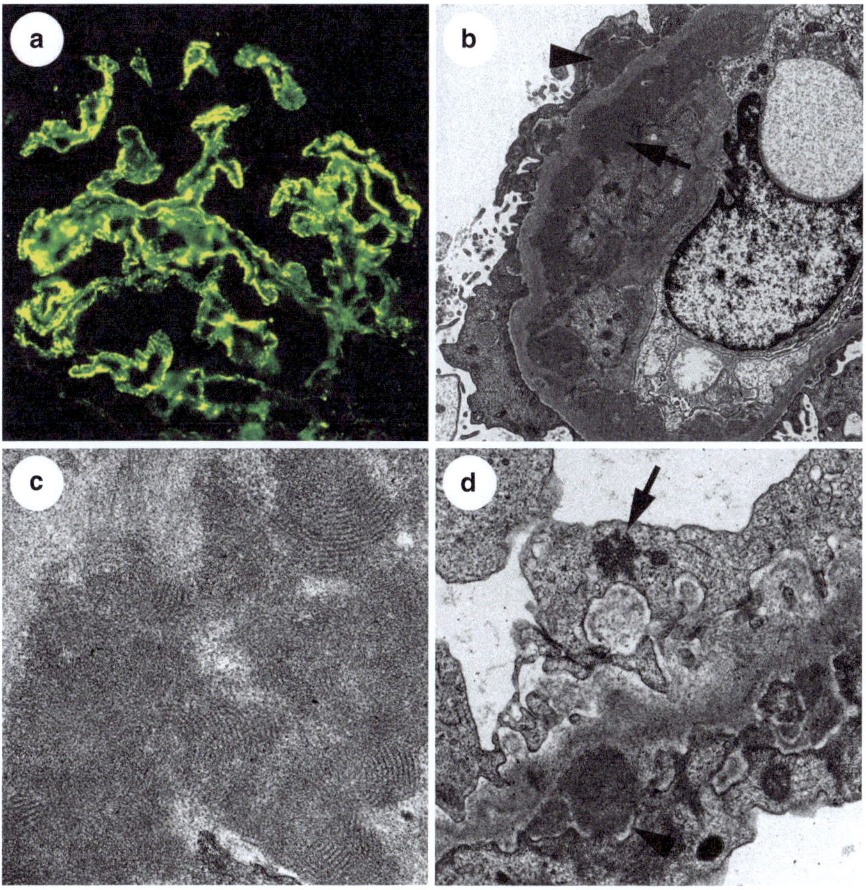

Fig. 9.2 Immunofluorescence and electron microscopy findings of lupus nephritis. (**a**) Strong positive immunofluorescent staining for IgG in a case of concurrent class IV diffuse lupus nephritis and class V membranous lupus nephritis. Note the fine granular pattern of subepithelial deposits as well as elongated curvilinear pattern of subendothelial deposits. (**b**) Electron microscopy demonstrating abundant subendothelial deposits (arrow) and limited subepithelial deposits (arrow head) in a patient with lupus nephritis. Extensive foot process effacement is present as well. (**c**) High-power electron micrograph of immune deposits with fingerprint-like pattern in lupus nephritis. (**d**) Electron micrograph of a tubuloreticular inclusion (arrow) within an endothelial cell of a patient with class V membranous lupus nephritis. Note the presence of subepithelial deposits (arrowhead)

ance, and in some cases fingerprint-like organized deposits may be present (Fig. 9.2c). Tubuloreticular inclusions are frequently detected within endothelial cells (Fig. 9.2d), a nonspecific finding that can be seen in patients with high interferon levels (irrespective of renal disease etiology). Variable foot process effacement can be present, and the degree usually correlates to the severity of the patient's proteinuria.

Biopsies with diffuse global disease and significant chronic injury are associated with adverse renal outcomes [22]. The biopsy result should be compared to the clinical and laboratory findings of the patient as variance may be present. For example, significant proteinuria in the presence of class I or II disease could indicate sampling error when the renal biopsy was performed. For patients with previously diagnosed lupus nephritis, a repeat renal biopsy should be considered if a patient develops new-onset proteinuria or kidney injury as this could indicate a change in the class of lupus nephritis, especially if the patient had a previous non-proliferative lesion [9, 21]. A repeat kidney biopsy may also detect chronic changes that may allow a reduction or cessation of immunosuppression [9].

The renal biopsy is not only essential in diagnosis of lupus nephritis but may help diagnose causes of renal injury aside from glomerulonephritis that significantly differ in treatment and prognosis [21]. SLE-associated tubulointerstitial nephritis has been rarely reported and appears to respond to corticosteroids alone, unlike lupus nephritis which requires heightened immunosuppression [23]. Lesions including thrombotic microangiopathy (TMA) can be detected in renal biopsies of patients with SLE. TMA in lupus nephritis is associated with antiphospholipid antibody syndrome, thrombotic thrombocytopenia purpura, hemolytic uremic syndrome, malignant hypertension, and calcineurin inhibitor therapy and is treated with plasma exchange [24, 25].

Treatment

General Principles

Management of SLE with renal involvement is based on the class of lupus nephritis. Therapy is generally aimed at treatment of extrarenal manifestations with appropriate immunosuppression if indicated. There is evidence that the antimalarial drug hydroxychloroquine may reduce the risk of lupus nephritis onset, relapse, and progression to chronic kidney disease [26, 27]. As a result, it is recommended as part of the treatment regimen for patients with lupus nephritis [26].

Hypertension and Proteinuria Control

Chronic kidney disease is a significant cardiovascular risk factor for patients with SLE [28, 29]. As a result, therapies are employed to maintain renal function in patients with lupus nephritis. Risk factors for chronic kidney disease include the presence of proteinuria and hypertension, and aggressive treatment of these risk factors is recommended [26, 28]. Angiotensin-converting enzyme inhibitors or angiotensin receptor blockers are favored due to their ability to lower both blood pressure and proteinuria. Renin-angiotensin aldosterone system (RAAS) blockade should be initiated as first-line treatment of hypertension [28]. In addition, RAAS blockade is recommended for proteinuria greater than 500 mg in 24 h [28].

Treatment of Class I and Class II Lupus Nephritis

Patients with class I and class II lupus nephritis are expected to maintain renal function with a favorable renal prognosis. Significant proteinuria should be treated with corticosteroids and calcineurin inhibitors [26, 30].

Treatment of Class III and Class IV Lupus Nephritis

Adolescents with nephrotic range proteinuria, class IV lupus nephritis, hypertension, and abnormal creatinine are at significant risk for progression to advanced chronic kidney disease [15, 31]. There is a favorable long-term renal prognosis for individuals that achieve remission with 5- and 10-year renal survival of 95% [32]. Complete remission is achieved when the estimated glomerular filtration rate is above 90 ml/min/1.73 m^2 without proteinuria or active urinary sediment. Rates of complete remission vary from 10% to 86% [33]. A partial remission is achieved when there is a 25% improvement in the estimated GFR, 50% reduction in proteinuria or urinary protein-to-creatinine ratio of 0.2–2 mg/mg, and a resolution of active urinary sediment [26]. A significant reduction in proteinuria has been demonstrated to be associated with increased long-term renal survival in patients with lupus nephritis [32, 33].

Treatment is divided into an induction and maintenance phase. Induction therapy generally lasts up to 6 months and is comprised of corticosteroids and cyclophosphamide (CYC) or mycophenolate mofetil (MMF) to decrease inflammation in the kidney and achieve remission. Maintenance therapy is comprised of a relatively reduced corticosteroid dosing and mycophenolate mofetil or azathioprine to maintain remission and minimize medication side effects. The duration of maintenance immunosuppression required remains unclear, but prolonged therapy is recommended for patients with significant risk of developing chronic kidney disease [34]. Immunosuppression therapies in juvenile-onset SLE are currently used off-label, and dosing is based on studies in patients with adult-onset lupus nephritis or other disease processes [8].

Corticosteroids are used for induction immunosuppression either as oral prednisone, as an intravenous administration of methylprednisolone 30 mg/kg (maximum dose 1000 mg) in severe cases, or a combination of intravenous and oral therapy [8, 26]. The dose should be slowly tapered during the induction phase and continued during maintenance. Corticosteroids alone are generally ineffective as sole treatment for proliferative lupus nephritis and should be used in combination with other immunosuppressive agents [26]. Combination therapy also allows the reduction of the corticosteroid dose which is of significant importance given the risk of steroid-related adverse effects including osteoporosis (see Sect. 7.3), weight gain, hirsutism, acne, striae, Cushingoid status, glucose intolerance, and growth retardation.

Intravenous CYC in combination with corticosteroids for induction therapy has been demonstrated to reduce the risk of ESRD in patients with lupus nephritis compared to steroids alone [35]. CYC is administered at 500–1000 mg/m^2/dose for six monthly doses (with dosage adjustment for renal insufficiency and leukopenia) [35]. CYC has significant adverse effects including the risk of gonadal failure, malignancy, infection, and hemorrhagic cystitis. Alternative dosing regimens which shorten the duration of cyclophosphamide exposure have been developed and studied in adult populations, such as the Euro-Lupus trial in which cyclophosphamide is administered at 500 mg biweekly for 6 weeks [35]. Adjuvant therapies such as 2-mercaptoethane sulfonate (MESNA) for hemorrhagic cystitis prevention, *Pneumocystis jirovecii* prophylaxis, and agents for ovarian protection (see Sect. 7.4) should be considered [8].

Mycophenolate mofetil has increasingly gained favor for use in both induction and maintenance phase of immunosuppression in proliferative lupus nephritis. MMF has been demonstrated to be similarly efficacious in induction treatment of proliferative lupus nephritis compared to cyclophosphamide in both adults and adolescents [35, 36]. It has been associated with increased renal and overall survival in children with lupus nephritis [15]. Black and Hispanic SLE patients have a better response to MMF than CYC induction [15, 35]. The *Aspreva Lupus Management Study (ALMS)* trial demonstrated a 53.9% versus 40% and 60.9% versus 38.8% treatment response rate for MMF versus intravenous CYC as induction therapy in Black and Hispanic patients, respectively [37]. MMF has been demonstrated to be superior to azathioprine in reducing the risk of relapse and maintaining renal function in individuals who had responded to induction therapy [34, 38]. While it does not carry the risk of gonadal toxicity, MMF has significant teratogenic effects (see Sect. 7.4). Gastrointestinal side effects, leukopenia, and an increased risk for infections are among the additional adverse effects seen with MMF therapy.

Given the variable rates of remission, additional therapies have been identified such as rituximab, a chimeric anti-CD20 monoclonal antibody. Though large-scale trials have not indicated a statistically significant clinical benefit with the addition of rituximab to conventional therapy, it is used by some clinicians to treat refractory cases of lupus nephritis [35, 39]. Calcineurin inhibitors have been used for refractory cases of lupus nephritis, but further investigation is required [26, 35, 40].

Treatment of Class V Lupus Nephritis

Patients with class V lupus nephritis may present with pure class V disease, consisting of the characteristic podocyte foot process effacement and subepithelial immune deposits on renal biopsy or mixed with class III or IV proliferative disease [41].

While the risk for progression to ESRD is only approximately 10% after 10 years, patients with pure class V disease are at risk for significant complications including thromboembolism due to hypoalbuminemia, particularly less than a serum level of 2.8 g/dL [41]. Patients with mixed disease have a significant risk for morbidity and mortality with a 49% overall survival rate and 20% renal survival at 10 years, with worsened survival among Blacks [41].

Recommended therapy consists of medical management of nephrotic syndrome. This includes diuretics, fluid, and sodium restriction [41]. Similar to other forms of nephrotic syndrome, hyperlipidemia control is recommended [41]. Renin-angiotensin-aldosterone (RAAS) blockade is recommended for hypertension and proteinuria control [41]. Rates of thromboembolism in patients with class V nephritis can range from 3% to 23%, and this risk is higher in patients with hypoalbuminemia and antiphospholipid antibody syndrome (APS) [41]. Thromboembolism prophylaxis is described further in this chapter.

Evidence regarding immunosuppressive treatments options is limited in both the adult and pediatric population. Clinicians should be aware that there may be a significant delay, up to 3–5 years, between treatment and remission of proteinuria due to residual structural defects in the glomerular basement membrane [41]. Patients with class V disease treated with a combination of corticosteroids and nonsteroidal immunosuppression had a positive response rate of 81% versus 60% with steroid monotherapy [42]. Steroids and cyclosporine (CsA) or intravenous CYC were demonstrated to have improved remission rates versus steroid therapy alone in class V disease [41]. Response rates between CYC, MMF, and azathioprine (AZA) appear to be similar, making the choice of optimal immunosuppressive therapy challenging [41]. Szeto and colleagues demonstrated a faster reduction of proteinuria and reduced 1-year relapse rate in patients with pure class V disease treated with tacrolimus induction versus historical controls [43]. However, current pediatric practice patterns tend to favor MMF for nonsteroidal immunosuppression in class V disease [44]. Current pediatric guidelines recommend the use of MMF with low-dose steroid for both induction and maintenance therapy of pure class V lupus nephritis [45].

Patients with concomitant class III and class IV proliferative lesions should be treated with combination immunosuppression given the risk of progression to chronic and end-stage renal disease [26, 46]. The combination of MMF and tacrolimus has been demonstrated to have a higher complete remission rate of 60% versus 15% with CYC therapy in adult patients with mixed disease [47].

Complications

Nephrotoxic Risk Factors

Clinicians should be aware of the nephrotoxic risk of commonly used medications in the treatment of SLE. This includes disease-modifying antirheumatic drugs (DMARDs) such as calcineurin inhibitors and nonsteroidal anti-inflammatory drugs

(NSAIDs) [29]. Switching to alternative medications with less nephrotoxic risk should be considered in patients with lupus nephritis that have advanced renal disease [29].

Cardiovascular Disease

Cardiovascular disease including accelerated atherosclerosis, myocardial infarction, and cerebrovascular disease are recognized as leading causes of premature death in patients with SLE [48]. Coronary artery disease can be seen at a young age and is thought to be related to atherosclerosis, arteritis, thromboembolism, spasm, or decreased perfusion [49]. Fatal myocardial infarction (MI) has been observed to be threefold higher in patients with SLE, with the risk of MI between 9 and 50 times that of the general population [49]. Coexisting chronic kidney disease is a risk factor for accelerated atherosclerotic disease. The presence of an abnormal creatinine or proteinuria further aggravates this risk [49]. Other risk factors include the presence of cytokines and other pro-inflammatory mediators [49]. Dyslipidemias are also frequently found in patients with lupus nephritis, and as a result patients should have screening and treatment of hyperlipidemia [28, 48]. Dietary and lifestyle modification such as reduction in dietary sodium, cessation of smoking, and avoidance of metabolic risk factors such as obesity and diabetes mellitus are recommended [28]. As patients with SLE are at higher risk for thromboembolic complications, they should be screened for antiphospholipid antibodies [50]. Prophylaxis with aspirin for patients with positive lupus anticoagulant or anticardiolipin antibodies is recommended [50]. Current guidelines recommend the use of warfarin in patients with idiopathic membranous nephropathy with a serum albumin level less than 2.5 g/dL [51]. As a result, thromboembolism prophylaxis should be considered in patients with significant hypoalbuminemia [41].

Bone Health

Children with SLE are at risk for decreased bone mass and osteoporosis. It is thought to be largely associated with chronic glucocorticoid use [52]. Bone mineral density can be assessed through bone densitometry or DEXA testing. It is recommended that patients with SLE on chronic glucocorticoids be supplemented if they have low levels of Vitamin D [53].

Pregnancy and Fertility

Infertility and adverse pregnancy outcomes are common concerns for patients with SLE. This includes adolescents who are making the transition from childhood to adulthood. The pregnancy rate decreases after the diagnosis of SLE [54]. There are both disease- and medication-related causes of infertility including primary ovarian failure, amenorrhea, and endometriosis. Chronic kidney disease itself can cause infertility due to hypothalamic-pituitary dysfunction. Patients with antiphospholipid antibody syndrome are at risk for spontaneous abortions, stillbirths, and premature births.

Cyclophosphamide is recognized for its gonadal toxicity [54, 55]. It can cause premature ovarian failure with depletion of oocytes. For males, CYC can affect both sperm quantity and quality. CYC gonadal toxicity is related to the cumulative dose of medication and age at administration. Patients are less likely to develop infertility if they receive CYC at a younger age, receive a lower total dose, and have regular menstrual cycles prior to or during treatment. It is recommended that patients receive counseling regarding the risk of infertility prior to commencement of CYC therapy. Strategies to prevent premature ovarian failure include prescribing the lowest effective dose of CYC with the shortest duration of therapy [54]. Leuprolide, a gonadotrophin-receptor hormone agonist, has been shown to reduce the risk of premature ovarian failure when administered before each dose of CYC [54].

Patients with lupus nephritis should be counseled regarding the risk of teratogenicity with their medication therapy, including MMF and ACE inhibitors. MMF therapy has been observed to be associated with an increased incidence of miscarriages and birth defects [56]. It is recommended that adolescent females receive counseling regarding pregnancy prevention including birth control prior to initiation of MMF. Should they conceive, MMF should be discontinued in favor of an alternative therapy such as azathioprine. In addition, ACE inhibitors should be discontinued if the patient becomes pregnant due to the risk of significant birth defects.

Psychological and Behavioral Issues

Young adults with SLE often report negative impacts of the disease on employment and personal relationships [57]. As a result, patients may have difficulty in school performance and maintaining peer and family relationships [1, 57]. Adolescents with SLE rate their quality of life as poor in domains including physical health, worry, self-esteem, and school performance [57]. Nonadherence to medications and recommended treatment plans can be seen early and throughout the course of disease. A comprehensive multidisciplinary care team including rheumatology, nephrology, adolescent medicine, psychiatry, and social work may help the adolescent patient address their medical and psychosocial needs [1]. Interventions aimed at improving the patient's knowledge of their disease, self-confidence and ability to manage their disease may be beneficial [57]. Similar to other chronic illnesses, effective transition of care to adult providers is important in ensuring patients enjoy continued health and well-being.

References

1. Levy DM, Kamphuis S. Systemic lupus erythematosus in children and adolescents. Pediatr Clin N Am. 2012;59(2):345–64.
2. Anders HJ, Rovin B. A pathophysiology-based approach to the diagnosis and treatment of lupus nephritis. Kidney Int. 2016;90(3):493–501.
3. Nowling TK, Gilkeson GS. Mechanisms of tissue injury in lupus nephritis. Arthritis Res Ther. 2011;13(6):250.
4. Tarr T, Derfalvi B, Gyori N, Szanto A, Siminszky Z, Malik A, et al. Similarities and differences between pediatric and adult patients with systemic lupus erythematosus. Lupus. 2015;24(8):796–803.
5. Hiraki LT, Feldman CH, Liu J, Alarcon GS, Fischer MA, Winkelmayer WC, et al. Prevalence, incidence, and demographics of systemic lupus erythematosus and lupus nephritis from 2000 to 2004 among children in the US Medicaid beneficiary population. Arthritis Rheum. 2012;64(8):2669–76.
6. Livingston B, Bonner A, Pope J. Differences in clinical manifestations between childhood-onset lupus and adult-onset lupus: a meta-analysis. Lupus. 2011;20(13):1345–55.
7. Tucker LB, Uribe AG, Fernandez M, Vila LM, McGwin G, Apte M, et al. Adolescent onset of lupus results in more aggressive disease and worse outcomes: results of a nested matched case-control study within LUMINA, a multiethnic US cohort (LUMINA LVII). Lupus. 2008;17(4):314–22.
8. Mina R, von Scheven E, Ardoin SP, Eberhard BA, Punaro M, Ilowite N, et al. Consensus treatment plans for induction therapy of newly diagnosed proliferative lupus nephritis in juvenile systemic lupus erythematosus. Arthritis Care Res (Hoboken). 2012;64(3):375–83.
9. Almaani S, Meara A, Rovin BH. Update on lupus nephritis. Clin J Am Soc Nephrol. 2016.
10. Bastian HM, Roseman JM, McGwin G Jr, Alarcon GS, Friedman AW, Fessler BJ, et al. Systemic lupus erythematosus in three ethnic groups. XII. Risk factors for lupus nephritis after diagnosis. Lupus. 2002;11(3):152–60.
11. Parikh SV, Rovin BH. Current and emerging therapies for lupus nephritis. J Am Soc Nephrol. 2016;27(10):2929–39.
12. Vachvanichsanong P, McNeil E. Pediatric lupus nephritis: more options, more chances? Lupus. 2013;22(6):545–53.
13. Balow JE. Clinical presentation and monitoring of lupus nephritis. Lupus. 2005;14(1):25–30.
14. Hiraki LT, Benseler SM, Tyrrell PN, Hebert D, Harvey E, Silverman ED. Clinical and laboratory characteristics and long-term outcome of pediatric systemic lupus erythematosus: a longitudinal study. J Pediatr. 2008;152(4):550–6.
15. Pereira T, Abitbol CL, Seeherunvong W, Katsoufis C, Chandar J, Freundlich M, et al. Three decades of progress in treating childhood-onset lupus nephritis. Clin J Am Soc Nephrol. 2011;6(9):2192–9.
16. Ayalon R, Beck LH Jr. Membranous nephropathy: not just a disease for adults. Pediatr Nephrol. 2015;30(1):31–9.
17. Hahn BH, McMahon MA, Wilkinson A, Wallace WD, Daikh DI, Fitzgerald JD, et al. American College of Rheumatology guidelines for screening, treatment, and management of lupus nephritis. Arthritis Care Res (Hoboken). 2012;64(6):797–808.
18. Petri M, Orbai AM, Alarcon GS, Gordon C, Merrill JT, Fortin PR, et al. Derivation and validation of the systemic lupus international collaborating clinics classification criteria for systemic lupus erythematosus. Arthritis Rheum. 2012;64(8):2677–86.
19. Weening JJ, D'Agati VD, Schwartz MM, Seshan SV, Alpers CE, Appel GB, et al. The classification of glomerulonephritis in systemic lupus erythematosus revisited. J Am Soc Nephrol. 2004;15(2):241–50.
20. Corwin HL, Schwartz MM, Lewis EJ. The importance of sample size in the interpretation of the renal biopsy. Am J Nephrol. 1988;8(2):85–9.

21. Rovin BH, Parikh SV, Alvarado A. The kidney biopsy in lupus nephritis: is it still relevant? Rheum Dis Clin N Am. 2014;40(3):537–52. ix
22. Marks SD, Sebire NJ, Tullus K. Classification of pediatric lupus nephritis. Kidney Int. 2007;72(7):897–8.
23. Michail S, Stathakis C, Marinaki S, Revenas C, Nakopoulou L, Vaiopoulos G. Relapse of predominant tubulointerstitial lupus nephritis. Lupus. 2003;12(9):728–9.
24. Song D, Wu LH, Wang FM, Yang XW, Zhu D, Chen M, et al. The spectrum of renal thrombotic microangiopathy in lupus nephritis. Arthritis Res Ther. 2013;15(1):R12.
25. Sun F, Wang X, Wu W, Wang K, Chen Z, Li T, et al. TMA secondary to SLE: rituximab improves overall but not renal survival. Clin Rheumatol. 2017;
26. Imran TF, Yick F, Verma S, Estiverne C, Ogbonnaya-Odor C, Thiruvarudsothy S, et al. Lupus nephritis: an update. Clin Exp Nephrol. 2016;20(1):1–13.
27. Pons-Estel GJ, Alarcon GS, McGwin G Jr, Danila MI, Zhang J, Bastian HM, et al. Protective effect of hydroxychloroquine on renal damage in patients with lupus nephritis: LXV, data from a multiethnic US cohort. Arthritis Rheum. 2009;61(6):830–9.
28. Griffin B, Lightstone L. Renoprotective strategies in lupus nephritis: beyond immunosuppression. Lupus. 2013;22(12):1267–73.
29. Anders HJ, Vielhauer V. Renal co-morbidity in patients with rheumatic diseases. Arthritis Res Ther. 2011;13(3):222.
30. Kidney Disease: Improving Global Outcomes (KDIGO) Glomerulonephritis Work Group. KDIGO clinical practice guideline for glomerulonephritis. Kidney Inter Suppl. 2012;2:139–274.
31. Couture J, Silverman ED. Update on the pathogenesis and treatment of childhood-onset systemic lupus erythematosus. Curr Opin Rheumatol. 2016;28(5):488–96.
32. Korbet SM, Lewis EJ, Schwartz MM, Reichlin M, Evans J, Rohde RD. Factors predictive of outcome in severe lupus nephritis. Lupus Nephritis Collaborative Study Group. Am J Kidney Dis. 2000;35(5):904–14.
33. Chen YE, Korbet SM, Katz RS, Schwartz MM, Lewis EJ, Collaborative Study G. Value of a complete or partial remission in severe lupus nephritis. Clin J Am Soc Nephrol. 2008;3(1):46–53.
34. Lenz O, Waheed AA, Baig A, Pop A, Contreras G. Lupus nephritis: maintenance therapy for lupus nephritis – do we now have a plan? Clin J Am Soc Nephrol. 2013;8(1):162–71.
35. Hogan J, Appel GB. Update on the treatment of lupus nephritis. Curr Opin Nephrol Hypertens. 2013;22(2):224–30.
36. Sundel R, Solomons N, Lisk L, Aspreva Lupus Management Study G. Efficacy of mycophenolate mofetil in adolescent patients with lupus nephritis: evidence from a two-phase, prospective randomized trial. Lupus. 2012;21(13):1433–43.
37. Isenberg D, Appel GB, Contreras G, Dooley MA, Ginzler EM, Jayne D, et al. Influence of race/ethnicity on response to lupus nephritis treatment: the ALMS study. Rheumatology (Oxford). 2010;49(1):128–40.
38. Dooley MA, Jayne D, Ginzler EM, Isenberg D, Olsen NJ, Wofsy D, et al. Mycophenolate versus azathioprine as maintenance therapy for lupus nephritis. N Engl J Med. 2011;365(20):1886–95.
39. Rovin BH, Furie R, Latinis K, Looney RJ, Fervenza FC, Sanchez-Guerrero J, et al. Efficacy and safety of rituximab in patients with active proliferative lupus nephritis: the lupus nephritis assessment with rituximab study. Arthritis Rheum. 2012;64(4):1215–26.
40. Cortes-Hernandez J, Torres-Salido MT, Medrano AS, Tarres MV, Ordi-Ros J. Long-term outcomes – mycophenolate mofetil treatment for lupus nephritis with addition of tacrolimus for resistant cases. Nephrol Dial Transplant. 2010;25(12):3939–48.
41. Ward F, Bargman JM. Membranous lupus nephritis: the same, but different. Am J Kidney Dis. 2016;68(6):954–66.
42. Swan JT, Riche DM, Riche KD, Majithia V. Systematic review and meta-analysis of immunosuppressant therapy clinical trials in membranous lupus nephritis. J Investig Med. 2011;59(2):246–58.

43. Szeto CC, Kwan BC, Lai FM, Tam LS, Li EK, Chow KM, et al. Tacrolimus for the treatment of systemic lupus erythematosus with pure class V nephritis. Rheumatology (Oxford). 2008;47(11):1678–81.
44. Boneparth A, Radhakrishna SM, Greenbaum LA, Yen E, Okamura DM, Cooper JC, et al. Approach to membranous lupus nephritis: a survey of pediatric nephrologists and pediatric rheumatologists. J Rheumatol. 2017;44(11):1619–23.
45. Groot N, de Graeff N, Avcin T, Bader-Meunier B, Brogan P, Dolezalova P, et al. European evidence-based recommendations for diagnosis and treatment of childhood-onset systemic lupus erythematosus: the SHARE initiative. Ann Rheum Dis. 2017;76(11):1788–96.
46. Beck LH Jr, Salant DJ. Treatment of membranous lupus nephritis: where are we now? J Am Soc Nephrol. 2009;20(4):690–1.
47. Bao H, Liu ZH, Xie HL, Hu WX, Zhang HT, Li LS. Successful treatment of class V+IV lupus nephritis with multitarget therapy. J Am Soc Nephrol. 2008;19(10):2001–10.
48. Tselios K, Koumaras C, Gladman DD, Urowitz MB. Dyslipidemia in systemic lupus erythematosus: just another comorbidity? Semin Arthritis Rheum. 2016;45(5):604–10.
49. Sinicato NA, da Silva Cardoso PA, Appenzeller S. Risk factors in cardiovascular disease in systemic lupus erythematosus. Curr Cardiol Rev. 2013;9(1):15–9.
50. Ruiz-Irastorza G, Cuadrado MJ, Ruiz-Arruza I, Brey R, Crowther M, Derksen R, et al. Evidence-based recommendations for the prevention and long-term management of thrombosis in antiphospholipid antibody-positive patients: report of a task force at the 13th International Congress on antiphospholipid antibodies. Lupus. 2011;20(2):206–18.
51. Hofstra JM, Wetzels JFM. Should aspirin be used for primary prevention of thrombotic events in patients with membranous nephropathy? Kidney Int. 2016;89(5):981–3.
52. Compeyrot-Lacassagne S, Tyrrell PN, Atenafu E, Doria AS, Stephens D, Gilday D, et al. Prevalence and etiology of low bone mineral density in juvenile systemic lupus erythematosus. Arthritis Rheum. 2007;56(6):1966–73.
53. Thakral A, Klein-Gitelman MS. An update on treatment and management of pediatric systemic Lupus erythematosus. Rheumatol Ther. 2016;3(2):209–19.
54. Hickman RA, Gordon C. Causes and management of infertility in systemic lupus erythematosus. Rheumatology (Oxford). 2011;50(9):1551–8.
55. Slater CA, Liang MH, McCune JW, Christman GM, Laufer MR. Preserving ovarian function in patients receiving cyclophosphamide. Lupus. 1999;8(1):3–10.
56. Coscia LA, Armenti DP, King RW, Sifontis NM, Constantinescu S, Moritz MJ. Update on the teratogenicity of maternal mycophenolate mofetil. J Pediatr Genet. 2015;4(2):42–55.
57. Tunnicliffe DJ, Singh-Grewal D, Chaitow J, Mackie F, Manolios N, Lin MW, et al. Lupus means sacrifices: perspectives of adolescents and young adults with systemic lupus erythematosus. Arthritis Care Res (Hoboken). 2016;68(6):828–37.

Chapter 10
Hemodialysis in Adolescents

Erica Winnicki, Paul Brakeman, Marsha Lee, and Stephanie Nguyen

Introduction

Hemodialysis is the most common initial end-stage renal disease (ESRD) treatment for children above 10 years of age in the United States [1]. The primary cause of ESRD for US children is cystic/hereditary/congenital disorders, followed by glomerular disease and secondary causes of glomerulonephritis [1]. The preferred treatment for all children with ESRD is kidney transplantation [2]. However, when kidney transplantation cannot occur preemptively, the decision of whether to initiate hemodialysis (HD) versus peritoneal dialysis (PD) must be individualized to the needs of the patient and family. PD has a number of advantages relative to HD, including the fact that it is a home-based therapy and is associated with preservation of renal function [3], which are discussed further in the chapter on PD. Relative to PD, the main advantage of HD is that the patient and family do not need to undergo training to perform dialysis, as HD is performed almost uniformly in-center for children in the United States [4]. The dialysis treatment duration is shorter for HD

E. Winnicki (✉)
Department of Pediatrics, Division of Nephrology, University of California San Francisco, San Francisco, CA, USA
e-mail: erica.winnicki@ucsf.edu

P. Brakeman
Department of Pediatrics, UCSF Benioff Children's Hospital San Francisco, University of California, San Francisco, San Francisco, CA, USA

M. Lee
UCSF Benioff Children's Hospital Pediatric Dialysis Unit, UCSF Benioff Children's Hospital, Pediatric Nephrology, San Francisco, CA, USA

S. Nguyen
Department of Pediatrics, UC Davis Children's Hospital, Sacramento, CA, USA
e-mail: stanguyen@ucdavis.edu

M. N. Haddad et al. (eds.), *Adolescents with Chronic Kidney Disease*,
https://doi.org/10.1007/978-3-319-97220-6_10

relative to PD and is generally performed thrice weekly. However these sessions are often disruptive to school, such that normal school attendance for adolescents on HD is precluded.

Initiation of Hemodialysis

The decision to initiate maintenance dialysis for a child or adolescent with CKD is based on multiple factors, both objective and subjective [4]. Objective measures used to determine when to initiate maintenance dialysis include the patient's estimated glomerular filtration rate (eGFR), the presence of fluid overload or electrolyte derangements (e.g., hyperkalemia, hyperphosphatemia, acidosis) that are refractory to medical therapy, and poor weight gain or malnutrition. Subjective measures used to determine when to initiate dialysis include patient fatigue, general weakness, and/or poor school functioning. While it is recommended that patients be counseled regarding renal replacement options when their eGFR has fallen below 30 ml/min/1.73m^2, there is no specific eGFR threshold at which maintenance dialysis must be commenced [5]. This is in part due to findings from the Initiating Dialysis Early and Late (IDEAL) trial, a study performed in adult patients with CKD who were randomized to early (defined as an eGFR 10–14 ml/min/1.73 m^2) versus late (defined as an eGFR 5–7 ml/min/1.73 m^2) initiation of dialysis, which did not find a survival benefit to the planned initiation of dialysis at higher levels of eGFR [6]. Additionally, estimation of kidney function in those with advanced kidney disease may be problematic as creatinine-based estimating equations will overestimate GFR in the setting of malnutrition and decreased creatinine production [7]. That stated, according to the survey of the European Society for Paediatric Nephrology/Transplant (ESPN/ERA-EDTA) Registry, the median eGFR at the start of RRT was 9 mL/min/1.73 m^2 [8]. During the years 1995–2002, 20% of US children with CKD initiated dialysis at an eGFR above 15 ml/min/1.73 m^2; adolescents were more likely to initiate dialysis earlier compared to younger children [9]. While there is a paucity of data on the effect of eGFR at initiation of dialysis in children with CKD and patient outcomes, it is reasonable to infer that the decision to initiate maintenance dialysis should not be based on eGFR alone.

Vascular Access for Adolescents on Hemodialysis

Vascular access decisions are critically important for children and adolescents with CKD. Given their long life expectancy and potential for repeated dialysis exposure during their lifetime, maintaining patent vasculature is necessary to ensure good long-term health outcomes. Choices for vasculature access include a central venous catheter (CVC) versus an arteriovenous fistula (AVF) or graft (AVG). There are clear advantages to AVF or AVG over a CVC. The latter are associated with increased risk for infection, stenosis, thrombosis, access failure, morbidity, and mortality in patients on dialysis [10–12]. It is recommended that an AVF or AVG be used for vascular access in adolescents weighing more than 20 kg on HD unless a kidney transplant is planned to occur within a year or HD is serving as a bridge to PD [13]. However, CVCs are used most often for children and adolescents on dialysis. According to the 2011 North American Pediatric Renal Trials and Collaborative Studies (NAPRTCS) data, 78.7% of children on HD had a CVC for access, 11.8% had an AVF, and 6.7% had an AVG [14]. The pros and cons of using CVCs for hemodialysis access in children and adolescents are shown in Table 10.1. When the decision is made to place a CVC for hemodialysis access, cuffed catheters are used and are tunneled under the skin. Attention should be paid to the location of placement and the size of the catheter. The preferred location of placement in order to decrease the rate of complications is the right internal jugular vein, followed (in order) by the right external jugular vein, left internal and external jugular veins, subclavian veins, femoral veins, and translumbar access to the inferior vena cava [15]. To achieve good blood flow rates, the largest diameter catheter for the patient's size should be chosen and the tip of the catheter should be placed in the right atrium. To prevent infectious complications, the Centers for Disease Control and Prevention (CDC) Dialysis Bloodstream Infection Prevention Collaborative recommends (in addition to reducing the number of CVCs) the following: (1) regular staff and patient training on proper catheter care (including hand hygiene and recognizing signs of infection); (2) cleaning the CVC exit site with an antiseptic agent, preferably alcohol-based chlorhexidine, during placement and dressing changes; (3) disinfecting the catheter hub every time the catheter is accessed or disconnected; and (4) applying an antimicrobial ointment, or povidone-iodine ointment, at the exit site with each dressing change [16]. Additionally, it has been shown that locking the catheter with an antimicrobial-containing citrate lock is better than heparin in preventing catheter-related infections [17].

Aside from planned termination of hemodialysis, catheter infection and thrombosis are the most common causes of CVC removal in children on dialysis [18]. Catheter-related infections can be categorized as catheter exit-site infection, tunnel

Table 10.1 Pros and cons of central venous catheter for hemodialysis in children and adolescents

Pros	Cons
Easily placed	Infection rates high
Can be used immediately	Failure rates and replacement rates high
Painless to the patient	Blood flow rates are variable, leading to potentially poor clearance
Requires little planning prior to placement	Permanent damage to central venous system (stenosis/thrombosis) may occur
Easily removed if used as "transitional" access for future PD or transplant patients	Damage to central vessels can prohibit future AVF/AVG placement in ipsilateral extremity
No vascular steal	Possible arrhythmia
Decreased risk of high-output cardiac failure	

Reprinted/adapted by permission from: Springer Nature, Chand et al. [15]

infection, catheter-related bloodstream infections (CRBSI), and metastatic infection (such as osteomyelitis, abscess formation, or endocarditis) [19]. Infection of the exit site is suspected when there is redness or drainage at the exit site; it is important to confirm that the infection does not extend beyond the exit site. Tunnel infections often present with redness, pain, and tenderness along the tunnel. Diagnosis of catheter-related infections is confirmed by culture of the exudate, blood, and/or catheter tip (in the case of catheter removal), and antibiotics are tailored according to culture results. When an infection is suspected, the patient should be treated empirically with vancomycin for Gram-positive organism coverage and a third-generation cephalosporin, carbapenem, or β-lactam/β-lactamase combination (based on local antibiogram) for Gram-negative organism coverage until culture results are known [20]. The catheter should be removed in cases of severe sepsis, tunnel-site infection, metastatic infection, bloodstream infection that continues despite >72 h of antimicrobial therapy to which the infecting microbes are susceptible, or infections due to *S. aureus*, *P. aeruginosa*, fungi, or mycobacteria [20]. Antibiotic lock therapy should be used in cases where the catheter is being salvaged. The duration of therapy depends on a number of factors, for which specific treatment guidelines exist [20].

In contrast to infants and young children whose blood vessels may be too small for successful AVF, adolescents have blood vessels that are large enough to realistically provide the option of AVF placement. As noted above, AVF is the optimal vascular access for hemodialysis. AVFs are placed in the nondominant arm if possible or the site with the largest venous diameter as determined by duplex ultrasound scanning or venography. The preferred sites for AVF placement are as follows (in order): radial artery to cephalic vein, brachial artery to cephalic vein, and brachial artery to basilic vein [15]. The potential complications of AVF include infection, thrombosis, stenosis, ischemia distal to anastomosis leading to steal syndrome, and aneurysm formation [21]. Patient-perceived complications related to AVFs may also include pain associated with cannulation and disfigurement [22]. AVG are the least frequent vascular access type used in children and adolescents on hemodialysis. The graft material most commonly used is polytetrafluoroethylene (PTFE) [15]. A comparison of the relative advantages and disadvantages of AVF versus AVG is shown in Table 10.2. While AVG are technically easier to create and can be used within a shorter time period relative to AVF, they are associated with a relatively higher

Table 10.2 Permanent vascular access options: AV fistula versus AV graft

AV fistula	AV graft
Lower infection rate	Higher infection rate
Lower thrombosis rate	Higher thrombosis rate
May take 3–6 months to mature	Usually able to be used within a few weeks
Primary failure rate is higher	Primary failure rate is lower
Secondary failure rates lower	Secondary failure rates higher

Reprinted/adapted by permission from: Springer Nature, Chand et al. [15]

complication rate including infection and thrombosis. Once placed, AVF and AVG require ongoing close visual inspection and surveillance of blood flow through the vascular access in order to detect and intervene early on complications [15].

Hemodialysis Prescription

The goal of the HD prescription is to achieve adequate removal of electrolytes, fluid, and toxins to maintain homeostasis, prevent side effects of hypervolemia, and prevent complications related to uremic toxins. Conventional HD in children and adolescents typically is delivered for 3–4 h per treatment three times a week. The adequacy of HD is usually measured in terms of urea clearance, recognizing that urea is a biomarker and not the only toxin, nor even the primary toxin, present in a uremic state [23, 24]. Despite these limitations in using the clearance of urea to determine dialysis adequacy, it remains the primary method to measure whether a dialysis prescription achieves adequate clearance of toxins.

There are multiple methods that can be used to estimate and model the removal of urea using serum samples obtained before and after hemodialysis treatments. The most commonly used model for estimating urea removal is the single-pool model for urea removal in which a pre- and post-dialysis urea serum level are used to estimate the total amount of urea removed during a HD treatment. The amount of urea removed is described as the "*Kt/V*" where *K* is the clearance of urea by the dialyzer, *t* is the time (duration) of the dialysis treatment, and *V* is the volume of distribution of urea which is approximately equal to patient's total body water [25]. Current guidelines recommend monthly measurement of the delivered dose of hemodialysis in children and adolescents, with a minimum single-pool *Kt/V* target of 1.2, although maintaining a measured *Kt/V* of >1.3 ensures that *Kt/V* of 1.2 is achieved for every treatment [4, 13]. There is some evidence in adults that the classic *Kt/V* equation overestimates urea removal for small patients due to inadequate estimation of the volume of distribution of urea by using weight to calculate *V* rather than body surface area (BSA), and thus care should be taken not to underdose smaller adolescents [26]. Additionally, while *Kt/V* >1.2 can be achieved in smaller patients with shorter treatments using a higher flux, larger dialyzer, it is generally not recommended to shorten HD treatments to less than 3 h [26].

Intensified HD may be prescribed for improved control of phosphate levels, anemia, blood pressure, fluid status, and/or growth/nutrition. Options for intensified hemodialysis in adolescents include short daily HD, intermittent nocturnal HD, and daily nocturnal HD [4]. However, if intensification of HD involves increased in-center HD sessions during the day, the benefits of HD intensification must be weighed against the drawbacks of missing on-site schooling and social interactions with peers. In addition it should be noted that for adults, the two largest randomized trials of frequent dialysis had conflicting results in terms of showing any benefit in terms of increased survival [27, 28].

Pediatric Hemodialysis Unit

In our experience, the pediatric hemodialysis unit has much to offer to the adolescent on chronic hemodialysis. Pediatric hemodialysis should provide a structured, age-appropriate environment with a multidisciplinary team with pediatric expertise usually consisting of a school teacher, social worker, pediatric dialysis nurses, pediatric renal dietician, and pediatric nephrologists [4]. This multifaceted, multidisciplinary pediatric team approach can lead to optimization of care for the adolescent hemodialysis patient and help facilitate kidney transplant readiness, specifically when there are challenging social situations and problems with medication nonadherence. During hemodialysis sessions, the adolescent hemodialysis patient is a captive audience to all of the age-specific, age-appropriate education the multidisciplinary pediatric team has to offer, including in-person teaching, education-level appropriate reading materials, online educational videos, and potential visits from the pediatric kidney transplant team. The many benefits of a pediatric hemodialysis unit must be taken into account when an adolescent hemodialysis patient is deciding between a pediatric hemodialysis and a local adult hemodialysis unit, which sometimes can accept older adolescents and may be geographically closer to the adolescent patient's home.

Complications of Hemodialysis

Well-known complications of, or conditions associated with, hemodialysis include hypertension, accelerated cardiovascular disease, and bone and mineral metabolism abnormalities [4], all of which are addressed below in this chapter. Another important side effect of being on dialysis with ESRD for children and adolescents is poor linear growth [29–31]. Other common side effects of HD include disequilibrium syndrome, fatigue, pruritus, pain, abnormal intestinal motility, disordered sleep, and abnormal pubertal development [32–36].

Poor linear growth is a known and common side effect of CKD and ESRD. Prior to the development of growth hormone, almost all patients who developed ESRD prior to skeletal maturity had abnormal linear growth. Despite the availability of growth hormone (GH), 40–60% of pediatric ESRD patients were still developing short stature as of 2010 [29, 31]. Some delays in linear growth may be related to poor nutrition and an associated catabolic state. All adolescent patients on HD should have a thorough nutritional evaluation and receive additional nutritional support if needed. In addition, acidosis should be adequately treated and eliminated by either intensifying the dialysis prescription or by the addition of oral sodium bicarbonate [29].

Uremia itself is associated with growth hormone resistance with both low IGF-1 levels possibly due to abnormalities in the JAK-stat signal pathway that triggers IGF-1 release in response to GH as well as end organ resistance to IGF-1 [31].

Adolescents on HD should be evaluated for linear growth potential with bone age radiographs of the nondominant hand or, if older, radiographs of the long bones to determine linear growth potential. Patients with growth potential, receiving adequate nutrition, and with well-controlled metabolic bone disease should be prescribed GH. In addition, patient and parent education should occur to attain the highest levels of adherence possible. In the situation where nutrition, acidosis, or bone and mineral metabolism may not be optimal, it is probably better to begin the process of prescribing GH while optimizing nutrition and metabolic control, as often insurance issues can delay obtaining GH in adolescents for several months when an adolescent may only have a small window of opportunity to maximize growth. In patients who are peri-pubertal with short stature with some growth potential, delaying puberty pharmacologically should be considered to allow for more time to achieve linear growth.

There are several relative contraindications for using GH in adolescents on HD including uncontrolled metabolic bone disease, hyperglycemia, and significant scoliosis [29]. Use of GH with uncontrolled metabolic bone disease (very elevated PTH) or significant scoliosis can lead to bone deformities. Use of GH in patients with hyperglycemia can lead to worse glycemic control; however, for the patient with diabetes mellitus and poor linear growth on HD, using GH with intensive management of glycemic control can achieve growth without significant morbidity from poor glycemic control. Absolute contraindications for GH include active malignancy and fusion of the epiphyses since GH will have no effect on linear growth if no further linear bone growth is possible [29].

One of the more acute intradialytic complications that can occur is disequilibrium syndrome. Disequilibrium syndrome can present with headache, muscle twitching, restlessness, and nausea and is associated with cerebral edema and raised intracranial pressure [33, 36]. This condition usually presents during the first HD session but can still develop in any patient undergoing HD. If unrecognized, it can progress to coma and even death. The risk of disequilibrium syndrome can be reduced by prescribing slower removal of urea concentration – particularly during initial treatments – and/or using osmotic agents such as mannitol for initial treatments [36].

Symptomatic complications of HD include fatigue, pain, and pruritus. The prevalence of fatigue in the adolescent HD population is high although exact numbers are not available. In the adult dialysis population, up to 80% patients report fatigue [37]. Some techniques for managing fatigue include supplementation with L-carnitine [35], evaluating and treating patients for disordered sleep and depression, and encouraging a healthy lifestyle including obtaining adequate exercise [38]. Chronic pain is quite common in the adult HD population with a reported prevalence of up to 90% [39, 40]. Types of pain include pain directly related to obtaining fistula access with needles, headache during dialysis, chronic headache, and chronic neuropathic pain of limbs, joints, and muscles [39]. Pharmacological management techniques include agents such as gabapentin, nonsteroidal anti-inflammatory agents, or, when required, opiates. Non-pharmacologic management techniques include transcutaneous electrical stimulation (TENS), topical thermal therapy, acupuncture, and mindfulness training [40]. Pruritus and other skin conditions are common in the dialysis population. Aggressive hydration is the most basic technique to help reduce skin symptoms. In addition, some patients benefit from the use of topical capsaicin or oral agents such as gabapentin [35]. Other skin complications can occur around sites of access including superficial bacterial and fungal infections and also hypersensitivity reactions to dressing materials.

Abnormal intestinal motility and function lead to complaints of abdominal pain, heartburn, dyspepsia, nausea, constipation, and/or diarrhea in many patients on hemodialysis [41–43]. These abdominal complaints, when combined with dietary restrictions, can severely limit calorie intake and contribute to undernutrition in HD patients. Chronic gastrointestinal complaints should prompt a complete evaluation and often require referral to a gastrointestinal specialist. Symptoms related to poor intestinal motility may respond to the use of erythromycin or other motility agents [44].

Hypertension and Cardiovascular Disease in Adolescent Hemodialysis Patients

Expectant remaining lifetime is reduced approximately by half in prevalent adolescent dialysis patients compared to transplant recipients and by two-thirds compared to the general population [45]. Pediatric mortality associated with renal failure is mainly due to cardiovascular causes; it accounted for 20–57% of deaths among children on hemodialysis and is the most common cause of death for adolescents receiving hemodialysis [46–48].

Sudden cardiac death is the most common cause of cardiovascular death in both adult and pediatric hemodialysis patients and is thought to be due to the cardiac stress from accumulation of toxins, electrolyte disequilibrium, and fluid overload [49]. The highest incidence of sudden cardiac death occurs on the day after a long intradialytic interval, which for in-center dialysis patients usually occurs on Monday [50, 51]. Longer intradialytic intervals were also associated with increased incidence of hospitalization for hypertension, fluid overload, or electrolyte disturbances in children on hemodialysis [52]. A similar increase in mortality or morbidity is not seen in peritoneal dialysis or in-home hemodialysis adult patients [53].

Hypertension is very common in ESRD and present in 79% of pediatric hemodialysis patients [54]. In children, hypertension and fluid status are the most important factors for the development of left ventricular hypertrophy (LVH). In the adult CKD and dialysis populations, LVH and dysfunction are important predictors of cardiovascular mortality and morbidity [55]. Blood pressure treatment goals for pediatric CKD patients vary between guidelines from less than the 50th to 90th percentile for age, sex, and height or less than 130/80 for older adolescents [56–58]. Blood pressure is frequently monitored during hemodialysis though intradialytic blood pressure as measured at home or by ambulatory blood pressure monitor has better predictive value on mortality than in-center measurements of adult hemodialysis patients. Additionally, ambulatory blood pressure monitoring has better predictive value for LVH in children than in-center pre- or post-dialysis blood pressure measurements [59]. Angiotensin-converting enzyme (ACE) inhibitors or angiotensin II receptor blockers (ARBs) are preferred for pediatric CKD patients for their renoprotective effects pre-dialysis [56, 58]. However, there are no pediatric studies to recommend any class of antihypertensive medication once on hemodialysis, though care should be taken to select for medications not extensively removed by hemodialysis [60]. In adult hemodialysis patients, reduction of blood pressure improved patient survival [61, 62], and an observational study of adult hemodialysis patients on ACE inhibitors or ARBs had lower mortality and cardiovascular morbidity [63]. However a meta-analysis of randomized controlled trials of ACE inhibitors and ARBs did not find a statistically significant difference in cardiovascular morbidity or mortality [64].

Extracellular volume expansion is an important contributor to elevated blood pressure, and achieving a dry weight to control blood pressure requires frequent monitoring in a growing adolescent [65]. Recommendations to control blood pressure include lowering dietary sodium intake to less than 2000 mg of sodium per day. For adolescents who are oliguric or anuric, fluid restriction is recommended to minimize intradialytic fluid accumulation. Noninvasive blood volume monitoring can be used as an aid for optimal fluid removal during hemodialysis [66, 67]. Noninvasive blood volume monitoring allows for "refill testing," where ultrafiltration is halted and hematocrit is monitored for change, indicating refilling of intravascular volume and availability of fluid for removal.

Chronic Kidney Disease-Mineral and Bone Disorder

Chronic kidney disease-mineral and bone disorder (CKD-MBD) encompasses a broad spectrum of clinical disorders that develop from the systematic dysregulation of mineral and bone metabolism due to chronic kidney disease [68]. These disorders include abnormalities of phosphate, calcium, parathyroid hormone (PTH), calcitriol (1,25-dihydroxyvitamin D3), and fibroblast growth factor (FGF-23) as well as renal osteodystrophy, a term now reserved for abnormal bone histology resulting from CKD. In addition the broader CKD-MBD term includes extra-skeletal and vascular calcifications which have important consequences on cardiovascular mortality.

The goal for adolescents on dialysis is to remain as close as possible to normal levels of calcium and phosphorus to minimize complications such as fractures, skeletal deformities, poor linear growth, and vascular and/or other soft tissue calcifications [69]. Practice guidelines recommend routine assessments of serum calcium, phosphorus, alkaline phosphatase, bicarbonate, intact PTH, and serum 25-hydroxyvitamin D levels [70, 71]. The goal of therapy is to maintain intact PTH targets levels to two to nine times the upper limits of normal. Supplementation with vitamin D_2 (ergocalciferol) or vitamin D_3 (cholecalciferol) is recommended for serum 25-hydroxyvitamin D levels less than 30 ng/ml [72].

As CKD progresses, phosphorus excretion decreases, and retention of serum phosphorus develops along with the many complications associated with CKD-MBD. Phosphorus is restricted to the recommended daily intake of phosphorus for adolescents, 1250 mg phosphorus per day [72]. For those with hyperphosphatemia and PTH levels above target range, phosphorus intake is reduced by 80%, 1000 mg phosphorus per day. The addition of oral phosphate-binding agents administered with meals and snacks is indicated for those with persistent hyperphosphatemia despite dietary phosphorus restriction. For adolescents, phosphate binders fall into two categories: calcium-based (calcium carbonate or calcium acetate) or non-calcium-containing phosphate binders (sevelamer hydrochloride or sevelamer carbonate) [73]. Aside from higher serum calcium with calcium-based binders, serum phosphorus levels decreased a similar amount between the categories of binders [74]. Calcium acetate and sevelamer carbonate improved metabolic acidosis compared to sevelamer hydrochloride in children on dialysis [75, 76]. Lanthanum carbonate, a non-calcium-containing phosphate binder approved for use in adults, is not recommended in pediatric patients due to evidence of its deposition in the bone and uncertain long-term safety [77, 78].

Ensuring adequate dietary calcium intake is necessary for skeletal development, including acquiring optimal peak bone mass in puberty. Calcium intake can be excessive or insufficient in adolescents with CKD. Endogenous production of calcitriol is decreased in CKD which impairs intestinal calcium absorption. Calcium supplementation or calcium-containing phosphate binder may be added when oral intake alone is not sufficient. The recommended daily intake for adolescents of elemental calcium is 1300 mg per day with an upper limit of 2500 mg elemental calcium per day from dietary sources and calcium-based phosphate binders for those on dialysis [72].

Active vitamin D sterols are a mainstay of treatment for secondary hyperparathyroidism in CKD. The goal of therapy for those on dialysis is to maintain intact PTH target levels between two and nine times the upper limits of normal to prevent hyperplasia of the parathyroid glands and maintain normal rates of bone turnover. Calcitriol, when used with calcium-based binders, results in decreased PTH levels; however concerns for hypercalcemia and its contribution to soft tissue calcification have led to interest in other active vitamin D analogues that minimize intestinal calcium and phosphorus absorption while still suppressing PTH [73, 79]. In a Cochrane meta-analysis of four randomized controlled trials for calcitriol, paricalcitol, and doxercalciferol, the authors found no difference in hypercalcemia compared to placebo or no treatment in children with CKD stages 2–5D [74]. Cinacalcet is a calcimimetic which halts parathyroid cell hyperplasia and is FDA approved for adult dialysis patients with secondary hyperparathyroidism. A Cochrane meta-analysis found cinacalcet effectively decreased PTH levels and decreased the need for surgical parathyroidectomy but had higher incidence of hypocalcemia in adults on dialysis [80]. Observational studies of pediatric dialysis patients found cinacalcet decreased intact PTH levels [81–84], but pediatric clinical studies were halted due to one death from hypocalcemia and low enrollment [85].

Anemia of Chronic Kidney Disease

Anemia of CKD becomes more prevalent in progressively advanced stages of CKD [86], and all adolescents on hemodialysis will receive treatment for anemia [87]. Causes of anemia of CKD are often multifactorial. Progressive renal parenchymal loss leads to decreased erythropoietin production by peritubular fibroblasts in the renal cortex, and decreased oxygen consumption by renal tubules increases renal tissue oxygen pressure above levels required for erythropoietin production [88]. There is also increased blood loss due to phlebotomy and retention in the dialyzer and dialysis blood lines. Iron deficiency from restrictive diets and anorexia as well as reduced dietary iron absorption due to systemic inflammation and medications such as phosphate binders and gastric acid inhibitors are other contributing factors [89, 90].

Anemia of CKD is associated with increased mortality and morbidity in adolescent hemodialysis patients. Pediatric hemodialysis patients with hemoglobin <11 g/dl have a higher risk of hospitalization and had a longer duration of hospitalization [91]. The risk of mortality declined by 69% for adolescents on hemodialysis with hemoglobin between 11 and 12 g/dl versus those with hemoglobin <10 g/dl. Unlike adults on hemodialysis where higher hemoglobin targets were associated with higher rates of mortality and cardiovascular events [92, 93], for children on dialysis and adolescents on hemodialysis, hemoglobin >12 g/dl is not associated with increased mortality, all-cause hospitalizations, or cardiovascular-related hospitalizations [94, 95]. For children and adolescents, attainment of higher hemoglobin levels is associated with higher quality-of-life measures and should be considered as important factors when assessing hemoglobin goals [96, 97].

Anemia is diagnosed based on age and sex and hemoglobin <12 g/dL for those ≥12 years old and <13 g/dL for males >15 years old [98]. Initial investigation for anemia should include complete cell count, absolute reticulocyte count, serum ferritin, serum transferrin saturation (TSAT), serum vitamin B_{12}, and folate levels. Serum transferrin saturation measures the availability of iron to support red blood cell production, while serum ferritin is a marker for iron storage and is an acute phase reactant which, for those on dialysis, needs to be interpreted with caution as it can be affected by inflammation [99]. Practice guidelines recommend maintaining hemoglobin levels between 11 and 12 g/dL with iron repletion and/or an erythropoiesis-stimulating agent (ESA) [98]. Patients with anemia resistant to iron and ESA therapy should be evaluated for occult blood loss, chronic infection or inflammation, deficiency of vitamin B12 or folate, hypothyroidism, and severe secondary hyperparathyroidism [4].

Intravenous (IV) iron administration is preferred in hemodialysis patients as randomized controlled trials in adult hemodialysis patients comparing IV iron with oral iron or placebo showed better attainment of hemoglobin goals and required lower ESA doses [100]. The readily available vascular access in hemodialysis patients makes IV iron more convenient and eliminates the potential issue of nonadherence. Iron studies should be routinely assessed monthly to guide therapy. It is recommended that pediatric hemodialysis patients be treated with iron to maintain TSAT >20% and ferritin >100 ng/ml. IV iron is associated with adverse reactions such as hypotension, dyspnea, and anaphylaxis; especially preparations of iron dextran, though adverse reactions can occur with any preparation [101].

ESA therapy is initiated after correction of other causes of anemia, such as iron deficiency and inflammatory status. ESA therapy helps avoid red cell transfusions especially for those eligible for renal transplantation to minimize risk for allosensitization [102]. The two most commonly used ESA therapies in pediatric hemodialysis patients are recombinant human erythropoietin (rHuEPO) and darbepoetin alfa. Recombinant human erythropoietin has a short half-life and is given via intravenous or subcutaneous routes several times per week. Darbepoetin alfa, an analogue of rHuEPO, has a three to four times longer half-life due to its increased glycosylation, thus can be given once every 1–2 weeks. The efficacy and safety of the darbepoetin alfa and rHuEPO are equivalently effective in CKD [103] and in pediatric ESRD patients [104]. Other ESAs (though much less studied) include peginesatide, new classes of continuous erythropoietin receptor activators, hypoxia-inducible transcription factor (HIF) stabilizers, as well as follow-on biologics or biosimilars that have proliferated following the expiration of patents for short-acting ESAs [105].

Outcome

The mortality rate for children and adolescents remains extremely high relative to the general pediatric population, with little change in mortality for pediatric dialysis patients over the past several years. The 1-year mortality rate for all children on hemodialysis between the years 1995 and 2010 was 4.3 per 100 patient-years, though this rate was relatively lower for adolescents in the 15–18 range at 3 per 100 patient-years [106]. The primary cause of death at 1 year for children of dialysis is cardiovascular disease. As kidney transplantation is associated with much lower mortality for children with ESRD compared to dialysis [107], the goal for children and adolescents on hemodialysis should be to get them to transplant as soon as possible.

References

1. Saran R, Li Y, Robinson B, Abbott KC, Agodoa LY, Ayanian J, et al. US renal data system 2015 annual data report: epidemiology of kidney disease in the United States. Am J Kidney Dis. 2016;67(3 Suppl 1):Svii. S1-305
2. Amaral S, Sayed BA, Kutner N, Patzer RE. Preemptive kidney transplantation is associated with survival benefits among pediatric patients with end-stage renal disease. Kidney Int. 2016;90(5):1100–8.
3. Moist LM, Port FK, Orzol SM, Young EW, Ostbye T, Wolfe RA, et al. Predictors of loss of residual renal function among new dialysis patients. J Am Soc Nephrol. 2000;11(3):556–64.

4. Warady BA, Neu AM, Schaefer F. Optimal care of the infant, child, and adolescent on dialysis: 2014 update. Am J Kidney Dis. 2014;64(1):128–42.
5. NKF. KDOQI clinical practice guideline for hemodialysis adequacy: 2015 update. Am J Kidney Dis. 2015;66(5):884–930.
6. Cooper BA, Branley P, Bulfone L, Collins JF, Craig JC, Fraenkel MB, et al. A randomized, controlled trial of early versus late initiation of dialysis. N Engl J Med. 2010;363(7):609–19.
7. Beddhu S, Samore MH, Roberts MS, Stoddard GJ, Pappas LM, Cheung AK. Creatinine production, nutrition, and glomerular filtration rate estimation. J Am Soc Nephrol. 2003;14(4):1000–5.
8. Chesnaye N, Bonthuis M, Schaefer F, Groothoff JW, Verrina E, Heaf JG, et al. Demographics of paediatric renal replacement therapy in Europe: a report of the ESPN/ERA–EDTA registry. Pediatr Nephrol. 2014;29(12):2403–10.
9. Atkinson MA, Oberai PC, Neu AM, Fivush BA, Parekh RS. Predictors and consequences of higher estimated glomerular filtration rate at dialysis initiation. Pediatr Nephrol. 2010;25(6):1153–61.
10. Rehman R, Schmidt RJ, Moss AH. Ethical and legal obligation to avoid long-term tunneled catheter access. Clin J Am Soc Nephrol. 2009;4(2):456–60.
11. Stevenson KB, Hannah EL, Lowder CA, Adcox MJ, Davidson RL, Mallea MC, et al. Epidemiology of hemodialysis vascular access infections from longitudinal infection surveillance data: predicting the impact of NKF-DOQI clinical practice guidelines for vascular access. Am J Kidney Dis. 2002;39(3):549–55.
12. Zaritsky JJ, Salusky IB, Gales B, Ramos G, Atkinson J, Allsteadt A, et al. Vascular access complications in long-term pediatric hemodialysis patients. Pediatr Nephrol. 2008;23(11):2061–5.
13. NKF. KDOQI clinical practice guidelines and clinical practice recommendations for 2006 updates: hemodialysis adequacy, peritoneal dialysis adequacy, and vascular access. Am J Kidney Dis. 2006;48(Suppl 1):S1–S322.
14. NAPTRCS. North American pediatric renal trials and collaborative studies annual dialysis report. 2011.
15. Chand DH, Valentini RP, Kamil ES. Hemodialysis vascular access options in pediatrics: considerations for patients and practitioners. Pediatr Nephrol. 2009;24(6):1121–8.
16. Control CfD. Core interventions.
17. Zhao Y, Li Z, Zhang L, Yang J, Yang Y, Tang Y, et al. Citrate versus heparin lock for hemodialysis catheters: a systematic review and meta-analysis of randomized controlled trials. Am J Kidney Dis. 2014;63(3):479–90.
18. Ramage IJ, Bailie A, Tyerman KS, McColl JH, Pollard SG, Fitzpatrick MM. Vascular access survival in children and young adults receiving long-term hemodialysis. Am J Kidney Dis. 2005;45(4):708–14.
19. Ramanathan V, Darouiche RO. Prevention and management of hemodialysis catheter infections. Expert Rev Anti-Infect Ther. 2012;10(12):1447–55.
20. Mermel LA, Allon M, Bouza E, Craven DE, Flynn P, O'Grady NP, et al. Clinical practice guidelines for the diagnosis and management of intravascular catheter-related infection: 2009 update by the Infectious Diseases Society of America. Clin Infect Dis. 2009;49(1):1–45.
21. Duronville JV, Diamantidis CJ. Medical safety in the care of the person with end-stage kidney disease. Semin Dial. 2018;31(2):140–8.
22. Casey JR, Hanson CS, Winkelmayer WC, Craig JC, Palmer S, Strippoli GF, et al. Patients' perspectives on hemodialysis vascular access: a systematic review of qualitative studies. Am J Kidney Dis. 2014;64(6):937–53.
23. Eloot S, Van Biesen W, Glorieux G, Neirynck N, Dhondt A, Vanholder R. Does the adequacy parameter Kt/V(urea) reflect uremic toxin concentrations in hemodialysis patients? PLoS One. 2013;8(11):e76838.
24. Lisowska-Myjak B. Uremic toxins and their effects on multiple organ systems. Nephron Clin Pract. 2014;128(3–4):303–11.
25. Gotch FA, Sargent JA. A mechanistic analysis of the National Cooperative Dialysis Study (NCDS). Kidney Int. 1985;28(3):526–34.

26. Daugirdas JT. Kt/V (and especially its modifications) remains a useful measure of hemodialysis dose. Kidney Int. 2015;88(3):466–73.
27. Group FHNT, Chertow GM, Levin NW, Beck GJ, Depner TA, Eggers PW, et al. In-center hemodialysis six times per week versus three times per week. N Engl J Med. 2010;363(24):2287–300.
28. Rocco MV, Lockridge RS Jr, Beck GJ, Eggers PW, Gassman JJ, Greene T, et al. The effects of frequent nocturnal home hemodialysis: the frequent hemodialysis network nocturnal trial. Kidney Int. 2011;80(10):1080–91.
29. Fine RN. Etiology and treatment of growth retardation in children with chronic kidney disease and end-stage renal disease: a historical perspective. Pediatr Nephrol. 2010;25(4):725–32.
30. Hodson EM, Willis NS, Craig JC. Growth hormone for children with chronic kidney disease. Cochrane Database Syst Rev. 2012;2
31. Ingulli EG, Mak RH. Growth in children with chronic kidney disease: role of nutrition, growth hormone, dialysis, and steroids. Curr Opin Pediatr. 2014;26(2):187–92.
32. Greenbaum LA, Warady BA, Furth SL. Current advances in chronic kidney disease in children: growth, cardiovascular, and neurocognitive risk factors. Semin Nephrol. 2009;29(4):425–34.
33. Haffner D, Zivicnjak M. Pubertal development in children with chronic kidney disease. Pediatr Nephrol. 2017;32(6):949–64.
34. Karunaratne K, Taube D, Khalil N, Perry R, Malhotra PA. Neurological complications of renal dialysis and transplantation. Pract Neurol. 2018;18(2):115–25.
35. Moledina DG, Perry WF. Pharmacologic treatment of common symptoms in dialysis patients: a narrative review. Semin Dial. 2015;28(4):377–83.
36. Zepeda-Orozco D, Quigley R. Dialysis disequilibrium syndrome. Pediatr Nephrol. 2012;27(12):2205–11.
37. Bossola M, Vulpio C, Tazza L. Fatigue in chronic dialysis patients. Semin Dial. 2011;24(5):550–5.
38. Kosmadakis GC, Bevington A, Smith AC, Clapp EL, Viana JL, Bishop NC, et al. Physical exercise in patients with severe kidney disease. Nephron Clin Pract. 2010;115(1):c7–c16.
39. Brkovic T, Burilovic E, Puljak L. Prevalence and severity of pain in adult end-stage renal disease patients on chronic intermittent hemodialysis: a systematic review. Patient Prefer Adherence. 2016;10:1131–50.
40. Pham PC, Khaing K, Sievers TM, Pham PM, Miller JM, Pham SV, et al. 2017 update on pain management in patients with chronic kidney disease. Clin Kidney J. 2017;10(5):688–97.
41. Ko CW, Chang CS, Lien HC, Wu MJ, Chen GH. Gastric dysrhythmia in uremic patients on maintenance hemodialysis. Scand J Gastroenterol. 1998;33(10):1047–51.
42. Salles Junior LD, Santos PR, dos Santos AA, de Souza MH. Dyspepsia and gastric emptying in end-stage renal disease patients on hemodialysis. BMC Nephrol. 2013;14:275.
43. Shirazian S, Radhakrishnan J. Gastrointestinal disorders and renal failure: exploring the connection. Nat Rev Nephrol. 2010;6(8):480–92.
44. Silang R, Regalado M, Cheng TH, Wesson DE. Prokinetic agents increase plasma albumin in hypoalbuminemic chronic dialysis patients with delayed gastric emptying. Am J Kidney Dis. 2001;37(2):287–93.
45. Neild GH. Life expectancy with chronic kidney disease: an educational review. Pediatr Nephrol. 2017;32(2):243–8.
46. Chesnaye NC, Schaefer F, Groothoff JW, Bonthuis M, Reusz G, Heaf JG, et al. Mortality risk in European children with end-stage renal disease on dialysis. Kidney Int. 2016;89(6):1355–62.
47. Mitsnefes MM, Laskin BL, Dahhou M, Zhang X, Foster BJ. Mortality risk among children initially treated with dialysis for end-stage kidney disease, 1990–2010. JAMA. 2013;309(18):1921–9.
48. McDonald SP, Craig JC. Long-term survival of children with end-stage renal disease. N Engl J Med. 2004;350(26):2654–62.
49. Banerjee D. Sudden cardiac death in haemodialysis: clinical epidemiology and mechanisms. J Electrocardiol. 2016;49(6):843–7.
50. Krishnasamy R, Badve SV, Hawley CM, McDonald SP, Boudville N, Brown FG, et al. Daily variation in death in patients treated by long-term dialysis: comparison of in-center hemodialysis to peritoneal and home hemodialysis. Am J Kidney Dis. 61(1):96–103.

51. Foley RN, Gilbertson DT, Murray T, Collins AJ. Long interdialytic interval and mortality among patients receiving hemodialysis. N Engl J Med. 2011;365(12):1099–107.
52. Springel T, Laskin B, Shults J, Keren R, Furth S. Longer interdialytic interval and cause-specific hospitalization in children receiving chronic dialysis. Nephrol Dial Transplant. 2013;28(10):2628–36.
53. McCullough PA, Chan CT, Weinhandl ED, Burkart JM, Bakris GL. Intensive hemodialysis, left ventricular hypertrophy, and cardiovascular disease. Am J Kidney Dis. 2016;68(5S1):S5–S14.
54. Chavers BM, Solid CA, Daniels FX, Chen S-C, Collins AJ, Frankenfield DL, et al. Hypertension in pediatric long-term hemodialysis patients in the United States. Clin J Am Soc Nephrol. 2009;4(8):1363–9.
55. Glassock RJ, Pecoits-Filho R, Barberato SH. Left ventricular mass in chronic kidney disease and ESRD. Clin J Am Soc Nephrol. 2009;4(Supplement 1):S79–91.
56. Flynn JT, Kaelber DC, Baker-Smith CM, Blowey D, Carroll AE, Daniels SR, et al. Clinical practice guideline for screening and management of high blood pressure in children and adolescents. Pediatrics. 2017;140(3):e20171904.
57. Dionne JM. Evidence-based guidelines for the management of hypertension in children with chronic kidney disease. Pediatr Nephrol. 2015;30(11):1919–27.
58. Lurbe E, Agabiti-Rosei E, Cruickshank JK, Dominiczak A, Erdine S, Hirth A, et al. 2016 European Society of Hypertension guidelines for the management of high blood pressure in children and adolescents. J Hypertens. 2016;34(10):1887–920.
59. Chaudhuri A, Sutherland SM, Begin B, Salsbery K, McCabe L, Potter D, et al. Role of twenty-four-hour ambulatory blood pressure monitoring in children on dialysis. Clin J Am Soc Nephrol. 2011;6(4):870–6.
60. KDOQI W. K/DOQI clinical practice guidelines for cardiovascular disease in dialysis patients. Am J Kidney Dis. 2005;45(4 Suppl 3):S1-153.
61. Agarwal R, Sinha AD. Cardiovascular protection with antihypertensive drugs in dialysis patients. Syst Rev Meta-Anal. 2009;53(5):860–6.
62. Heerspink HJL, Ninomiya T, Zoungas S, de Zeeuw D, Grobbee DE, Jardine MJ, et al. Effect of lowering blood pressure on cardiovascular events and mortality in patients on dialysis: a systematic review and meta-analysis of randomised controlled trials. Lancet. 2009;373(9668):1009–15.
63. Efrati S, Zaidenstein R, Dishy V, Beberashvili I, Sharist M, Averbukh Z, et al. ACE inhibitors and survival of hemodialysis patients. Am J Kidney Dis. 2002;40(5):1023–9.
64. Tai DJ, Lim TW, James MT, Manns BJ, Tonelli M, Hemmelgarn BR, et al. Cardiovascular effects of angiotensin converting enzyme inhibition or angiotensin receptor blockade in hemodialysis: a meta-analysis. Clin J Am Soc Nephrol. 2010;5(4):623–30.
65. Sorof JM, Brewer ED, Portman RJ. Ambulatory blood pressure monitoring and interdialytic weight gain in children receiving chronic hemodialysis. Am J Kidney Dis. 1999;33(4):667–74.
66. Candan C, Sever L, Civilibal M, Caliskan S, Arisoy N. Blood volume monitoring to adjust dry weight in hypertensive pediatric hemodialysis patients. Pediatr Nephrol. 2009;24(3):581–7.
67. Patel HP, Goldstein SL, Mahan JD, Smith B, Fried CB, Currier H, et al. A standard, noninvasive monitoring of hematocrit algorithm improves blood pressure control in pediatric hemodialysis patients. Clin J Am Soc Nephrol. 2007;2(2):252–7.
68. Moe S, Drueke T, Cunningham J, Goodman W, Martin K, Olgaard K, et al. Definition, evaluation, and classification of renal osteodystrophy: a position statement from kidney disease: improving global outcomes (KDIGO). Kidney Int. 2006;69(11):1945–53.
69. Hanudel MR, Salusky IB. Treatment of pediatric chronic kidney disease-mineral and bone disorder. Curr Osteoporos Rep. 2017;15(3):198–206.
70. Kidney Disease: Improving Global Outcomes (KDIGO) CKD-MBD Update Work Group. KDIGO 2017 clinical practice guideline update for the diagnosis, evaluation, prevention, and treatment of Chronic Kidney Disease–Mineral and Bone Disorder (CKD-MBD). Kidney Int Suppl. 2017;7:1–59.
71. NKF. K/DOQI clinical practice guidelines for bone metabolism and disease in children with chronic kidney disease. Am J Kidney Dis. 2005;46:S1–S122.

72. NKF. K/DOQI clinical practice guidelines for nutrition in children with chronic kidney disease: 2008 update. Am J Kidney Dis. 2009;53:S1–123.
73. Wesseling-Perry K, Salusky IB. Phosphate binders, vitamin D and calcimimetics in the management of chronic kidney disease–mineral bone disorders (CKD-MBD) in children. Pediatr Nephrol. 2013;28(4):617–25.
74. Hahn D, Hodson EM, Craig JC. Interventions for metabolic bone disease in children with chronic kidney disease. Cochrane Database Syst Rev 2015;(11): CD008327. DOI: https://doi.org/10.1002/14651858.CD008327.pub2. p. 1–92.
75. Gonzalez E, Schomberg J, Amin N, Salusky IB, Zaritsky J. Sevelamer carbonate increases serum bicarbonate in pediatric dialysis patients. Pediatr Nephrol. 2010;25(2):373–5.
76. Pieper AK, Haffner D, Hoppe B, Dittrich K, Offner G, Bonzel KE, et al. A randomized crossover trial comparing sevelamer with calcium acetate in children with CKD. Am J Kidney Dis. 2006;47(4):625–35.
77. Fosrenol (lanthanum carbonate) [package insert]. Wayne: Shire US; 2011.
78. Spasovski GB, Sikole A, Gelev S, Masin-Spasovska J, Freemont T, Webster I, et al. Evolution of bone and plasma concentration of lanthanum in dialysis patients before, during 1 year of treatment with lanthanum carbonate and after 2 years of follow-up. Nephrol Dial Transplant. 2006;21(8):2217–24.
79. Salusky IB, Goodman WG, Sahney S, Gales B, Perilloux A, Wang HJ, et al. Sevelamer controls parathyroid hormone-induced bone disease as efficiently as calcium carbonate without increasing serum calcium levels during therapy with active vitamin D sterols. J Am Soc Nephrol. 2005;16(8):2501–8.
80. Ballinger AE, Palmer SC, Nistor I, Craig JC, Strippoli GFM. Calcimimetics for secondary hyperparathyroidism in chronic kidney disease patients. Cochrane Database Syst Rev 2014;(12): CD006254. DOI: https://doi.org/10.1002/14651858.CD006254.pub2. p. 1–84.
81. Muscheites J, Wigger M, Drueckler E, Fischer DC, Kundt G, Haffner D. Cinacalcet for secondary hyperparathyroidism in children with end-stage renal disease. Pediatr Nephrol. 2008;23(10):1823–9.
82. Padhi D, Langman CB, Fathallah-Shaykh S, Warady BA, Salusky IB, Lee E, et al. An open-label study to evaluate a single-dose of cinacalcet in pediatric dialysis subjects. Pediatr Nephrol. 2012;27(10):1953–9.
83. Platt C, Inward C, McGraw M, Dudley J, Tizard J, Burren C, et al. Middle-term use of cinacalcet in paediatric dialysis patients. Pediatr Nephrol. 2010;25(1):143–8.
84. Silverstein DM, Kher KK, Moudgil A, Khurana M, Wilcox J, Moylan K. Cinacalcet is efficacious in pediatric dialysis patients. Pediatr Nephrol. 2008;23(10):1817–22.
85. Kim J, Ross JS, Kapczynski A. Pediatric exclusivity and regulatory authority: implications of amgen v hhs. JAMA. 2018;319(1):21–2.
86. Wong H, Mylrea K, Feber J, Drukker A, Filler G. Prevalence of complications in children with chronic kidney disease according to KDOQI. Kidney Int. 2006;70(3):585–90.
87. Chavers BM, Roberts TL, Herzog CA, Collins AJ, St Peter WL. Prevalence of anemia in erythropoietin-treated pediatric as compared to adult chronic dialysis patients. Kidney Int. 2004;65(1):266–73.
88. Donnelly S. Why is erythropoietin made in the kidney? The kidney functions as a critmeter. Am J Kidney Dis. 2001;38(2):415–25.
89. Atkinson MA, Furth SL. Anemia in children with chronic kidney disease. Nat Rev Nephrol. 2011;7(11):635–41.
90. Nissenson AR, Strobos J. Iron deficiency in patients with renal failure. Kidney Int Suppl. 1999;69:S18–21.
91. Warady BA, Ho M. Morbidity and mortality in children with anemia at initiation of dialysis. Pediatr Nephrol. 2003;18(10):1055–62.
92. Besarab A, Bolton WK, Browne JK, Egrie JC, Nissenson AR, Okamoto DM, et al. The effects of normal as compared with low hematocrit values in patients with cardiac disease who are receiving hemodialysis and epoetin. N Engl J Med. 1998;339(9):584–90.

93. Parfrey PS, Foley RN, Wittreich BH, Sullivan DJ, Zagari MJ, Frei D. Double-blind comparison of full and partial anemia correction in incident hemodialysis patients without symptomatic heart disease. J Am Soc Nephrol. 2005;16(7):2180–9.
94. Amaral S, Hwang W, Fivush B, Neu A, Frankenfield D, Furth S. Association of mortality and hospitalization with achievement of adult hemoglobin targets in adolescents maintained on hemodialysis. J Am Soc Nephrol. 2006;17(10):2878–85.
95. Rheault MN, Molony JT, Nevins T, Herzog CA, Chavers BM. Hemoglobin of 12 g/dl and above is not associated with increased cardiovascular morbidity in children on hemodialysis. Kidney Int. 2017;91(1):177–82.
96. Gerson A, Hwang W, Fiorenza J, Barth K, Kaskel F, Weiss L, et al. Anemia and health-related quality of life in adolescents with chronic kidney disease. Am J Kidney Dis. 2004;44(6):1017–23.
97. Van Damme-Lombaerts R, Broyer M, Businger J, Baldauf C, Stocker H. A study of recombinant human erythropoietin in the treatment of anaemia of chronic renal failure in children on haemodialysis. Pediatr Nephrol. 1994;8(3):338–42.
98. Kidney Disease: Improving Global Outcomes (KDIGO) Anemia Work Group. KDIGO clinical practice guideline for anemia in chronic kidney disease. Kidney Int. 2012;2:279–335.
99. Rambod M, Kovesdy CP, Kalantar-Zadeh K. Combined high serum ferritin and low iron saturation in hemodialysis patients: the role of inflammation. Clin J Am Soc Nephrol. 2008;3(6):1691–701.
100. Albaramki J, Hodson EM, Craig JC, Webster AC. Parenteral versus oral iron therapy for adults and children with chronic kidney disease. Cochrane Database Syst Rev (Online). 2012;1:CD007857.
101. Pandey R, Daloul R, Coyne DW. Iron treatment strategies in dialysis-dependent CKD. Semin Nephrol. 2016;36(2):105–11.
102. Obrador GT, Macdougall IC. Effect of red cell transfusions on future kidney transplantation. Clin J Am Soc Nephrol. 2013;8(5):852–60.
103. Warady BA, Arar MY, Lerner G, Nakanishi AM, Stehman-Breen C. Darbepoetin alfa for the treatment of anemia in pediatric patients with chronic kidney disease. Pediatr Nephrol. 2006;21(8):1144–52.
104. De Palo T, Giordano M, Palumbo F, Bellantuono R, Messina G, Colella V, et al. Clinical experience with darbepoetin alfa (NESP) in children undergoing hemodialysis. Pediatr Nephrol. 2004;19(3):337–40.
105. Warady BA, Silverstein DM. Management of anemia with erythropoietic-stimulating agents in children with chronic kidney disease. Pediatr Nephrol. 2014;29(9):1493–505.
106. Chavers BM, Molony JT, Solid CA, Rheault MN, Collins AJ. One-year mortality rates in US children with end-stage renal disease. Am J Nephrol. 2015;41(2):121–8.
107. Samuel SM, Tonelli MA, Foster BJ, Alexander RT, Nettel-Aguirre A, Soo A, et al. Survival in pediatric dialysis and transplant patients. Clin J Am Soc Nephrol. 2011;6(5):1094–9.

Chapter 11
Peritoneal Dialysis in Adolescents with End-Stage Renal Disease

Maha N. Haddad and Arundhati Kale

Introduction

Adolescents with end-stage renal disease (ESRD) who are in need of renal replacement therapy have a choice between renal transplantation, hemodialysis (HD), and peritoneal dialysis (PD). Preemptive renal transplantation is the best option for treatment of ESRD in children and adolescents as it is associated with a survival benefit [1]. However, dialysis may have to be initiated in some patients who are not ready for transplant. Hemodialysis is the most common initial dialysis modality in older children. Peritoneal dialysis use has a lot of advantages. Despite that, not every patient is a candidate for peritoneal dialysis. To qualify for peritoneal dialysis, the patient's peritoneal membrane must have an adequate surface area for diffusion and ultrafiltration, the patient must have a support person or family member at home who can learn PD, and the house environment must have adequate space for the patient and the supplies.

There are pros and cons for choosing PD, especially in this age group. The pros of PD include maintenance of a regular day schedule, ability to attend school and participate in sports activities, laxity in diet restrictions compared to hemodialysis, avoidance of vascular access (which may be easily visible to friends), and better preservation of residual renal function [2]. The need for nightly dialysis treatments which may interfere in late-night social activities and the patient's freedom to attend sleepovers are cons of this treatment. The decision to start PD is made after involving

M. N. Haddad (✉)
Department of Pediatric Nephrology, UC Davis Medical Center, Sacramento, CA, USA
e-mail: mnhaddad@ucdavis.edu

A. Kale
Section of Nephrology, UC Davis Medical Center, Sacramento, CA, USA

M. N. Haddad et al. (eds.), *Adolescents with Chronic Kidney Disease*,
https://doi.org/10.1007/978-3-319-97220-6_11

the patient and family in a frank discussion of these advantages and constraints. This chapter will review the epidemiology of peritoneal dialysis, the physiologic basis and practical aspects of this treatment, and the potential complications and patient outcomes.

Epidemiology

According to the 2016 US Renal Data System (USRDS) annual report, the incidence of ESRD in children declined between 2008 and 2014 [3]. In 2014, newly diagnosed patients with ESRD were 6% less than the previous year. The point prevalence of children with ESRD as of December 31, 2014, was 9721, a 1.6% decline from the previous year. Peritoneal dialysis is the most common initial treatment modality in children younger than 9 years and those who weigh less than 20 kg [4], whereas hemodialysis is the most common initial modality for children 9.5 years and older [3].

Transplant has become the most prevalent ESRD treatment modality in children. Of the 9721 children and adolescents between the ages of 0 and 21 years with prevalent ESRD as of December 31, 2013, kidney transplant was the most common modality (70.2%), followed by hemodialysis (18.0%) and peritoneal dialysis (11.5%) [3]. This was a similar pattern from the previous year [5].

Anatomy and Physiology of the Peritoneal Membrane

The surface area of the peritoneal membrane is close to the body surface area; hence solute and water exchange between the capillaries supplying the epithelium and dialysate is relatively easily accomplished in most patients. Peritoneal capillary blood flow is between 100 and 150 ml/min in adults. Physiologically, the exchange of solutes and water occurs by three mechanisms: diffusion, convection, and osmosis. Diffusion occurs via pores in the peritoneal membrane which are of three sizes; the largest are >20 nm in diameter and few in number, the small pores (4–6 nm) are the majority and are responsible for solute clearance, the ultrasmall pores are the fewest in number and responsible for >50% of water clearance [6]. Diffusion depends on the surface area of the peritoneum, the size of the molecules, and the permeability of the membrane. Diffusion of solutes from higher concentration in the blood to dialysate occurs during an exchange, and water is excreted by creating an osmotic gradient between the dialysate and blood. The osmotic agent in most dialysis fluids is dextrose; however, a glucose polymer like icodextrin can also be used. There is a two-way exchange between the blood and dialysate, and movement of solutes and water stops when equilibrium is reached; the time at which this occurs depends on the transport characteristics of the peritoneal membrane and determines the optimal dwell time for the patient. Net ultrafiltration (UF) is the difference between water absorbed by the peritoneum via the capillaries and lymphatics and dialysate volume at the end of a cycle. This can be expressed by the following equation [7]:

$$J_F = K_f\left(\left[P_c + s_f\right] - \left[p_c + P_f\right]\right)$$

where:

K_f = peritoneal membrane permeability coefficient
P_c = hydraulic pressure in the capillary
s_f = osmotic pressure of the peritoneal fluid
p_c = oncotic pressure in the capillary
P_f = hydraulic pressure of the fluid under flux

Both osmotic and concentration gradients are maintained by frequent exchange of dialysate. Since the surface area of the peritoneum is important in this exchange, any process that limits this will decreases the efficacy of the treatment. Such processes include the presence of adhesions or fibrosis, which may occur secondary to peritonitis or long-term dialysis (especially with higher dextrose solutions).

Equipment

Catheters For the performance of efficient peritoneal dialysis, of utmost importance is a properly placed catheter. Catheters of various sizes are available; however the choice is somewhat limited in the pediatric age group. The best success is achieved when the catheter is placed by an experienced surgeon; at many institutions, a few dedicated surgeons are identified for dialysis access placement. Patients with ostomies require planning to make sure that the exit site is farthest from the ostomy in order to prevent infection of the catheter. From the cosmetic point of view in teenagers, an exit site below the belt line will be more acceptable to the patient. A downward-facing exit site and the use of double-cuffed Swan neck tunnel along with a preoperative dose of antibiotics have been shown to decrease the incidence of peritonitis [8]. Laparoscopy is frequently used to place the catheter under direct visualization. Typically, partial or complete omentectomy is performed at the same time to avoid catheter occlusion; more recently other procedures like omental folding have been successful [9]. Preoperative antibiotic prophylaxis is generally recommended to decrease the risk of peritonitis. The catheter should be flushed in the OR to ensure good function. Transfer sets with luer-lock connections are safer than spike and port.

Postoperative Care

It is recommended that the dressing on the exit site be left intact for at least 1 week unless it is soiled. The rationale for this is that catheter immobilization allows for a good seal to form which is essential to prevent both exit site and tunnel infections

[8]. Prematurely starting PD before a seal forms results in leakage of fluid that predisposes the patient to infections. The dressing should be changed once a week for the initial 2–3 weeks after the catheter is placed, and PD start should also be delayed for 2 weeks if possible. Occasionally, it is necessary to initiate PD early after catheter placement in which case low dwell volumes are recommended.

Cyclers In a majority of pediatric patients, automated PD is prescribed since most patients in this age group have transport characteristics that require hourly exchanges. Newer cyclers such as the Home Choice Pro® come equipped with memory cards to record treatment data including alarms and missed treatments and provide helpful tools to check compliance in this vulnerable age group.

PD Solutions Commercially available solutions are suitable for achieving clearance and ultrafiltration; most use dextrose as the osmotic agent. Electrolyte and mineral balance is maintained with appropriate composition of these in the dialysate. However, with long-term use, very high glucose concentrations along with glucose degradation products (GDP) and lactate can harm not only the peritoneum but also affect residual renal function [10]. More biocompatible solutions are available in some countries and are generally more expensive than glucose-based solutions.

Training and Support

Once a patient is identified as a candidate for peritoneal dialysis and a catheter has been placed, intensive training for home dialysis is begun. If the patient is an older adolescent and has the capacity to be trained, he/she can be the primary person performing the procedure. However, if the patient is unable to do it, one parent is trained, and home dialysis is not started until both trainer and trainee are confident about the trainee's ability to independently perform the procedure without supervision. It is our recommendation that another family member also be trained as backup for the primary person. Training includes care of the catheter exit site and usually takes 1–2 weeks to complete. A home visit is usually performed by the training nurse prior to catheter placement to ensure that the home is suitable and to make suggestions on storing supplies. The patient/parent is not only trained in the dialysis procedure but also in recognizing common complications of the treatment such as dehydration/fluid overload, exit site or tunnel infection, and, most importantly, early signs of peritonitis. Simple troubleshooting skills are also imparted during the training process to address cycler issues.

PD Types and Treatment Options

PD can be performed in several ways. These can be broadly divided into manual PD and automated PD; a cycler is utilized for the latter. Continuous ambulatory PD or CAPD, which does not require a cycler, is performed by manual exchange of the

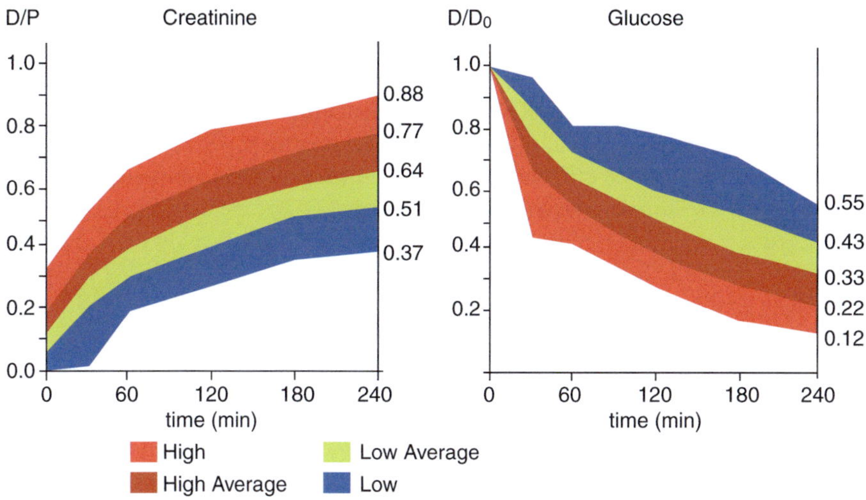

Fig. 11.1 Transporter characteristics plotted according to the standardized peritoneal equilibration test. Clearance of creatinine on the left and glucose on the right that depict high, high average, low average and low transport. D/P: dialysate/plasma ratio; D/D0: actual dialysate to initial dialysate glucose concentration ratio. (With permission from [12])

dialysis solution four to five times a day. CAPD is typically used in the adult population. Most pediatric centers in the USA use CCPD or continuous cycling PD that utilizes an automated machine. With the cycler, many options are available depending on the needs of the patient and based on the transport characteristics of the peritoneal membrane. The transport characteristics are determined by the peritoneal equilibration test (PET), which measures both solute and water transport in a 4-h period. The test has been standardized with the use of 2.5% dextrose at a volume of 1100 ml/m^2 BSA. Dialysate-to-plasma (D/P) ratios of urea, glucose, and creatinine are measured at specific points in time to determine the rate of transport of these chemicals. Baseline levels are drawn at time 0 and then at 2 h and 4 h in plasma and dialysis fluid. Based on these ratios, the patients are determined to be high, high average, low average, and low transporters (Fig. 11.1). While the concentration of urea and creatinine is expected to rise in the dialysate, the opposite occurs with glucose transport. The high transporters require less time to equilibrate, and the low transporters need more time. Based on the ratio, the ideal dwell time can be determined so that maximal efficiency is ascertained.

PD Dose

The standardized dose of the dwell volume is generally 1100 ml/m^2/cycle. Volumes higher than this may increase intra-abdominal pressure leading to discomfort, inguinal hernias, or hydrothorax. Increased hydrostatic pressure in the abdominal cavity may also interfere with transport. Treatment time can be anywhere between 8 and 10 h. Dwell time is determined by the transport characteristics determined by the PET. Approximately 4 weeks after the target prescription is reached, adequacy is determined by calculating the Kt/V_{urea}. For calculating the adequacy, the dialysis effluent is collected in a bag during the prescribed treatment period and thoroughly mixed. Samples from the effluent and blood are then sent for determining the urea, glucose, and creatinine concentrations. Per the KDOQI guidelines, target total Kt/V_{urea} (dialysate + renal) must be at least 1.7 per week [11]. Weekly Kt/V_{urea} can be calculated using the following formula:

$$\left(24\,\mathrm{h}\,D/P\,\mathrm{urea}\times 24\,\mathrm{h}\,\mathrm{dialysate\ volume}\times 7\right)/V$$

where V is the volume of distribution for urea which can be presumed to equal total body water (TBW), D is concentration of urea in the dialysate, and P is plasma urea. For those patients who have urine output >100 ml/day, residual renal clearance of urea is also calculated with a 24-h urine collection.

In addition to the above measurement, determinants of adequate dialysis include a normal hemodynamic state, adequate growth and nutrition, normal electrolyte and mineral balance, school attendance/performance, and a good quality of life for the patient and family.

Complications of Peritoneal Dialysis

Infectious complications are the most common cause for hospitalization [5]. Hospitalizations secondary to peritonitis have increased by 16.5% in 2008–2012 from the preceding 4 years. Infectious complications include exit-site infections, tunnel infections, and peritonitis.

Exit-site infections are infections of the skin and subcutaneous tissue where the catheter exits the abdomen. They are usually caused by bacteria, mostly commonly *Staphylococcus aureus* followed by pseudomonas species [13].

Tunnel infection occurs when the infection extends below and is between the two cuffs. Some centers get an ultrasound evaluation of the tunnel to look for signs of tunnel infection.

Examination of the exit site should include examining for swelling, crust formation, redness of the skin, pain on pressure, and secretion. It is recommended to use an objective score when assessing the exit site. If no swelling, crust, redness, pain on pressure, or secretion is present, each would score a 0, and the total score would be a 0. The score would be a "1" for each measure examined when swelling involves the exit site only, crust is less than 0.5 cm, redness is less than 0.5 cm, there is a presence of slight pain on pressure, and the secretion is serous. The score would be a "2" for each measure examined when swelling includes the tunnel, crust is >0.5 cm, redness is >0.5 cm, pain is severe in pressure, and the secretion is purulent. Thus, the total score can range from 0 to 10 [13].

If the exit site looks normal and the total score is 0, then there is no infection. Exit sites are often colonized with *Staphylococcus epidermidis*, and a positive culture with this bacterium without an inflamed exit site should not be considered an infection.

Treatment of Exit-Site Infections

Prompt diagnosis and treatment of exit-site infections are crucial to prevent peritonitis. If there is erythema of the skin without drainage, extensive exit-site care alone with careful assessment of the exit site may suffice. However, if there is drainage, it is should be sent for culture and gram stain before starting the treatment with oral antibiotics that should then be tailored based on culture and sensitivity results. Antibiotics should be continued till the exit site is back to normal, usually for 2 weeks, or longer if it is caused by pseudomonas species, which is harder to treat, and requires at least 3 weeks of oral antibiotics. The initial choice of the oral antibiotic is based on previous infections and whether or not there is history of MRSA.

Chronic exit-site care should be done using a sterile antiseptic solution. There are differences in practices in chronic exit-site care among centers including the choice of the topical antiseptic cleansing agents and the topical antibiotic used. At our center, we advise patients to do daily exit-site care after taking a shower. We use 3% saline or ExSept (0.114% sodium hypochlorite) followed by the application of the antibacterial agent (mupirocin cream) to prevent infections caused by *S. aureus*. Due to the increased risk of infections with *Pseudomonas aeruginosa* with this practice, some centers opt to use gentamicin as the topical antibacterial agent as it is active against both *S. aureus* and *P. aeruginosa*. However, using gentamicin may result in increased gram-positive peritonitis rates, in addition to the concerns of emerging gentamicin-resistant bacteria.

Acute Peritonitis

Infectious peritonitis is the most frequent complication of peritoneal dialysis in the pediatric population. Peritonitis is the leading cause of hospitalization for patients on PD and is associated with mortality and morbidity, such as having to change the modality to hemodialysis due to irreversible technique failure and the need to change the peritoneal dialysis catheter. There is significant variation in peritonitis rates among centers [14, 15]. The rate of peritonitis has declined over the past several decades. According to the North American Pediatric Renal Trials and Collaborative Studies (NAPRTCS) annual report 2011, the annualized rate of peritonitis was 0.64, or one episode every 18.8 months, and decreased with age to 0.57, or one episode every 21.1 months, in patients over 12 years. The rate of peritonitis is less with the use of double cuffs, swan neck tunnels, and downward exit-site orientation. The risk of peritonitis is also less in nightly PD with no day dwell, as a dry abdomen has the potential of enhancing local peritoneal host defense [16]. The risk of peritonitis is higher in patients on ambulatory peritoneal dialysis compared to automated peritoneal dialysis [16]. Other risk factors for peritonitis include malnutrition, use of gastrostomy tubes, exit-site infection, and touch contamination [15, 17].

Prevention

Care providers of patients on peritoneal dialysis should make every effort to prevent acute peritonitis. In the USA, and in a collaborative effort to reduce peritoneal dialysis complications including peritonitis, SCOPE (Standardizing Care to improve Outcomes in Pediatric End-Stage Renal Disease) was introduced in 2011 [18]. The SCOPE guidelines are comprehensive and include bundle guidelines for surgical insertion of the catheter, patient and caregiver training, and follow-up care (see Tables 11.1, 11.2, and 11.3) [18]. The guidelines recommend using a single dose of first-generation cephalosporin prior to surgery, exit-site orientation in the lateral or downward position, and avoidance of surgical sutures. After surgery, the recommendation is to avoid changing the dressing at the exit site for 7 days after catheter insertion unless it is soiled, to use a sterile procedure for all exit-site dressing changes until the exit site is healed, and to not use the PD catheter for dialysis for at least 14 days postoperatively (Table 11.1). For training, it is recommended that a qualified nurse perform the training and that there be one trainer per trainee. Training should be comprehensive and should cover all elements of aseptic connection and hand hygiene. It should be followed by repeat concept demonstration in follow-up visits (Table 11.2). Follow-up should include emphasis on previously taught techniques (Table 11.3). In a follow-up study on peritonitis rates 36 months after commencing SCOPE guidelines at 24 participating centers, a marked reduction of monthly peritonitis rates was found following compliance with those guidelines. The mean monthly peritonitis rate decreased from 0.63 episodes per patient year

Table 11.1 Peritoneal dialysis catheter insertion bundle

Intraoperative care
PD catheter exit-site orientation is in the lateral or downward position
A single dose of a first-generation cephalosporin is given prior to incision
No sutures are placed at catheter exit site
Postoperative care
Exit-site dressing is not changed for the first 7 postoperative days, unless soiled, loose, or damp and, if changed, conducted by a healthcare professional
Sterile procedure is used for all exit-site dressing changes until the exit site is healed
PD catheter is immobilized until exit site is healed
PD catheter is not used for peritoneal dialysis for at least 14 postoperative days

PD peritoneal dialysis
Adapted from Neu et al. with permission [18].

Table 11.2 Peritoneal dialysis patient and caregiver training bundle

Training performed by a qualified registered nurse
Trainer to trainee (or family) ratio 1:1
Appropriate teaching aides such as photographs, mannequin, or apron used during training
Training should cover all elements specified in ISPD guidelines [8]
Training should include specific procedures for:
Hand hygiene according to the World Health Organization guidelines [31]
Exit-site care
Aseptic connection technique
Post-training concept and demonstration test administered at completion of training and again at 1-month post-training visit
Home visit performed

ISPD International Society of Peritoneal Dialysis
Adapted from Neu et al. with permission [18]

Table 11.3 Peritoneal dialysis catheter/exit-site follow-up care bundle

Objective score of exit site using the International Pediatric Peritoneal Dialysis Network (IPPN) scoring tool
Review key aspects of each of the following:
Hand hygiene
Exit-site care
Aseptic technique
Query for touch contaminations or other break in aseptic technique and whether they were treated according to ISPD guidelines
Repeat concept and demonstration test administered every 6 months
Patient/caregiver receives training after a peritonitis episode

Items to be included at each monthly visit
Adapted from Neu et al. with permission [18]

prelaunch to 0.43 episodes per patient year postlaunch [19]. A similar conclusion was reported when studying 734 children from 29 centers [17].

In addition, the Consensus Guidelines for the Prevention and Treatment of Catheter-Related Infections and Peritonitis in Pediatric Patients Receiving Peritoneal Dialysis (International Society of Peritoneal Dialysis (ISPD) guidelines) were published in 2012 [8]. These recommendations echo the SCOPE guidelines and include guidelines on training, catheter type and treatment, early exit-site care, chronic exit-site care, connectology, contamination, care of ostomy patients, diagnosis of PD-related peritonitis, antibiotic treatment, and the use of adjunctive prophylactic antibiotic therapy [8].

Causative Organisms of Peritonitis

There are global variations in the causative agents and their antibiotic susceptibility [14]. This should be taken into consideration when initiating empiric antibiotic therapy while waiting for culture results. The majority of peritonitis episodes in children are caused by gram-positive bacteria, followed by gram-negative bacteria and culture-negative peritonitis, though the order is different in different studies [20]. Fungal peritonitis is rare accounting for 5–7% of peritonitis episodes, whereas culture-negative peritonitis accounts for about 20% of all peritonitis episodes [17].

Presentation and Diagnosis of Peritonitis Clinicians should have high suspicion for peritonitis, and it should be ruled out as soon as possible. It should be ruled out on the sole basis of a cloudy effluent and if the patient develops signs and symptoms, such as abdominal pain, vomiting, anorexia, chills, and fever. If left untreated, peritonitis can result in septic shock. The peritoneal sample should be sent for cell count, gram stain, and culture. Empiric diagnosis should be made if the white cell count of the effluent is over 100/mm3 and over 50% of the WBCs are polymorphonuclear cells [8].

Other causes for cloudy effluent include eosinophilia, chemical peritonitis, hemoperitoneum, and rarely chylous effluent or if the specimen is taken from a dry peritoneum [21].

Treatment of Acute Peritonitis

Intraperitoneal antibiotics should be used when possible to treat infectious peritonitis as intraperitoneal administration results in higher antibiotic concentration in the peritoneal cavity. Initial antibiotic choice should cover gram-positive and gram-negative organisms. ISPD guidelines recommend the use of cefepime monotherapy as a starting agent if it is available [8]. Other choices include using a combination of a first-generation cephalosporin and a third-generation cephalosporin or an aminoglycoside. If there is history of previous methicillin-resistant *S. aureus*, use of vancomycin plus a third-generation cephalosporin or an aminoglycoside is recommended. When vancomycin and aminoglycosides are used, drug levels should be monitored to prevent toxicity due to systemic absorption. Intraperitoneal antibiotics can be given intermittently with a long dwell (4–6 h) or continuously by adding them to each exchange [8].

If the gram stain is positive for fungus, antifungal therapy should be promptly initiated, with preparation for catheter removal.

Fungal prophylaxis is recommended for the duration of the antibiotic therapy to reduce the risk of fungal peritonitis. This can be accomplished by the use of either oral nystatin or oral fluconazole.

Antibiotic therapy should be tailored according to the results of culture and sensitivity of the organism.

Removal of the catheter is indicated in relapsing peritonitis, in fungal or mycobacterial peritonitis, or if the peritonitis is not responding to treatment.

In a study examining data from the International Pediatric Peritonitis Registry (IPPR), 11% of non-fungal peritonitis episodes were followed by a relapse [22]. Peritonitis relapse was defined as recurrence of peritonitis with the same organism within 4 weeks after completion of antibiotic treatment. No significant difference was found in the spectrum of causative organisms in relapsing peritonitis and non-relapsing peritonitis episodes [22].

Noninfectious Complications of PD

Noninfectious complications include hemoperitoneum, herniation (including incisional, inguinal, and umbilical) from the increased intraperitoneal pressure, fluid leaks, and hydrothorax [23]. Hydrothorax results from a communication between the peritoneal and pleural spaces. It is recommended to surgically fix the hernias once identified and use small fill volumes in the postoperative period until the incision heals.

In adolescent females, the effluent can become bloody during menses. Adolescent females should be reassured if they experience that.

Peritoneal Access Complications

Peritoneal dialysis revisions are common in pediatric patients. Mechanical dysfunction of the peritoneal catheter is a major cause for access revision and can occur due to omental obstruction, migration of the catheter tip, or catheter blockage by fibrin or blood clots. In a study examining data from the International Pediatric Peritoneal Dialysis Network Registry (IPDN), the overall access revision was 0.14 per treatment year, and the majority of access revisions were reported within the 1st year of peritoneal dialysis treatment with good catheter survival rates [24]. Young age, presence of ostomies, the use of swan neck catheter with curled intraperitoneal portion, and the diagnosis of congenital anomalies of the kidney and urinary tract were risk factors for access revision [24]. Other complications include leak, catheter cracking and erosion, and cuff extrusion. Overall complications were associated with longer presence of the PD catheter [25]. While some studies suggested that omentectomy decreased the risk of obstruction, other studies found that obstruction occurred independent of omentectomy [26].

Encapsulating peritoneal sclerosis, where the peritoneal membrane becomes thickened and fibrotic, is a rare but serious complication that is associated with significant morbidity and mortality. It is characterized by loss of mesothelial cells, thickening of the submesothelial layer, and angiogenesis. In a survey study done over 10 years by the European Pediatric Dialysis working group, the prevalence was 1.5% or 8.7 per 1000 patient years on PD. [27] Encapsulating peritoneal sclerosis can result in membrane failure and intestinal obstruction. It is thought to be caused by inflammation triggered by chronic exposure of the peritoneal membrane to the hypertonic dialysis solutions, although the exact cause remains unclear [28].

Outcome

The 1-year all-cause mortality rate for patients with ESRD has improved with time [5]. For the 2008–2012 era, the mortality rate was 36/1000 years for 18–21-year-olds and was 14 and 12 for the 14–17-year-olds and 10–13 year-olds, respectively. When adjusted to modality, the mortality rate was 35/1000 years for patients on peritoneal dialysis and 11 and 46 for transplant patients and hemodialysis patients, respectively, demonstrating the transplant has superior survival than either of the dialysis modalities.

In a study that examined the survival of adolescents (age 12–19 years) who began ESRD therapy during adolescence from 1978 to 2002, the authors found that the 10-year survival was better for later cohorts, younger adolescents, transplant recipients and preemptive transplant recipients, males, and Caucasian and Asian patients [29].

The 1-year cardiovascular mortality is 3/1000 patient years for PD patients, and the infection mortality is 2/1000 patient years. The risk of mortality due to infection is highest in infants, while the risk of cardiovascular mortality increases with age [30].

References

1. Amaral S, Sayed BA, Kutner N, Patzer RE. Preemptive kidney transplantation is associated with survival benefits among pediatric patients with end-stage renal disease. Kidney Int. 2016;90(5):1100–8.
2. Fischbach M, Terzic J, Menouer S, Soulami K, Dangelser C, Helmstetter A, et al. Effects of automated peritoneal dialysis on residual daily urinary volume in children. Adv Perit Dial. 2001;17:269–73.
3. United States Renal Data System USRDS Chapter 8: ESRD among children, adolescents, and young adults. 2016.
4. Saran R, Robinson B, Abbott KC, Agodoa LYC, Albertus P, Ayanian J, et al. US renal data system 2016 annual data report: epidemiology of kidney disease in the United States. Am J Kidney Dis. 2017;69(3)
5. United States Renal Data System. 2015 USRDS annual data report: epidemiology of kidney disease in the United States. National Institute of heath; National Institute of Diabetes and Digestive and Kidney Diseases. 2015. Bethesda, MD.
6. Haraldsson B. Assessing the peritoneal dialysis capacities of individual patients. Kidney Int. 1995;47(4):1187–98.
7. Ahmad S. Manual of clinical dialysis. London: Science Press; 1999.
8. Warady BA, Bakkaloglu S, Newland J, Cantwell M, Verrina E, Neu A, et al. Consensus guidelines for the prevention and treatment of catheter-related infections and peritonitis in pediatric patients receiving peritoneal dialysis: 2012 update. Perit Dial Int. 2012;32(Suppl 2):S32–86.
9. Goh YH. Omental folding: a novel laparoscopic technique for salvaging peritoneal dialysis catheters. Perit Dial Int. 2008;28(6):626–31.
10. Haag-Weber M, Kramer R, Haake R, Islam MS, Prischl F, Haug U, et al. Low-GDP fluid (Gambrosol trio) attenuates decline of residual renal function in PD patients: a prospective randomized study. Nephrol Dial Transplant. 2010;25(7):2288–96.

11. Neu AM, Ho PL, McDonald RA, Warady BA. Chronic dialysis in children and adolescents. The 2001 NAPRTCS annual report. Pediatr Nephrol. 2002;17(8):656–63.
12. Warady BA, Alexander SR, Hossli S, Vonesh E, Geary D, Watkins S, et al. Peritoneal membrane transport function in children receiving long-term dialysis. J Am Soc Nephrol. 1996;7(11):2385–91.
13. Schaefer F, Klaus G, Muller-Wiefel DE, Mehls O. Intermittent versus continuous intraperitoneal glycopeptide/ceftazidime treatment in children with peritoneal dialysis-associated peritonitis. The Mid-European Pediatric Peritoneal Dialysis Study Group (MEPPS). J Am Soc Nephrol. 1999;10(1):136–45.
14. Schaefer F, Feneberg R, Aksu N, Donmez O, Sadikoglu B, Alexander SR, et al. Worldwide variation of dialysis-associated peritonitis in children. Kidney Int. 2007;72(11):1374–9.
15. North American Pediatric Renal Trials and Collabortive Studies 2011. NAPRTCS 2011 Annual Dialysis Report. https://web.emmes.com/study/ped/annlrept/annualrept2011.pdf
16. Ramalakshmi S, Bernardini J, Piraino B. Nightly intermittent peritoneal dialysis to initiate peritoneal dialysis. Adv Perit Dial. 2003;19:111–4.
17. Sethna CB, Bryant K, Munshi R, Warady BA, Richardson T, Lawlor J, et al. Risk factors for and outcomes of catheter-associated peritonitis in children: the SCOPE collaborative. Clin J Am Soc Nephrol. 2016;11(9):1590–6.
18. Neu AM, Miller MR, Stuart J, Lawlor J, Richardson T, Martz K, et al. Design of the standardizing care to improve outcomes in pediatric end stage renal disease collaborative. Pediatr Nephrol. 2014;29(9):1477–84.
19. Neu AM, Richardson T, Lawlor J, Stuart J, Newland J, McAfee N, et al. Implementation of standardized follow-up care significantly reduces peritonitis in children on chronic peritoneal dialysis. Kidney Int. 2016;89(6):1346–54.
20. Warady BA, Feneberg R, Verrina E, Flynn JT, Muller-Wiefel DE, Besbas N, et al. Peritonitis in children who receive long-term peritoneal dialysis: a prospective evaluation of therapeutic guidelines. J Am Soc Nephrol. 2007;18(7):2172–9.
21. Li PK, Szeto CC, Piraino B, Bernardini J, Figueiredo AE, Gupta A, et al. Peritoneal dialysis-related infections recommendations: 2010 update. Perit Dial Int. 2010;30(4):393–423.
22. Lane JC, Warady BA, Feneberg R, Majkowski NL, Watson AR, Fischbach M, et al. Relapsing peritonitis in children who undergo chronic peritoneal dialysis: a prospective study of the international pediatric peritonitis registry. Clin J Am Soc Nephrol. 2010;5(6):1041–6.
23. van Asseldonk JP, Schroder CH, Severijnen RS, de Jong MC, Monnens LA. Infectious and surgical complications of childhood continuous ambulatory peritoneal dialysis. Eur J Pediatr. 1992;151(5):377–80.
24. Borzych-Duzalka D, Aki TF, Azocar M, White C, Harvey E, Mir S, et al. Peritoneal Dialysis access revision in children: causes, interventions, and outcomes. Clin J Am Soc Nephrol. 2017;12(1):105–12.
25. Stewart CL, Acker SN, Pyle LL, Kulungowski A, Cadnapaphornchai M, Bruny JL, et al. Factors associated with peritoneal dialysis catheter complications in children. J Pediatr Surg. 2016;51(1):159–62.
26. Radtke J, Schild R, Reismann M, Ridwelski RR, Kempf C, Nashan B, et al. Obstruction of peritoneal dialysis catheter is associated with catheter type and independent of omentectomy: a comparative data analysis from a transplant surgical and a pediatric surgical department. J Pediatr Surg 2018;53(4):640–3.
27. Shroff R, Stefanidis CJ, Askiti V, Edefonti A, Testa S, Ekim M, et al. Encapsulating peritoneal sclerosis in children on chronic PD: a survey from the European Paediatric Dialysis Working Group. Nephrol Dial Transplant. 2013;28(7):1908–14.
28. Brown EA, Bargman J, van Biesen W, Chang MY, Finkelstein FO, Hurst H, et al. Length of time on peritoneal dialysis and encapsulating peritoneal sclerosis – position paper for ISPD: 2017 update. Perit Dial Int. 2017;37(4):362–74.
29. Ferris ME, Gipson DS, Kimmel PL, Eggers PW. Trends in treatment and outcomes of survival of adolescents initiating end-stage renal disease care in the United States of America. Pediatr Nephrol. 2006;21(7):1020–6.

30. Weaver DJ, Somers MJG, Martz K, Mitsnefes MM. Clinical outcomes and survival in pediatric patients initiating chronic dialysis: a report of the NAPRTCS registry. Pediatr Nephrol. 2017;32(12):2319–30.
31. Pittet D, Allegranzi B, Boyce J. World Health Organization world alliance for patient safety first global patient safety challenge Core Group of E. The World Health Organization guidelines on hand hygiene in health care and their consensus recommendations. Infect Control Hosp Epidemiol. 2009;30(7):611–22.

Chapter 12
Kidney Transplant in Adolescents: Medical Aspects

Jessica Brennan and Paul Brakeman

Introduction

In the United States, 783 patients ages 11–17 were transplanted in 2017 representing about 40% of all pediatric kidney transplants [1]. For these adolescent patients with end-stage renal disease (ESRD), renal transplantation usually represents the best treatment modality in terms of cognitive and social outcomes, as well as survival [2, 3]. Recent data demonstrates that an 11–17-year-old on the kidney transplant waiting list is approximately twice as likely to die as an 11–17-year-old with a kidney transplant [4]. In addition, evaluation of the quality of life of adolescent kidney transplant recipients post-transplant demonstrates a quality of life that is similar to healthy controls and substantially higher than adolescent patients with chronic kidney disease (CKD) [5, 6]. However, an unsuccessful transplant that fails after only a few years represents a missed medical opportunity as well as ultimately likely shortening the lifespan of an adolescent patient. Here we describe strategies for pre-, peri-, and post-transplant care directed at achieving medically and socially successful transplant outcomes for adolescent patients.

J. Brennan
Division of Transplant, Department of Surgery, University of California, San Francisco, CA, USA
e-mail: Jessica.Brennan@ucsf.edu

P. Brakeman (✉)
Department of Pediatrics, UCSF Benioff Children's Hospital San Francisco, University of California, San Francisco, San Francisco, CA, USA
e-mail: Paul.Brakeman@ucsf.edu

M. N. Haddad et al. (eds.), *Adolescents with Chronic Kidney Disease*,
https://doi.org/10.1007/978-3-319-97220-6_12

Pre-transplant Medical Considerations

Pre-transplant Evaluation

Renal transplantation generally is indicated for adolescents with end-stage renal disease on dialysis and referral to a pediatric transplant center for evaluation for kidney transplant should occur for all pediatric patients on dialysis. Adolescent patients with chronic kidney should be evaluated and listed to accrue wait-list time and to prepare the patient medically, socially, and psychologically with a goal to perform preemptive transplantation thereby avoiding dialysis. At our center, we generally evaluate and list patients with chronic kidney disease once their estimated or measured glomerular filtration rate (GFR) drops below 30 ml/min/1.73 m^2. Some kidney disease progresses very rapidly, and those patients with very rapid decline of GFR should be evaluated while their GFR is >30 ml/min/1.73 m^2 to allow for pre-emptive transplantation. The speed at which a center can prepare a living kidney donor for donation also factors into when patients should be evaluated to achieve preemptive transplantation. Early evaluation of donors may help to achieve preemptive transplantation; however, if performed too soon, some donor work-up testing may need to be repeated with increased expense and potentially with some increased risk to the donor if the donor evaluation occurs well before a recipient is ready for transplantation.

The pre-transplant work-up for the adolescent patient shares many similarities with the work-up for an adult candidate. The goals of the pre-transplant evaluation are to educate the teen and family about the entire renal transplant process and identify and treat any comorbid conditions that may affect patient or graft survival. Some variations exist among transplant centers about who makes up the transplant team. The Centers for Medicare and Medicaid Services (CMS) mandates that a pediatric nephrologist, surgeon, nurse, social worker, and dietician evaluate potential candidates. In addition, pediatric centers may enlist help from child psychology, infectious disease, pharmacy, and anesthesia during the evaluation process. A multidisciplinary approach is indispensable to provide complete care for adolescent patients and their families.

Specific attention must be paid to the unique cognitive-behavioral characteristics of the adolescent patient with advanced CKD approaching kidney transplant. Neurocognitive maturation is not yet complete in the adolescent brain; in addition, ESRD patients are at a risk for cognitive impairment and lower intellectual function [7]. A thorough assessment by a medical social worker and child psychologist is essential to better understand the intellectual abilities of the teen and to estimate the ability to achieve adherence and success with a kidney transplant. Teaching should be at the appropriate level for both the teen and caregivers. Adolescents have a greater understanding of their prognosis compared to younger patients; yet they may not have the coping skills of adult patients. Providing age-appropriate education can help alleviate anxiety and foster the initiation of positive health-related proficiencies [8].

A pre-transplant assessment of predictors for medication nonadherence, including African-American race, male gender, close proximity to the transplant center, and legal issues, can be used to identify high-risk patients who require intensive support [9]. It is also important to evaluate for substance use or abuse during the pre-transplant process. In our program, active substance use is a contraindication for transplantation. The topic of medication nonadherence is addressed in further detail in a different chapter.

The recipient will undergo multiple laboratory tests and studies to test for suitability. Standard lab tests are listed in Table 12.1. A standard panel of tests includes chest X-ray, EKG, and echocardiogram for hypertensive patients or known cardiac abnormalities. Additionally every candidate should have a PPD or QuantiFERON®-TB Gold testing to ensure no active tuberculosis. Standard blood typing, human leukocyte antigen typing, and a calculated panel of reactive antibody (cPra) testing are performed by immunogenetic laboratories. Any teen with a history of congenital posterior valves or other congenital urological anomalies should undergo a urological evaluation to determine whether their bladder is an adequate conduit to the allograft prior to surgery as well as the potential need for urine drainage via catheterization. Concomitant health problems may require additional referrals to specialists.

A thorough exam of the patients' immunization status should be completed. All standard childhood vaccines should be complete [10, 11]. Whenever possible, vaccines should be completed prior to transplant because immunosuppressive medications given after transplantation may decrease vaccine effectiveness. Most centers

Table 12.1 Suggested pre-transplant laboratory evaluation and screening for hypercoagulability

General pre-transplant testing	Infectious disease testing
CBC + differential	CMV IgG, IgM
Basic metabolic panel	Hepatitis A IgM
Liver function testing: AST, ALT, total bilirubin, GGT, albumin, uric acid, INR, PTT	Hepatitis B core antibody, surface antibody, surface antigen
Iron, transferrin, and % saturation	Hepatitis C antibody
Magnesium, phosphorous	HIV antigen/antibody
Alkaline phosphatase	Varicella antibody
IgA, IgG, IgM	Herpes simplex viruses 1 and 2, IgM, IgG
Complements for lupus patients	EBV antibodies
HLA typing, single antigen classes I and II	
ABO × 2	
Urinalysis, urine protein-to-creatinine ratio	
Hypercoagulability testing	
Anti-cardiolipin antibody IgG, IgM	Russell viper venom test
Factor V Leiden mutation	RPR
Protein C activity	Antithrombin III activity
Protein S activity	Prothrombin (20210) mutation
Homocysteine	Methylenetetrahydrofolate reductase mutations

aim for completing vaccines at least 6 weeks prior to transplantation to allow for clearance of attenuated organisms and as to not interfere with final cross-match testing. Older teens who received the pneumococcal vaccine before 2010 may have received vaccine containing protection from only seven strains of the bacterium, 7-valent pneumococcal conjugate vaccine (PCV7). After 2010, the standard changed to Prevnar, a 13-valent pneumococcal conjugate vaccine (PCV13), which broadened protection against additional pneumococcal strains. Adolescents who completed PCV7 should also receive PCV 13. Adolescents with CKD are also recommended to receive the 23-valent pneumococcal polysaccharide vaccine (PPSV23).

Pre-transplant patients are also eligible for additional vaccines under the CDC guidelines for high-risk populations. In addition to the standard meningococcal conjugate vaccine that protects against four serogroups (A, C, W, and Y), an additional meningococcal B vaccine may also be appropriate for patients with complement component deficiencies, taking eculizumab (Soliris®), functional asplenia, or those living in communities with active outbreaks.

Lastly, the human papilloma virus vaccine (HPV) became available in 2006, and the 9-valent HPV vaccine was added to the standard schedule of childhood vaccines in 2016 for both males and females. Older teens may have missed this vaccine due to the recent changes in recommendations. The number of vaccines necessary for the HPV vaccine differs by the age of the patient so should be evaluated closely.

Evaluation for Hypercoagulability

Allograft thrombosis is a well-known and sometimes catastrophic complication after kidney transplant affecting approximately 1.4% of pediatric transplants [12]. Hypercoagulability due to genetic and acquired conditions is associated with an increased risk of graft thrombosis in the adult population [13]. While most of the published information on evaluation for and treatment of hypercoagulable risk factors to prevent graft thrombosis is in adults, there are a few published case series in pediatric patients [14–16]. While no randomized trials have been performed to determine the utility of evaluating patients for risk factors that can contribute to thrombosis of the renal allograft, most centers routinely perform some pre-transplant testing to identify risk factors for thrombosis in all patients awaiting kidney transplant.

The inherited conditions most commonly investigated include factor V Leiden (FVL) mutation, prothrombin 20210 G>A mutation, protein C deficiency, protein S deficiency, tissue plasminogen activator inhibitor-1 (PAI-1) promoter mutation, and methylenetetrahydrofolate reductase (MTHFR) mutations. Acquired conditions that are routinely evaluated include the presence of antiphospholipid (APL) antibodies and hyperhomocysteinemia. Of these conditions, FVL mutation is the most common inherited condition with a prevalence of 5–8% of the general population and up to 50% in patients with a personal or family history of recurrent thrombosis. FVL mutations confer a fourfold increased risk of allograft thrombosis and thrombotic complications post-transplant in the adult population. APL antibodies are the most commonly acquired thrombophilia with a prevalence of 1–3% in the general population [13].

When a hypercoagulable risk is identified in a pediatric patient, treatment and thrombosis prevention may include perioperative heparin followed by aspirin [17], perioperative heparin followed by low molecular weight heparin (LMWH) for 2 months post-transplant and aspirin long term [18], or perioperative heparin and conversion to either warfarin or LMWH long term for the highest-risk patients [14]. It is important to recognize that long-term anticoagulation with warfarin or LMWH does carry significant risk in young active adolescent patients who may be developmentally unable to understand completely the risks of anticoagulation and are prone to risk-taking behavior [19]. These complications can include superficial bruising, hemarthrosis, or even clinically significant subdural hematomas as a result of regular childhood play and activities.

Evaluation for Pharmacologic Risk Pre-transplant

The United Network for Organ Sharing and the Centers for Medicare and Medicaid Services have written mandates requiring transplantation programs to document the participation of a pharmacist on multidisciplinary teams caring for transplant patients. In the near future, CMS has indicated that pre-transplant evaluation should include the participation of a transplant pharmacist. Evaluation by a transplant pharmacist can help identify and evaluate pharmacological risk factors including issues with drug absorption, use of herbal supplements, preexisting medications effecting immunosuppressant drug metabolism, use of estrogen containing oral contraceptives, and medication allergies [20]. For example, adolescents using oral contraceptives should stop the medication 4–6 weeks prior to their surgery to reduce clotting risk. In addition, there is accumulating evidence for the potential utility of identifying specific alleles in cytochrome P-450 isoenzyme 3A (CYP3A) associated with variations in tacrolimus metabolism [21].

Post-transplant Medical Considerations

Standard of care for all pediatric and adolescent transplant recipients should include close follow-up with a multidisciplinary team approach. General post-transplant care for kidney transplant patients is well summarized in published guidelines [22, 23]. A thorough assessment of the adolescent post-transplant patient includes physical exam, laboratory exam, nutrition and growth monitoring, compliance monitoring, and psychosocial follow-up. Adolescent patients need to maintain close follow-up even when they are years out from transplant, as young adults are at the highest risk of medication nonadherence compared with other age groups [24].

Screening for Infections and the Use of Prophylactic Medications

Cytomegalovirus (CMV) is a significant cause of morbidity for all ages of transplant recipients. It most often occurs during the first year of transplant, and the onset is delayed by the use of antiviral therapy [25]. Currently, limited data exist regarding the efficacy of preemptive therapy in pediatric patients. According to the American Society of Transplantation (AST) Infectious Disease Community of Practice, no single standard for treatment or duration of appropriate CMV prophylaxis exists [25]. CMV disease risk is highest in those patients who have no CMV antibodies (AB) and receive a CMV seropositive donor kidney, a situation more common in children and adolescents. CMV disease risk is lowest for those with both a negative CMV AB recipient and donor. AST guidelines for adults recommend screening for CMV monthly for the first 6 months [25], but no randomized studies have directly compared screening strategies in children. At our center, all transplant recipients are screened for CMV monthly for the first 6 months and then every 3 months for the 1st year post-transplant. After the 1st year, patients are screened every 6 months until 3 years post-transplant. Viremia may be asymptomatic or cause system-wide disease and can be treated with intravenous ganciclovir or valganciclovir with or without reduction in immunosuppression.

Transplant patients are at risk for both primary infections and reactivation of Epstein-Barr virus (EBV). By adulthood, 90% of individuals become seropositive for EBV, a human herpes virus 4, which can be particularly detrimental to children and adolescents who are often antibody negative at the time of transplant. A wide continuum of EBV disease exists. The virus may lead to the neoplastic transformation known as post-transplant lymphoproliferative disorder (PTLD). In addition to EBV antibody status, age less than 18 years and intensive immunosuppression regimens are known risk factors for EBV infections [26, 27]. As with CMV, frequent monitoring for the virus is crucial for transplant recipients. KDIGO guidelines recommend screening once in the 1st week for seronegative recipients who receive kidneys from seropositive donors followed by monthly screening for the first 3–6 months and then every 3 months for the 1st year post-transplant [22]. Quantitative EBV PCR is the most commonly used assay at most transplant centers. An international reference standard doesn't exist for this virus adding to the challenge of monitoring [26]. At our center, EBV quantitative PCR is screened monthly for the first 6 months and then every 3 months for the 1st year post-transplant. After the 1st year, patients are screened every 6 months until 3 years post-transplant and then annually thereafter. Latent cases of PTLD may occur in pediatric patients many years out from transplant. Adolescents should be screened regularly for symptoms of PTLD including presence of lymphadenopathy, weight loss, fever, and malaise, particularly in the highest-risk groups (EBV-negative recipients or those patients receiving multiple courses of lymphocyte-depleting agents to treat rejection).

Other monitoring strategies for adults include screening for EBV every 2–4 weeks during the first 3 months post-transplant and then monthly until 6 months post-transplant. This strategy takes into account that most primary EBV infections occur in the first 3–6 months after transplant in the seronegative patients [22]. However, this strategy does not allow for preemptive identification of late infection, and there are no randomized studies directly comparing screening strategies in pediatric patients.

BK polyomavirus is an opportunistic and ubiquitous virus that commonly infects renal transplant patients and in severe infections may cause BK nephropathy (BKN) and graft loss. The primary BK infection usually occurs in the first decade of life, and the virus remains quiescent in the transitional urothelium of the urinary tract thereafter [28]. Therefore, in adolescent transplant patients, BK polyomavirus infections usually represent a reactivation of quiescent virus. There are no adolescent-specific protocols for the management of BK polyomavirus. The AST Infectious Disease Community of Practice recommends screening for the virus every 3 months during the first 2 years post-transplant, as the virus is most likely to appear in the first 2 years after transplant [22]. If the BK virus is present in the urine and not the serum, the risk to the allograft is much lower. When BK virus is detected in the blood, the primary treatment is careful reduction of immunosuppression, usually lowering the mycophenolate dose or reducing the target levels of tacrolimus, cyclosporine, sirolimus, or everolimus. Vigilant monitoring of serum BK viral titers is necessary as once BK viral titers subside, immunosuppression should be increased to prior target levels [28, 29]. Additionally, a transplant renal biopsy may be helpful to direct therapy if serum creatinine increases to determine BKN or transplant rejection.

Additional therapies for persistent BK polyomavirus infections include replacing mycophenolate with a mechanistic target of rapamycin (mTOR) inhibitor and in severe cases of BKN using intravenous immunoglobulin (IVIG) [30, 31]. While there is in vitro evidence that mTOR inhibitors have an antiproliferative effect on BK polyomavirus [32] and observational evidence that patients on mTOR inhibitors have less BK polyomavirus infection [33], there is no definitive clinical evidence that mTOR inhibitors reduce the risk for BKN [34]. In general, the mainstay of treatment of BKN is immunosuppression reduction.

The risk of Pneumocystis jirovecii pneumonia has significantly lessened by the use of antibacterial prophylaxis. In the adult population, the risk of PJP may be as high as 3–5% in solid organ transplant (SOT) recipients. For this reason, the AST guidelines recommend prophylaxis for all recipients for at least 6–12 months depending on risk factors [35]. The most common choice is trimethoprim-sulfamethoxazole, but other acceptable alternatives include dapsone, atovaquone, and intravenous pentamidine.

Additional Post-transplant Monitoring

Due to the known increased risk for cardiovascular disease in SOT patients, adolescents should have lipid profile monitoring post-transplant. The National Kidney Foundation Kidney Disease Outcomes Quality Initiative (NKF-KDOQI) dyslipidemia guidelines recommend adolescents be screened 2–3 months after transplant or 2–3 months after a change in treatment or condition known to cause dyslipidemia [22]. These guidelines also recommend a higher LDL-C target goal than in adults due to uncertainty of benefits of dyslipidemia treatment in younger patients. Any patient on mTOR inhibitors (e.g., sirolimus or everolimus) should have lipids monitored carefully since more than 60% of adult transplant recipients on mTOR inhibition develop lipid abnormalities [36, 37]. Our center monitors fasting lipid profiles at 1 and 6 months post-transplant and annually thereafter.

Tobacco including e-cigarette use should be screened for annually and discouraged due to the increase risk of cardiovascular disease, cancers, and premature death [38].

Additionally, transplant patients may develop transaminitis secondary to medications including but not limited to mycophenolate, and transaminases should be monitored every 6–12 months. Some centers monitor mycophenolic acid (MPA) levels or the area under the curve to monitor immunosuppression, although there have been no large randomized trials demonstrating a benefit for this in children. In addition, in adults, two randomized trials using 12-h trough levels to direct dosing showed no benefit on graft survival [39, 40]; however, in pediatric patients, a low 12-h trough level of MPA has been associated with the development of donor-specific antibodies [41].

Surveillance Biopsies

Many pediatric transplant centers rely solely on a decrease in estimated glomerular filtration rate (eGFR) to identify patients with possible rejection and who need a renal transplant biopsy, while other centers routinely perform surveillance biopsies at predetermined intervals in all transplant recipients. In the adult transplant population, the use of surveillance biopsies is center-dependent. A recent UNOS survey of transplant centers determined that of 121 responding centers, only 17% performed surveillance biopsies on all patients [42].

Surveillance biopsies are used to identify subclinical rejection (SCR) for which children are at an increased theoretical risk due to a large adult donor kidney for their relative size. Based on retrospective studies, there are high rates of SCR in pediatric kidney transplant patients: 8–25% of pediatric protocol biopsies demonstrate Banff type 1A or greater rejection, and 28–44% demonstrate borderline changes or meet criteria for Banff rejection [43–45]. In the pediatric transplant population, there are only two controlled trials and no randomized controlled trials evaluating the utility of surveillance biopsies [46, 47]. Seikku and colleagues compared pediatric recipients receiving surveillance biopsies at 3 months followed prospectively to a historical control group [48]. Subclinical rejection (Banff score 1A or higher) at 3 months was detected and treated in 39% of the patient receiving surveillance biopsies. The surveillance biopsy group experienced fewer acute rejection episodes, and eGFR was significantly higher at 18 months compared to controls (87 vs. 68 mL/min/1.73 m^2). However, there were important differences between the surveillance biopsy group and the historical control group including the transplant era, differences in immunosuppression, and HLA mismatches. Kanzelmeyer and colleagues compared pediatric recipients receiving surveillance biopsies at 6 months to a nonrandomized control group transplanted concurrently and controlled for differences in immunosuppression and HLA mismatches [49]. Subclinical rejection (Banff score 1A) was detected and treated in 16% of the patients receiving surveillance biopsies. In addition, 7% of biopsies identified borderline changes, and immunosuppression was intensified for those patients. Overall 33% of patients had immunosuppression modified as a result of the surveillance biopsy either for rejection or evidence of medication toxicity. The surveillance biopsy group had significantly higher eGFR at 3.5 years post-transplant compared to controls (57 vs. 46 mL/min/1.73 m^2, $p = 0.036$). However, there was no difference in eGFR at 1.5 or 2.5 years post-transplant indicating a relatively distant potential benefit that is somewhat difficult to explain mechanistically. Overall, surveillance biopsies appear to be safe with a reported intervention or transfusion rate of less than 0.5% [43]. In the future, surveillance biopsies may become obsolete as commercially available blood tests become available for evaluating patients noninvasively for acute cellular rejection [50, 51].

Reproductive Health Post-transplant

Sexually active teens have a reduced chance of becoming pregnant while on dialysis or with advanced CKD due to fertility issues including oligomenorrhea, amenorrhea, and hormonal dysregulation of the hypothalamic-pituitary-ovarian axis [52]. Post-transplantation there is rapid improvement in the hypothalamic-pituitary-ovarian axis and fertility within 1–6 months [53], and all patients of childbearing age should be counseled on the risk of pregnancy and encouraged to use contraception.

One recent study from a single pediatric transplant center with 49 patients 13–23 years of age demonstrated that 15% of males and 53% of females self-reported sexual activity. In their population, they reported no unplanned pregnancies; however, 30% of the sexually active adolescents reported having at least one sexually transmitted infection (STI) [54]. Various methods of post-transplant contraception are well described elsewhere [53, 55, 56]. In our center, we generally recommend low-estrogen oral contraceptive medications combined with a barrier method for pregnancy and STI prevention. Some patients opt for long-acting reversible methods such as intrauterine devices or subdermal implants such as depot medroxyprogesterone acetate (DMPA) to enhance adherence. Alternate contraception methods include the use of two barrier methods for contraception. Standard preventive care for adults includes a semiannual pap test; however, pap tests are not typically a standard of practice until 21 years of age.

It is important to note that in the adult transplant population, 56.9% of male and 93.4% of female patients report sexual dysfunction of some type, although this is less prevalent than in the adult dialysis population [57]. Issues reported include difficulty achieving arousal, orgasm, and/or orgasm satisfaction. It is important for providers to identify these issues and work with adolescent patients to improve sexual function. In the adult transplant population, sexual dysfunction has a clear correlation with depression which may or may not be causative.

Dermatology Care Post-transplant

Issues of body image are of particular importance in the adolescent transplant population. Necessary transplant medications cause known cosmetic side effects. Some of the known side effects include acne in 20% of patients on prednisone [58], hirsutism in 21–45% of patients on cyclosporine [59], alopecia in less than 15% of patients on tacrolimus [60], gingival hyperplasia in 4–16% of patients on cyclosporine [59], and some types of skin cancer [60]. In particular changes to the skin can be bothersome and negatively affect body image. Moloney and colleagues studied quality of life related to dermatological complications. In the adult population, both younger adults and females felt that skin-related complications negatively affected their quality of life. In cases of severe cutaneous human papillomavirus infections, conversion to sirolimus may help control the lesions [61–63]. Transplant patients should be referred to dermatology for skin-related side effects, and all patients should have baseline screening for cancers.

Mental Health Care for the Adolescent Patient

Many studies have identified and described the burden of chronic kidney disease and kidney transplant on the adolescent quality of life and mental health. While quality of life in adolescents is improved post-transplant [64], several groups have reported high rates of abnormal body image, depression, anxiety, and behavioral disorders post-kidney transplant. In a case-controlled study by Berney-Martinet and colleagues, the rates of depression, anxiety, and behavioral disorders in adolescents post-kidney transplant were 35%, 22.5%, and 30%, respectively, which were all higher compared to a control population of adolescents [65]. In another series at a single center, only 17% of adolescent kidney transplant patients and/or parents reported depressive symptoms [66]. In addition, these conditions are associated and contribute to medication nonadherence. It is therefore critical that adolescents be routinely evaluated and treated for mental health conditions. All adolescent patients should be seen by a social worker for routine screening for psychosocial dysfunction and referred to a trained transplant psychologist or counselor if mental health issues are identified. In addition, it is critical to have the appropriate support of a psychiatrist for the medical management of any identified mental health disorders.

In addition, body image can be negatively affected by surgical scars [66]. While any surgical scar can be viewed as disfiguring by patients, adolescents who undergo bilateral nephrectomy may have larger or more numerous surgical scars than for a kidney transplant alone. Midline scars on the abdomen may also be perceived as more disfiguring than laparoscopic scars. Laparoscopic nephrectomy should be utilized when possible to avoid larger scars, and teens should be fully informed of the type of surgical approach and the associated scars prior to surgery.

Long-Term Outcomes for Adolescent Kidney Transplant Patients

The difficulty of performing a successful kidney transplantation and maintaining allograft function in adolescent patients is highlighted by the persistently poorer long-term graft survival in adolescents versus other pediatric patients (Fig. 12.1) [4, 67]. The Organ Procurement and Transplantation Network (OPTN) and Scientific Registry of Transplant Recipients (SRTR) data demonstrates that the 5-year allograft survival for adolescent patients is only 81% for living-donor kidneys and 72% for deceased-donor kidneys which is substantially lower than the youngest pediatric group [4]. In addition, on average, pediatric patients have poorer outcomes than adult patients for living-related kidney transplants [68]. The factors driving these

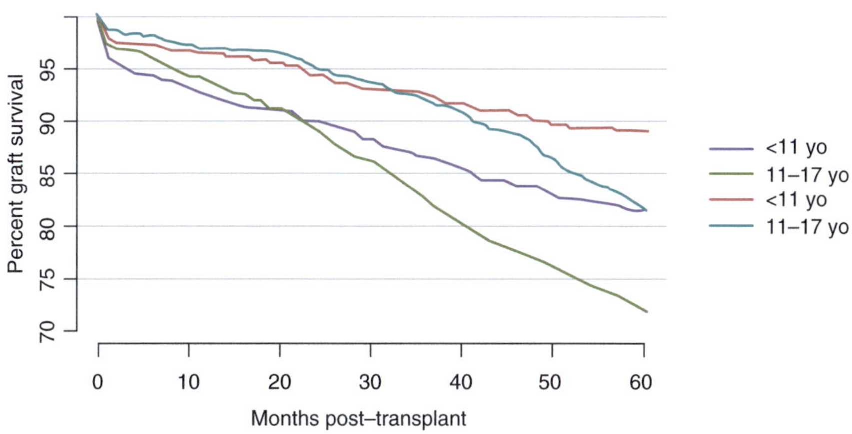

Fig. 12.1 Allograft survival of kidney transplants for adolescents versus younger recipients. Graft survival among pediatric kidney transplant recipients by age and donor type, 2006–2010, demonstrates reduced graft survival time for adolescents compared to younger pediatric patients [4]. Graft survival was estimated using unadjusted Kaplan-Meier methods. DD deceased donor, LD living donor

poor outcomes are likely multifactorial and include poor medication adherence among adolescent patients and the shifting of responsibility for care that occurs in adolescence. In addition, biologic factors related to the pubertal growth spurt or changes in immunosuppression metabolism may be potentially important in these poor outcomes. The burden of having a chronic medical condition is high for adolescent patients, but with the dedicated support of their families and a multidisciplinary transplant team, we can facilitate the success of kidney transplantation for even the most challenging adolescent patients.

References

1. https://unos.org/data/transplant-trends/
2. Hebert SA, Swinford RD, Hall DR, Au JK, Bynon JS. Special considerations in pediatric kidney transplantation. Adv Chronic Kidney Dis. 2017;24(6):398–404.
3. Verghese PS. Pediatric kidney transplantation: a historical review. Pediatr Res. 2017;81(1–2):259–64.
4. Hart A, Smith JM, Skeans MA, Gustafson SK, Stewart DE, Cherikh WS, Wainright JL, Kucheryavaya A, Woodbury M, Snyder JJ, Kasiske BL, Israni AKOPTN. SRTR 2015 annual data report: kidney. Am J Transplant. 2017;17(Suppl 1):21–116.
5. Tong A, Tjaden L, Howard K, Wong G, Morton R, Craig JC. Quality of life of adolescent kidney transplant recipients. J Pediatr. 2011;159(4):670–5.
6. Tong A, Wong G, McTaggart S, Henning P, Mackie F, Carroll RP, Howard K, Craig JC. Quality of life of young adults and adolescents with chronic kidney disease. J Pediatr. 2013;163(4):1179–85.
7. Reed-Knight B, Lee JL, Cousins LA, Mee LL. Intellectual and academic performance in children undergoing solid organ pretransplant evaluation. Pediatr Transplant. 2015;19(2):229–34.
8. Korus M, Stinson JN, Pool R, Williams A, Kagan S. Exploring the information needs of adolescents and their parents throughout the kidney transplant continuum. Prog Transplant. 2011;21(1):53–60.
9. Connelly J, Pilch N, Oliver M, Jordan C, Fleming J, Meadows H, Baliga P, Nadig S, Twombley K, Shatat I, Taber D. Prediction of medication non-adherence and associated outcomes in pediatric kidney transplant recipients. Pediatr Transplant. 2015;19(5):555–62.
10. Recommended immunization schedule for children and adolescents aged 18 years or younger, United States, 2017. https://www.cdc.gov/vaccines/schedules/hcp/imz/child-adolescent.html
11. Neu AM. Immunizations in children with chronic kidney disease. Pediatr Nephrol. 2012;27(8):1257–63.
12. Winnicki E, Dharmar M, Tancredi D, Butani L. Comparable survival of en bloc versus standard donor kidney transplants in children. J Pediatr. 2016;173:169–74.
13. Parajuli S, Lockridge JB, Langewisch ED, Norman DJ, Kujovich JL. Hypercoagulability in kidney transplant recipients. Transplantation. 2016;100(4):719–26.
14. Dick AA, Lerner SM, Boissy AR, Farrell CE, Alfrey EJ. Excellent outcome in infants and small children with thrombophilias undergoing kidney transplantation. Pediatr Transplant. 2005;9(1):39–42.
15. Gülhan B, Tavil B, Gümrük F, Aki TF, Topaloglu R. Renal transplantation experience in a patient with factor V Leiden homozygous, MTHFR C677T heterozygous, and PAI heterozygous mutation. Pediatr Transplant. 2015;19(5):E126–9.
16. Oh J, Schaefer F, Veldmann A, Nowak G, Nowak-Göttl U, Tönshoff B, Kreuz W. Heterozygous prothrombin gene mutation: a new risk factor for early renal allograft thrombosis. Transplantation. 1999;68(4):575–8.

17. Nagra A, Trompeter RS, Fernando ON, Koffman G, Taylor JD, Lord R, Hutchinson C, O'Sullivan C, Rees L. The effect of heparin on graft thrombosis in pediatric renal allografts. Pediatr Nephrol. 2004;19(5):531–5.
18. Kranz B, Vester U, Nadalin S, Paul A, Broelsch CE, Hoyer PF. Outcome after kidney transplantation in children with thrombotic risk factors. Pediatr Transplant. 2006;10(7):788–93.
19. Qu Y, Galvan A, Fuligni AJ, Lieberman MD, Telzer EH. Longitudinal changes in prefrontal cortex activation underlie declines in adolescent risk taking. J Neurosci. 2015;35(32):11308–14.
20. Maldonado AQ, Tichy EM, Rogers CC, Campara M, Ensor C, Doligalski CT, Gabardi S, Descourouez JL, Doyle IC, Trofe-Clark J. Assessing pharmacologic and nonpharmacologic risks in candidates for kidney transplantation. Am J Health Syst Pharm. 2015;72(10):781–93.
21. Lunde I, Bremer S, Midtvedt K, Mohebi B, Dahl M, Bergan S, Åsberg A, Christensen H. The influence of CYP3A, PPARA, and POR genetic variants on the pharmacokinetics of tacrolimus and cyclosporine in renal transplant recipients. Eur J Clin Pharmacol. 2014;70(6):685–93.
22. Kidney Disease: Improving Global Outcomes (KDIGO) Transplant Work Group. KDIGO clinical practice guideline for the care of kidney transplant recipients. Am J Transplant. 2009 Nov;9(Suppl 3):S1–155.
23. Baker RJ, Mark PB, Patel RK, Stevens KK, Palmer N. Renal association clinical practice guideline in post-operative care in the kidney transplant recipient. BMC Nephrol. 2017;18(1):174.
24. Nevins TE, Nickerson PW, Dew MA. Understanding medication nonadherence after kidney transplant. J Am Soc Nephrol. 2017;28(8):2290–301.
25. Razonable RR, Humar A. AST infectious diseases community of practice. Cytomegalovirus in solid organ transplantation. Am J Transplant. 2013;13(Suppl 4):93–106.
26. Le J, Durand CM, Agha I, Brennan DC. Epstein-Barr virus and renal transplantation. Transplant Rev. 2017;31(1):55–60. https://doi.org/10.1016/j.trre.2016.12.001. Epub 2016 Dec 29
27. Höcker B, Fickenscher H, Delecluse HJ, Böhm S, Küsters U, Schnitzler P, Pohl M, John U, Kemper MJ, Fehrenbach H, Wigger M, Holder M, Schröder M, Billing H, Fichtner A, Feneberg R, Sander A, Köpf-Shakib S, Süsal C, Tönshoff B. Epidemiology and morbidity of Epstein-Barr virus infection in pediatric renal transplant recipients: a multicenter, prospective study. Clin Infect Dis. 2013;56(1):84–92. https://doi.org/10.1093/cid/cis823. Epub 2012 Oct 5
28. Hirsch HH, Brennan DC, Drachenberg CB, Ginevri F, Gordon J, Limaye AP, Mihatsch MJ, Nickeleit V, Ramos E, Randhawa P, Shapiro R, Steiger J, Suthanthiran M, Trofe J. Polyomavirus-associated nephropathy in renal transplantation: interdisciplinary analyses and recommendations. Transplantation. 2005;79(10):1277–86.
29. Pham PT, Schaenman J, Pham PC. BK virus infection following kidney transplantation: an overview of risk factors, screening strategies, and therapeutic interventions. Curr Opin Organ Transplant. 2014;19(4):401–12.
30. Sharma AP, Moussa M, Casier S, Rehman F, Filler G, Grimmer J. Intravenous immunoglobulin as rescue therapy for BK virus nephropathy. Pediatr Transplant. 2009;13(1):123–9.
31. Shah T, Vu D, Naraghi R, Campbell A, Min D. Efficacy of intravenous immunoglobulin in the treatment of persistent BK viremia and BK virus nephropathy in renal transplant recipients. Clin Transpl. 2014:109–16.
32. Hirsch HH, Yakhontova K, Lu M, Manzetti JBK. Polyomavirus replication in renal tubular epithelial cells is inhibited by Sirolimus, but activated by tacrolimus through a pathway involving FKBP-12. Am J Transplant. 2016;16(3):821–32.
33. Thangaraju S, Gill J, Wright A, Dong J, Rose C, Gill J. Risk factors for BK polyoma virus treatment and association of treatment with kidney transplant failure: insights from a paired kidney analysis. Transplantation. 2016;100(4):854–61.
34. Mallat SG, Tanios BY, Itani HS, Lotfi T, McMullan C, Gabardi S, Akl EA, Azzi JR. CMV and BKPyV infections in renal transplant recipients receiving an mTOR inhibitor-based regimen versus a CNI-based regimen: a systematic review and meta-analysis of randomized, controlled trials. Clin J Am Soc Nephrol. 2017;12:1321.
35. Martin SI, Fishman JA, AST Infectious Diseases Community of Practice. Pneumocystis pneumonia in sold organ transplantation. Am J Transplant. 2013;13(Suppl 4):272–9. https://doi.org/10.1111/ajt.12119.

36. Favi E, Spagnoletti G, Salerno MP, Pedroso JA, Romagnoli J, Citterio F. Tacrolimus plus mycophenolate mofetil vs. cyclosporine plus everolimus in deceased donor kidney transplant recipients: three-yr results of a single-center prospective clinical trial. Clin Transpl. 2013;27(4):E359–67.
37. Ichimaru N, Yamanaka K, Kato T, Kakuta Y, Abe T, Imamura R, Nonomura N, Kaimori JY, Takahara S. Risk factors and incidence for lipid abnormalities in kidney transplant patients. Transplant Proc. 2015;47(3):672–4.
38. Nogueira JM, Haririan A, Jacobs SC, Cooper M, Weir MR. Cigarette smoking, kidney function, and mortality after live donor kidney transplant. Am J Kidney Dis. 2010;55(5):907–15.
39. van Gelder T, Silva HT, de Fijter JW, Budde K, Kuypers D, Tyden G, Lohmus A, Sommerer C, Hartmann A, Le Meur Y, Oellerich M, Holt DW, Tönshoff B, Keown P, Campbell S, Mamelok RD. Comparing mycophenolate mofetil regimens for de novo renal transplant recipients: the fixed-dose concentration-controlled trial. Transplantation. 2008;86(8):1043–51.
40. Gaston RS, Kaplan B, Shah T, Cibrik D, Shaw LM, Angelis M, Mulgaonkar S, Meier-Kriesche HU, Patel D, Bloom RD. Fixed- or controlled-dose mycophenolate mofetil with standard- or reduced-dose calcineurin inhibitors: the Opticept trial. Am J Transplant. 2009;9(7):1607–19.
41. Filler G, Todorova EK, Bax K, Alvarez-Elías AC, Huang SH, Kobrzynski MC. Minimum mycophenolic acid levels are associated with donor-specific antibody formation. Pediatr Transplant. 2016;20(1):34–8.
42. Mehta R, Cherikh W, Sood P, Hariharan S. Kidney allograft surveillance biopsy practices across US transplant centers: a UNOS survey. Clin Transpl. 2017;31(5).
43. Aoun B, Decramer S, Vitkevic R, Wannous H, Bandin F, Azema C, Callard P, Brocheriou I, Ulinski T. Protocol biopsies in pediatric renal transplant recipients on cyclosporine versus tacrolimus-based immunosuppression. Pediatr Nephrol. 2013;28(3):493–8.
44. Birk PE, Stannard KM, Konrad HB, Blydt-Hansen TD, Ogborn MR, Cheang MS, Gartner JG, Gibson IW. Surveillance biopsies are superior to functional studies for the diagnosis of acute and chronic renal allograft pathology in children. Pediatr Transplant. 2004;8(1):29–38.
45. Hymes LC, Greenbaum L, Amaral SG, Warshaw BL. Surveillance renal transplant biopsies and subclinical rejection at three months post-transplant in pediatric recipients. Pediatr Transplant. 2007;11(5):536–9.
46. Birk PE. Surveillance biopsies in children post-kidney transplant. Pediatr Nephrol. 2012;27(5):753–60.
47. Rose EM, Kennedy SE, Mackie FE. Surveillance biopsies after paediatric kidney transplantation: a review. Pediatr Transplant. 2016;20(6):748–55.
48. Seikku P, Krogerus L, Jalanko H, Holmberg C. Better renal function with enhanced immunosuppression and protocol biopsies after kidney transplantation in children. Pediatr Transplant. 2005;9(6):754–62.
49. Kanzelmeyer NK, Ahlenstiel T, Drube J, Froede K, Kreuzer M, Broecker V, Ehrich JH, Melk A, Pape L. Protocol biopsy-driven interventions after pediatric renal transplantation. Pediatr Transplant. 2010;14(8):1012–8.
50. Roedder S, Sigdel T, Salomonis N, Hsieh S, Dai H, Bestard O, Metes D, Zeevi A, Gritsch A, Cheeseman J, Macedo C, Peddy R, Medeiros M, Vincenti F, Asher N, Salvatierra O, Shapiro R, Kirk A, Reed EF, Sarwal MM. The kSORT assay to detect renal transplant patients at high risk for acute rejection: results of the multicenter AART study. PLoS Med. 2014;11(11):e1001759.
51. Erpicum P, Hanssen O, Weekers L, Lovinfosse P, Meunier P, Tshibanda L, Krzesinski JM, Hustinx R, Jouret F. Non-invasive approaches in the diagnosis of acute rejection in kidney transplant recipients, part II: omics analyses of urine and blood samples. Clin Kidney J. 2017;10(1):106–15.
52. Nadeau-Fredette AC, Hladunewich M, Hui D, Keunen J, Chan CT. End-stage renal disease and pregnancy. Adv Chronic Kidney Dis. 2013;20(3):246–52.
53. Yousif ME, Bridson JM, Halawa A. Contraception after kidney transplantation, from myth to reality: a comprehensive review of the current evidence. Exp Clin Transplant. 2016;14(3):252–8.

54. Ashoor I, Aviles D, Pasternak R, Vehaskari VM. Sexually transmitted infections in pediatric renal transplant recipients: time to take notice. Pediatr Transplant. 2015;19(6):584–7.
55. Centers for Disease Control and Prevention (CDC). U S. Medical eligibility criteria for contraceptive use, 2010. MMWR Recomm Rep. 2010 Jun 18;59(RR-4):1–86.
56. Godfrey EM. Helping clinicians prevent pregnancy among sexually active adolescents: U.S. medical eligibility criteria for contraceptive use and U.S. selected practice recommendations for contraceptive use. J Pediatr Adolesc Gynecol. 2015;28(4):209–14.
57. Josephson MA, McKay DB. Women and transplantation: fertility, sexuality, pregnancy, contraception. Adv Chronic Kidney Dis. 2013;20(5):433–40.
58. Khosravi M, Golchai J, Mokhtari G. Muco-cutaneous manifestations in 178 renal transplant recipients. Clin Transpl. 2011;25(3):395–400.
59. Product Information: Sandimmune(R) oral soft gelatin capsules, oral solution, intravenous injection, cyclosporine oral soft gelatin capsules, oral solution, intravenous injection. East Hanover: Novartis Pharmaceuticals Corporation (per FDA); 2013.
60. Product Information: PROGRAF(R) oral capsules, IV injection, tacrolimus oral capsules, IV injection. Deerfield: Astellas Pharma US (per manufacturer); 2011.
61. Moloney FJ, Keane S, O'Kelly P, Conlon PJ, Murphy GM. The impact of skin disease following renal transplantation on quality of life. Br J Dermatol. 2005;153(3):574–8.
62. Shahidi S, Moeinzadeh F, Mohammadi M, Gholamrezaei A. Sirolimus-based immunosuppression for treatment of cutaneous warts in kidney transplant recipients. Iran J Kidney Dis. 2011;5(5):351–3.
63. Dharancy S, Catteau B, Mortier L, Boleslawski E, Declerck N, Canva V, Piette F, Mathurin P, Pruvot FR. Conversion to sirolimus: a useful strategy for recalcitrant cutaneous viral warts in liver transplant recipient. Liver Transpl. 2006;12(12):1883–7.
64. Dobbels F, Decorte A, Roskams A, Van Damme-Lombaerts R. Health-related quality of life, treatment adherence, symptom experience and depression in adolescent renal transplant patients. Pediatr Transplant. 2010;14(2):216–23.
65. Berney-Martinet S, Key F, Bell L, Lépine S, Clermont MJ, Fombonne E. Psychological profile of adolescents with a kidney transplant. Pediatr Transplant. 2009;13(6):701–10.
66. Kärrfelt HM, Berg UB. Long-term psychosocial outcome after renal transplantation during childhood. Pediatr Transplant. 2008;12(5):557–62.
67. Dharnidharka VR, Lamb KE, Zheng J, Schechtman KB, Meier- Kriesche H-U. Across all solid organs, adolescent age recipients have worse transplant organ survival than younger age children: a US national registry analysis. Pediatr Transplant. 2015;19:471–6.
68. Torkaman M, Khalili-Matin-Zadeh Z, Azizabadi-Farahani M, Moghani-Lankarani M, Assari S, Pourfarziani V, Saadat SH, Kavehmanesh Z, Afshar-Payman S. Outcome of living kidney transplant: pediatric in comparison to adults. Transplant Proc. 2007;39(4):1088–90.

Chapter 13
Kidney Transplantation in Children and Adolescents: Surgical Aspects

Andrew Perry, Jakub Woloszyn, and Chandrasekar Santhanakrishnan

Introduction

Pediatric kidney transplantation has become highly successful in the modern era and is the treatment of choice for children with end-stage renal disease (ESRD). In addition to an overall survival benefit, kidney transplantation also improves cognitive function, social adjustment, growth, and quality of life [1, 2]. In 2016, 728 kidney transplants were performed in children under 18 years of age in the United States, and this has remained relatively stable over the past 10 years, based on data from the Organ Procurement and Transplantation Network (OPTN) as of March 22, 2017. This chapter discusses surgical aspects of renal transplantation in children, including preoperative planning, operative technique, and perioperative management.

Preoperative Management

Recipient Selection

A thorough evaluation is performed by a multidisciplinary team prior to kidney transplantation. This evaluation process is discussed in detail in the prior chapter. From a surgical perspective, size considerations are important in deciding when to transplant children. We have tended to wait for children to be a minimum of 8 kg

A. Perry · J. Woloszyn
Department of Surgery, University of California, Davis, Sacramento, CA, USA
e-mail: perry@ucdavis.edu; jwoloszyn@ucdavis.edu

C. Santhanakrishnan (✉)
Department of Surgery, Division of Transplant Surgery, University of California, Davis, Sacramento, CA, USA
e-mail: cskrishnan@ucdavis.edu

M. N. Haddad et al. (eds.), *Adolescents with Chronic Kidney Disease*,
https://doi.org/10.1007/978-3-319-97220-6_13

prior to proceeding with transplantation. This is a decision that is made on a case by case basis and taking into consideration individual circumstances. In concert with optimal body weight, timing of transplantation should follow the growth curve of the recipient. More specifically, optimal timing for renal transplantation should take place as the growth curve of the child begins to plateau.

Donor Selection

Living donors are generally preferred over deceased donors due to better long-term graft survival. Five-year graft survival for all living donor renal transplants is 85.5%, compared to 74.3% for those from deceased donors, based on OPTN data as of March 22, 2017. In 2004, 50% of pediatric transplants were from living donors; however, in October 2005, UNOS implemented a revised allocation policy dedicating renal allografts from young deceased donors preferentially to pediatric recipients. Following this change, there has been a shift toward deceased donor transplantations in the pediatric population, and by 2016, only 34% were from living donors.

Potential living donors must undergo a rigorous screening process, which includes medical, physical, and psychosocial evaluations. The evaluation process aims to identify a healthy donor organ for the recipient but more importantly executes a moral and ethical responsibility to ensure the health and well-being of a donor after organ donation. ABO compatibility and HLA compatibility are used to identify potential living donors, related or unrelated. Potential donors then undergo an evaluation process to ensure healthy renal function and the absence of prohibitive medical and social problems. Radiographic imaging is an important component of the screening process. At our center, CT angiography of the abdomen and pelvis is used to (1) ensure normal renal and urologic anatomy and (2) delineate the renal vascular anatomy.

Generally, the left kidney is favored for living donation, as its longer renal vein facilitates the implantation procedure. However, the presence of certain lesions within the kidney or anomalous renal vasculature may affect organ selection. For instance, when multiple renal arteries are present to one kidney, the contralateral kidney may be selected to facilitate implantation. Another common scenario arises when a cystic lesion is identified within one kidney. These lesions are characterized for malignant potential using imaging (CT or MRI) and occasionally require biopsy. A lesion with malignant potential is prohibitive for living donation. However, if a benign lesion with little to no malignant potential is identified, the kidney with the lesion is often favored for transplantation to minimize future risk to the donor.

Preoperative Planning

Hemodynamics, intravascular volume status, and electrolyte disturbances should be addressed prior to surgery. Blood typing and a cross-match for the recipient should be performed, with three units of packed red blood cells available for surgery.

Laboratory work-up should include complete blood count, chemistry panel, and liver function assay. Additionally, a prothrombin time (PT) and partial thromboplastin time (PTT) should be obtained to ensure the absence of coagulopathy. Dialysis may be required to address electrolyte disturbances and uremia, but fluid removal should be limited (see section on "Intraoperative Anesthesia" (Sect. 3.3)). Recipients with a high panel reactive antibody (PRA) should undergo a cross-match with donor plasma. In addition to laboratory work-up, obtaining a chest x-ray is a routine component of the perioperative work-up. For those at risk for or with a known cardiac issue, a transthoracic echocardiogram is routinely performed to ensure adequate function.

There are circumstances when native nephrectomies are indicated prior to transplantation. This is most likely in scenarios where patients have severe nephrotic syndrome and have profound hypoalbuminemia. In these cases, we recommend native nephrectomies and allow the patient to recover until they achieve acceptable serum albumin levels prior to transplantation. This would necessitate the need for dialysis until the time of transplantation. Recipients with recurrent urinary tract infections from chronic vesicoureteral reflux should also undergo native nephrectomy to mitigate the risk of postoperative infections in the immunosuppressed state. In the setting of renal failure with polyuria, posttransplant fluid management can present difficulties for the clinician and the patient. Native nephrectomy is therefore indicated to mitigate risks of hypotension and electrolyte disturbances which could complicate the patient's recovery and posttransplant course. Other indications for native nephrectomy include size limitations due to polycystic kidney disease, refractory hypertension, and urolithiasis.

Managing Urological Disorders

Congenital anomalies of the kidney and urinary tract including renal dysplasia/aplasia, obstructive uropathy, and reflux nephropathy are the primary cause of ESRD in up to 36% of pediatric kidney transplants in North America [3], making this group of diagnoses the most common cause of ESRD in children and adolescents. Urological abnormalities such as posterior urethral valves, congenital urogenital sinus anomalies, and the prune belly syndrome are major contributors to these causes of ESRD in children. Renal transplantation into children with such lower urinary tract abnormalities and/or bladder dysfunction may be associated with a reduction in graft function and graft survival [4] if urologic management is unaddressed prior to transplantation.

Work-up for children with renal failure should always include an investigation for lower urinary tract abnormalities. An in-depth history and physical exam should be done focusing on history and frequency of urinary tract infections, examination of genitalia and perineum, and a neurological exam. A detailed history of voiding practices, including frequencies and volumes, can also be helpful. A post-void renal ultrasound is useful to assess residual urine volumes and delineate abnormal anatomy. When urological abnormalities are suspected or there is an abnormal ultrasound finding, a voiding cystourethrogram (VCUG) is the radiological study of choice. This should be done in all children with a history of urinary tract infections as well. This study provides anatomic details of the lower urinary tract and provides functional information on vesicoureteral reflux and bladder emptying. In patients with confirmed or suspected neurogenic abnormalities, a urodynamic evaluation should be performed to more specifically evaluate neurogenic bladder dysfunction.

The goal for managing lower urinary tract disorders is to ensure adequate ureteral drainage into a sterile, low-pressure reservoir that can be easily emptied. Management of urological disorders prior to renal transplantation requires a highly individualized approach involving consultation with a pediatric urologist. Low-grade vesicoureteral reflux without a history of urinary tract infections can be left untreated. However, recurrent urinary tract infections or high-grade vesicoureteral reflux requires surgical management. In the absence of significantly dilated native ureters, correcting the reflux by reimplanting the native ureters (ureteroneocystostomy) is one option. Nephrectomy or nephroureterectomy are alternative options and are more appropriate in the setting of high-grade reflux with megaureters.

Bladder dysfunction can manifest as diminished compliance, incomplete voiding, or small bladder volumes. Primary management should include catheterization and medical management with anticholinergic therapy. If catheterization is intended posttransplant, this should be practiced prior to transplantation to ensure patient/family tolerance and cooperation with such frequent invasive instrumentation, especially with younger children. Surgical management is directed toward establishing a compliant bladder or urinary reservoir that easily empties. There are a variety of augmentation procedures that use native ureter or bowel to reduce intravesical pressure, increase bladder volume, and dampen contractions from bladder spasticity in the case of neurogenic bladders. Lastly, a complete urinary diversion procedure may be necessary, such as an ileal conduit. In this case, a segment of ileum is used to create a neobladder, which is externalized to the skin by a urostomy for drainage.

Surgical Approach

The operative approach is either through an intra-abdominal approach through a midline incision using the recipient aorta and inferior vena cava (IVC) for vascular anastomosis (Figs. 13.1 and 13.6) or a pelvic extraperitoneal approach using the recipient iliac vessels (Fig. 13.2). The intra-abdominal approach requires a right medial visceral rotation of the right hemi-colon (Catelle-Brassch maneuver), which exposes the retroperitoneum, IVC, and aorta. Due to size limitations with the extraperitoneal approach in children, recipients weighing less than 10 kg should undergo an intra-abdominal renal transplantation. An extraperitoneal approach is generally favored in patients weighing greater than 20 kg. For recipients weighing 10–20 kg, consideration of body habitus and size of the kidney ultimately determines the operative approach.

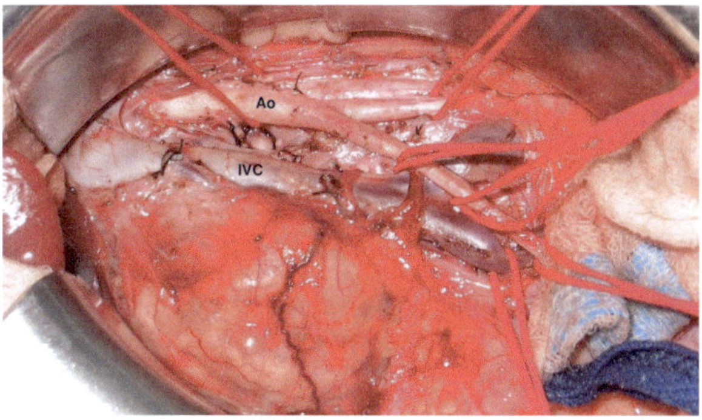

Fig. 13.1 Exposure of the aorta (labeled **Ao**) and inferior vena cava (labeled IVC) for an intra-abdominal kidney transplantation. The patient's head is toward the left, and the patient's feet are toward the right. Red rubber vessel loops on the right of the image are wrapped around the patient's common iliac veins and arteries. (Photo courtesy of Richard Perez, MD)

Fig. 13.2 Exposure of the external iliac artery (labeled **A**) and external iliac vein (labeled **V**) for a pelvic extraperitoneal kidney implantation. These are the patient's left iliac vessels. The patient's head is to the right of the image and the feet are to the left of the image. (Photo taken by Andrew Perry, MD)

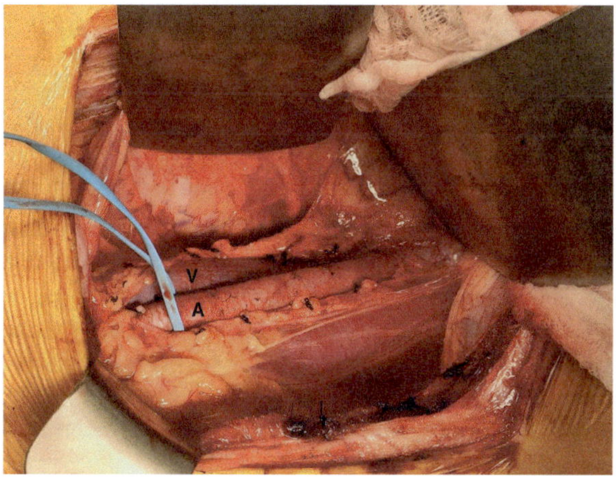

Back-table preparation of the kidney is performed prior to implantation (Fig. 13.3). Perinephric adipose tissue is stripped from the graft, and the renal artery and vein are isolated to prepare for the vascular anastomosis. The gonadal vessels and small peri-hilar vessels are ligated. Careful attention is paid to the ureter during back-table dissection, as extensive skeletonization of the ureter increases the risk of ischemic injury after implantation. With deceased donor grafts, the graft is typically placed on hypothermic pulsatile perfusion using preservation solution to assist in organ assessment and aid in organ preservation. Hypothermic pulsatile perfusion has been shown to improve graft survival and decrease rates of delayed graft function (DGF) in deceased donor renal transplants [5].

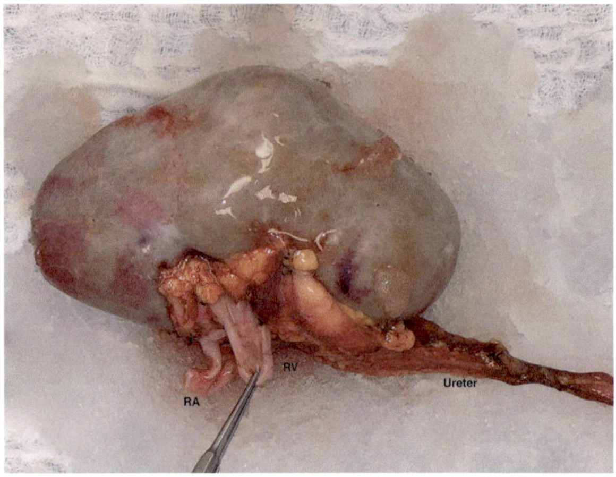

Fig. 13.3 Kidney in preparation for implantation after back-table dissection. The renal artery (RA), renal vein (RV), and ureter are labeled. (Photo taken by Andrew Perry, MD)

Multiple renal arteries or veins can present a technical challenge for the surgeon. A very small artery or vein may simply be ligated with a negligible impact on organ perfusion. One caveat to this is an accessory artery supplying the inferior pole, which likely contributes to the bloody supply of the ureter. Any disruption of the blood supply to the ureter increases the risk of ischemic stricture.

Larger accessory vessels typically require a vascular reconstruction. There are a variety of reconstructive strategies used to manage multiple vessels. If there are multiple renal arteries originating from the aorta in close proximity, in the case of deceased donor organs, a common aortic patch that includes the origins of both arteries may be used for the anastomosis. In living donor grafts, one artery can be implanted onto the other in an end-to-side fashion, or a side-to-side "pantaloon" anastomosis may be performed using the origin of each artery (Fig. 13.4). The latter creates a large common channel for reimplantation into the recipient. Lastly, each artery may be reimplanted into the recipient separately. This is less favorable, as it requires an additional anastomosis and longer warm ischemia time while sewing in the graft.

Vascular Anastomosis

To begin the vascular anastomosis, systemic heparin (weight-based dosing) is administered and the vessels are clamped. Both the venous and arterial anastomoses are performed in an end-to-side fashion. The venous anastomosis is typically performed first, followed by the arterial anastomosis. A longitudinal venotomy or arteriotomy is performed with a #11 scalpel. The venotomy is extended to an appropriate length to match the renal vein, while the arteriotomy is matched to the renal artery using an arterial punch. The arterial punch creates an elliptical opening that optimizes arterial blood flow across the anastomosis by keeping the stiff arterial wall

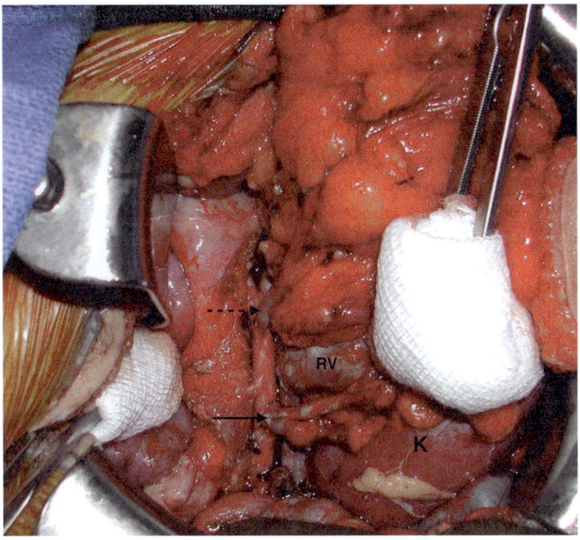

Fig. 13.4 An intra-abdominal kidney transplantation with multiple renal arteries is shown after reperfusion. The solid arrow denotes an arterial reconstruction employing the "pantaloon" side-to-side reconstruction, implanted onto the recipient's aorta. The segmented arrow shows a third artery separately implanted into the recipient's aorta. The renal vein (labeled RV) is shown as it connects to the recipient's inferior vena cava. The kidney (labeled K) is partially visible in the bottom right of the image. (Photo courtesy of Richard Perez, MD)

splayed open. At this point, corner sutures are placed at either end of the arteriotomy or venotomy using 5-0 or 6-0 polypropylene suture (Fig. 13.5). The vessels are then sutured in a running fashion from each corner, meeting in the middle. Throughout the implantation process, the graft is kept cold by wrapping the kidney with ice-cold gauze and periodically applying topical ice-cold saline. Once the anastomoses are complete, clamps are released and the graft is re-perfused. In the case of bleeding at the suture lines, additional sutures can be placed to achieve hemostasis.

Ureteral Reimplantation

After renal reperfusion, the ureter is anastomosed to the bladder (ureteroneocystostomy). The most commonly performed technique is a modified Lich-Gregoir extravesical ureteroneocystostomy, which is based on described techniques to minimize vesicoureteral reflux [6–8]. The urinary catheter is clamped, and small volume of crystalloid containing gentamicin is infused to distend the bladder. This aids in exposing the bladder when selecting a suitable location to make a cystotomy. The end of the ureter is typically spatulated by incising the ureter longitudinally (~1 cm), which creates a larger opening to facilitate the anastomosis. Using 5-0 polydioxanone suture (monofilament, absorbable), the anastomosis of full-thickness ureter to

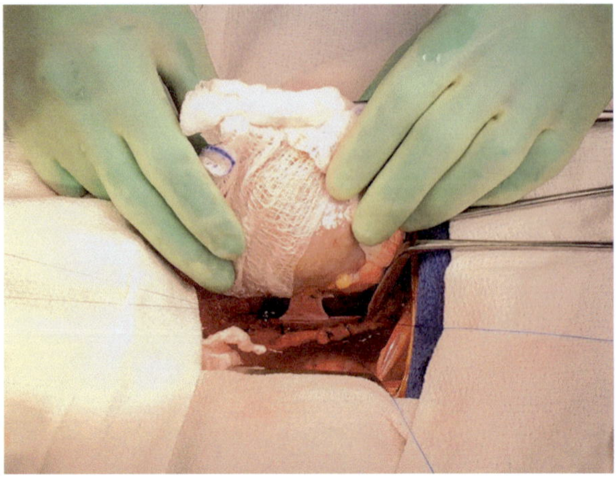

Fig. 13.5 Kidney during implantation at the beginning of the venous anastomosis to the recipient's external iliac vein. Thin blue sutures can be seen, which are securing the "corners" of the anastomosis. The kidney is shown wrapped in ice-cold gauze to keep the graft cold while out of cold storage. (Photo taken by Andrew Perry, MD)

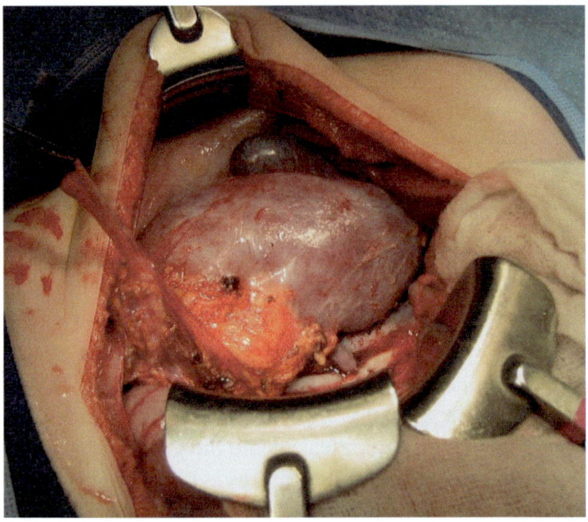

Fig. 13.6 An intra-abdominal kidney transplant in a pediatric recipient after reperfusion. The ureter is being held by forceps in the top left of the image. The gallbladder and liver edge can be seen in the top right of the image. (Photo courtesy of Richard Perez, MD)

bladder mucosa is performed in a running fashion. The detrusor is then re-approximated over a short segment of ureter using 4-0 polydioxanone to create a submucosal tunnel, which is intended to provide an anti-reflux mechanism.

Alternative techniques to the Lich-Gregoir are the Leadbetter technique [9] and a "single-stitch" technique described by Taguchi [10]. The Leadbetter involves incising the bladder and performing a ureteroneocystostomy from the inside of the bladder. Taguchi's "single-stitch" technique uses a single mattress suture to secure the ureter to bladder mucosa. This technique is often used for small ureters from small pediatric kidneys to minimize the risk of ischemic stricture.

Although some centers do not use ureteral stents, it is our practice to use stents in all our recipients. In adult and large adolescent patients, a double J stent extends from the renal pelvis and terminates in the bladder. The stent is typically left in place for 4–6 weeks as the anastomosis matures and is removed by cystoscopy. In order to limit instrumentation in the pediatric population, however, we instead use a pediatric feeding tube to stent the ureteroneocystostomy. The tube extends from the renal pelvis of the transplanted kidney, across the anastomosis, and exits through the urethra, where it is secured to the Foley catheter. The catheter and stent are then removed on postoperative day 7, at the time of discharge from the hospital.

Intraoperative Anesthesia

Communication between the surgeon and anesthesia team is crucial for successful outcomes in pediatric renal transplantation. The most important anesthetic concerns include careful attention to the patient's hemodynamics, optimization of intravascular volume, and maintaining adequate perfusion pressure to the graft. Since the blood volume of an adult kidney is significant in proportion to the intravascular volume of a small child, reperfusion of the transplanted kidney in pediatric patients effectively causes a rapid loss in systemic intravascular volume. Additionally, the introduction of an adult kidney to the pediatric circulation redirects a significant proportion of the patient's total cardiac output to the graft. If not managed appropriately, these changes can cause catastrophic hypotension and an inadequate perfusion pressure to the graft, risking graft thrombosis.

Several measures can be done in anticipation of this dramatic hemodynamic shift prior to reperfusion. First, if preoperative dialysis is necessary to correct electrolyte disturbances and uremia, fluid removal should be limited. During the operation, an arterial line and central venous catheter should be placed for hemodynamic monitoring. Fluid loading using crystalloid, albumin, and/or blood products should be done to maintain a CVP of 8–12 cm H20 and a mean arterial pressure (MAP) of 60–70 mm Hg. Lastly, infusion of a vasopressor such as dopamine can be initiated if the target MAP cannot be achieved, but this should only be done after adequate volume loading.

A major concern in transplantation is ischemia-reperfusion injury. In order to mitigate this, 20% mannitol (a free radical scavenger) at 1 g/kg and sodium bicarbonate are administered prior to release of the vascular clamps. It is also administered along with furosemide (1 mg/kg) in order to promote immediate urine output.

Aortic cross clamping during the arterial anastomosis leads to the accumulation of lactic acid due to hypoperfusion of the lower extremities. When the aorta is unclamped and blood flow is reestablished, the lactic acid is "washed out," which can cause acidosis and hypotension. These consequences can be mitigated with the administration of sodium bicarbonate at the time of reperfusion.

Immunosuppression

Induction immunosuppression is administered at the commencement of the operation. At our center, this consists of anti-thymocyte globulin (ATG), methylprednisolone, and mycophenolate mofetil (MMF). The cumulative dose of ATG depends on the immunologic risk of the recipient and is typically administered in divided doses over 3–5 days. Tacrolimus is then initiated on postoperative day 1, which, along with mycophenolate mofetil, comprises the majority of maintenance immunosuppression.

Posttransplant Management

Early Postoperative Management

In the early postoperative period, careful attention to hemodynamics and intravascular volume continues to be crucial. If a central venous catheter is placed, a chest x-ray is obtained to confirm appropriate position of the catheter tip at the atriocaval junction. An ultrasound is typically obtained to establish baseline perfusion measurements of the kidney and assess for any technical problems that could be rectified with immediate re-exploration. In the first 48 h after transplantation of an adult kidney in a pediatric patient, urine output can be large. In this setting, urine output is replaced in a 1:1 ratio with normal saline, in addition to standard maintenance fluid rate. A chemistry panel should be obtained frequently within the first 24 h of transplantation to monitor for electrolyte disturbances. A complete blood count should be obtained at least every 12 h in the early postoperative period to monitor for hemorrhage and dilutional anemia.

Surgical Complications

Intra-abdominal transplantation of renal grafts requires mobilization of the bowel to expose the large vessels for implant. This predisposes the pediatric patient to ileus. Ileus manifests as abdominal distension, nausea, bilious emesis, and failure to pass flatus or bowel movement. Initial management consists of NPO, nasogastric tube decompression, limitation of narcotics, and correction of any underlying electrolyte abnormalities. An early postoperative bowel obstruction presents similar to an ileus and should similarly be managed with nasogastric tube decompression and supportive measures. Operative management should be reserved for cases that fail to resolve with nonoperative management, as there is significant morbidity associated with re-exploration within 4–6 weeks of surgery.

A bowel injury should always be in the differential diagnosis of perioperative gastrointestinal dysfunction, especially in the setting of an intra-abdominal graft implantation. Typically, a bowel injury with perforation presents with fever, tachycardia, leukocytosis, abdominal tenderness, and distension and can progress toward sepsis and shock. However, the immunosuppressed transplant recipient can have a dampened response to injury and inflammation that would potentially mask an underlying bowel injury.

Early Graft Dysfunction

Oligoanuria in the early postoperative period can represent an emergency, and it is critical to identify causes that require urgent intervention. Causes of early graft dysfunction include hypovolemia, hemorrhage, catheter obstruction, acute rejection, thrombosis, acute tubular necrosis (ATN), and urological problems such as urine leak or ureteral obstruction. Early recurrence of certain systemic diseases from the donor in the transplanted graft, such as the case with FSGS, can also manifest in early graft dysfunction in the postoperative period.

The clinician should assess the patient to address issues needing immediate intervention (hypovolemia, sepsis, or catheter obstruction). Work-up should include blood work including complete blood count, chemistry panel, and urinalysis to assess for infectious etiologies, hemorrhage, and electrolyte disturbances. Ultrasound with Doppler assessment is critical in the work-up for oligoanuria. A perigraft fluid collection can manifest from bleeding or a urine leak. Hydronephrosis on ultrasound indicates potential urinary obstruction at the ureteral anastomosis or ureteropelvic junction. Lastly, Doppler assessment is crucial to ensure adequate graft perfusion and rule out arterial or venous thrombosis.

Vascular Complications

There is a higher risk for graft thrombosis in pediatric renal transplantation, especially in small children. In fact, graft thrombosis is responsible for up to 35% of early graft loss in the pediatric population [1], with an overall incidence of 0.7–5% [11]. Perioperative graft thrombosis should be suspected in the setting of sudden oligoanuria in a previously functioning kidney. Immediate ultrasound with Doppler assessment of vascular flow should be performed for a quick and easy diagnostic assessment.

Primary risk factors for graft thrombosis include pretransplant peritoneal dialysis, donor age less than 6 years old, recipient age less than 2 years old, ATN, a history of previous renal transplantation, and cold ischemia time >24 h [11, 12]. Technical issues with the vascular anastomosis and systemic hypotension causing poor perfusion pressure to the graft are also felt to contribute to thrombosis. Thrombophilic disorders also increase the risk for graft thrombosis (protein C and S deficiencies, factor V Leiden, antiphospholipid antibodies, and prothrombin mutation). Patients with thrombophilic risk factors should be initiated on systemic anticoagulation and/or aspirin therapy soon after transplantation.

Unfortunately, arterial thrombosis is often an irrecoverable complication, as any intervention to salvage the kidney accompanies excessive warm ischemia. On the other hand, venous thrombosis merits urgent intervention because it may be salvageable. Surgical exploration with thrombectomy, in association with systemic heparinization, can be attempted to salvage the graft.

Postoperative bleeding may require re-exploration to achieve hemostasis and evacuate the hematoma. A small perigraft hematoma in a hemodynamically stable patient can be observed safely without further intervention. Indications to surgically explore a perigraft hematoma include bleeding that requires blood transfusion or is associated with hemodynamic compromise. A large hematoma can also diminish perfusion to the kidney if there is mass effect or compression on the kidney, in which case evacuation of the hematoma is necessary. Lastly, a large hematoma is often discomforting to the patient, and evacuation will provide significant symptomatic relief.

Renal artery stenosis can cause graft dysfunction or worsening hypertension. This is a complication that typically presents later in the posttransplant period. Ultrasound with Doppler assessment can establish the diagnosis, while angiography is the gold standard. Treatment initially involves balloon angioplasty with or without stenting. If this is unsuccessful, autotransplantation of the graft with revision of the arterial anastomosis is indicated.

Urologic Complications

Urologic injuries can present as both early and late complications. A urinary leak most commonly presents in the acute postoperative period. A typical presentation is a graft having slow or delayed graft function, as urine leaking into the abdomen results in reabsorption of creatinine, potassium, and other metabolites. The patient may have abdominal discomfort at the graft site from a urinoma, which can be detected by ultrasonography. The definitive studies to confirm a urine leak are a nuclear medicine scan or a diagnostic nephrostogram of the transplant kidney. Management consists of radiologically guided drainage of the urinoma and a nephrostomy with or without nephroureteral stent placement for urinary drainage. After 4–6 weeks, the urinary tract can be interrogated with a nephrostogram to evaluate for persistence of urinary extravasation. Large defects that do not heal with minimally invasive strategies require surgical revision of the ureteroneocystostomy.

Urinary obstruction can present both early and late in the postoperative period. Early obstruction from ureteral edema at the ureteroneocystostomy can be prevented with routine stent placement at the time of transplantation. Ureteral stents are typically removed 4–6 weeks after transplantation, after which urinary obstruction from strictures can present. Ureteral obstruction after stent removal is typically due to ischemic injury to the ureter or technical issues with the anastomosis between the ureter and the bladder. Initial management focuses on establishing urinary drainage. This is best achieved with a nephrostomy tube. Short segment strictures are typically managed nonoperatively with multiple rounds of balloon dilation and nephroureteral stent placement. If normal ureteral flow is not achieved after multiple dilations at the strictured segment of ureter, a surgical revision is warranted. Surgical options include reimplantation of donor ureter into the bladder or reimplantation of the donor ureter into native ureter (if available).

Conclusion

Kidney transplantation is the most effective treatment for children with ESRD, but successful outcomes require a dedicated multidisciplinary approach. Healthy communication and coordination between pediatric nephrologists, transplant surgeons, pediatric urologists, pediatric anesthesiologists, pharmacists, and a dedicated pediatric nursing team are essential.

Acknowledgment This work was supported in part by Health Resources and Services Administration contract 234-2005-37011C. The content is the responsibility of the authors alone and does not necessarily reflect the views or policies of the Department of Health and Human Services, nor does mention of trade names, commercial products, or organizations imply endorsement by the US government.

References

1. Smith JM, Stablein D, Singh A, Harmon W, McDonald RA. Decreased risk of renal allograft thrombosis associated with interleukin-2 receptor antagonists: a report of the NAPRTCS. Am J Transplant Off J Am Soc Transplant Am Soc Transplant Surg. 2006;6(3):585–8.
2. Smith JM, Martz K, Blydt-Hansen TD. Pediatric kidney transplant practice patterns and outcome benchmarks, 1987–2010: a report of the North American Pediatric Renal Trials and Collaborative Studies. Pediatr Transplant. 2013;17(2):149–57.
3. North American Pediatric Renal Trials and Collaborative Studies. 2014 annual transplant report. 2014.
4. Ellis D, Gilboa N, Bellinger M, Shapiro R. Renal transplantation in infants and children. In: Shapiro R, Simmons RL, Starzl TE, editors. Renal transplantation. Stamford: Appleton & Lange. 1997, p. 427–69.
5. Moers C, Smits JM, Maathuis MH, Treckmann J, van Gelder F, Napieralski BP, et al. Machine perfusion or cold storage in deceased-donor kidney transplantation. N Engl J Med. 2009;360(1):7–19.
6. Lich RHL, Davis LA. Recurrent urosepsis in children. J Urol. 1961;86:554–8.
7. Gregoir W. The surgical treatment of congenital vesico-ureteral reflux. Acta Chir Belg. 1964;63:431–9.
8. Gregoir W, Vanregemorter G. Congenital vesico-ureteral reflux. Urol Int. 1964;18:122–36.
9. Politano VA, Leadbetter WF. An operative technique for the correction of vesicoureteral reflux. J Urol. 1958;79(6):932–41.
10. Taguchi Y, Klauber GT, MacKinnon KJ. Implantation of transplant ureters: a technique. J Urol. 1971;105(2):194–5.
11. Singh A, Stablein D, Tejani A. Risk factors for vascular thrombosis in pediatric renal transplantation: a special report of the North American Pediatric Renal Transplant Cooperative Study. Transplantation. 1997;63(9):1263–7.
12. Gulati A, Sarwal MM. Pediatric renal transplantation: an overview and update. Curr Opin Pediatr. 2010;22(2):189–96.

Chapter 14
Immunosuppressive Medications in Kidney Transplantation

Lavjay Butani

Introduction

In today's era a large variety of immunosuppressive agents are available to the pediatric transplant nephrologist to choose from. The choice of immunosuppression varies considerably based on factors such as physician and center preference and on patient and transplant characteristics such as sensitization, prior rejection episodes, and comorbidities such as diabetes and heart disease. However, as a general rule, most protocols, both adult and pediatric, include an induction agent such as an antithymocyte antibody (like thymoglobulin) or an IL-2 receptor blocker (such as basiliximab) along with maintenance immunosuppression including various combinations of corticosteroids, calcineurin inhibitors (CNI) (either cyclosporine or tacrolimus), and antiproliferative agents such as mycophenolate mofetil (MMF), azathioprine, or sirolimus. This next section briefly discusses the key features of these agents, their unique contribution, and their toxicities.

Corticosteroids

Until recently, steroids have constituted the backbone of all induction and maintenance immunosuppressive protocols due to their potent and nonspecific immunosuppressive effects [1]. Steroids, after binding to their cytosolic receptor, translocate into the nucleus and inhibit the transcription of genes involved in T-cell activation such as IL-1, IL-2, IL-3, IL-6, γ-IF, and TNF-α. At high dose steroids may also reduce the expression of IL-2 receptors. However, the disadvantages of chronic

L. Butani
Department of Pediatrics, University of California Davis Medical Center,
Sacramento, CA, USA
e-mail: lbutani@ucdavis.edu

M. N. Haddad et al. (eds.), *Adolescents with Chronic Kidney Disease*,
https://doi.org/10.1007/978-3-319-97220-6_14

steroid use are well recognized. Their cosmetic side effects such as acne, cushingoid facies, abdominal striae, and hirsutism are a disincentive to adolescents and young adults and may contribute to nonadherence. Other adverse effects include hyperglycemia, hyperlipidemia, hypertension, osteopenia, growth failure, cataracts, and increased susceptibility to infections. In an attempt to minimize these toxicities, most immunosuppressive protocols include a taper of the steroid dose over time. Some pediatric centers also convert stable patients who are perceived to be at a lower risk of rejection (based on factors such as tissue typing and long-standing adherence to the medication regimen) onto alternate day therapy or even toward a steroid-free regimen. Both of these approaches have been tried with variable degrees of success but even in the CNI era are associated with a higher risk of acute rejection [2]. This may be due to the rebound increase in T-cell activation as a consequence of the upregulation of the IL receptors in response to a decrease in their gene transcription. As will be discussed later, there has been a resurgence of interest in avoiding steroids in renal transplant recipients by steroid avoidance or by steroid minimization (using only 3–5 days of steroid therapy in the immediate posttransplant period); data from the most recent North American Pediatric Renal Trials And Collaborative Studies (NAPRTCS) report show that only about 50% of children are receiving maintenance steroids at day 30 posttransplant [3].

Induction Immunosuppression

Induction therapy refers to the use of T-cell depleting or modulating agents that are used in the immediate peri-transplant period. The 2009 Kidney Disease Improving Global Outcomes clinical practice guidelines state that induction therapy should be used in all renal transplant recipients due to their favorable risk-benefit and cost-benefit ratios [4]. Interestingly, the 2014 NAPRTCS annual report describes that only about 40% of children receiving renal transplants were administered some form of induction immunosuppressive therapy; however, this number excludes those transplant patients who received induction agents for the first time, later than the first posttransplant day. While the use of monoclonal and polyclonal anti-T-cell antibodies for induction was much more common in the mid to late 1990s, their use has declined due, in part, to the availability of the less toxic IL-2 receptor blockers. In recent years, no pediatric renal transplant recipient registered with the NAPRTCS received the monoclonal antibody OKT3, 26% received antithymocyte globulin (ATG), and 8% were treated with the IL-2 receptor blockers. The use of induction agents is driven by their efficacy in reducing acute rejection especially during the postoperative period when maintenance immunosuppressive medications are being initiated and target therapeutic drug levels achieved; while several studies have demonstrated a reduction in acute rejection with these agents, this may come at the cost of increased infections and without unequivocal long-term benefits, at least in immunologically low-risk recipients [5, 6]. Each of the commonly used induction agents will now be discussed briefly.

IL-2 Receptor Blockers

Currently, the only commercially available IL-2 receptor blocker is basiliximab, a humanized chimeric monoclonal IgG antibody directed against the α-subunit of the IL-2 receptor which is expressed on *activated* T and B cells. The humanization of this antibody makes it less immunogenic and increases its half-life. Use of the IL-2 blockers has been demonstrated to reduce the risk of acute rejection by as much as 40% in the 1st year, with a possible benefit on graft survival [7] and without an increased risk of malignancies. Another major advantage that the IL-2 blockers have over the antilymphocyte antibodies is their relative lack of side effects. No cytokine release syndrome (such as was common with OKT3) is seen with basiliximab. Basiliximab is administered intravenously as an infusion, the first dose being administered in the immediate preoperative period. There are data that suggest that the IL-2 blockers are at least as effective, if not somewhat more effective, than horse ATG induction in preventing acute rejection while at the same time being more convenient to administer and associated with a lower risk of adverse events [8, 9]. In a recent randomized controlled trial comparing basiliximab to rabbit ATG induction, in low-risk adults receiving a steroid-minimization immunosuppression regimen, 1-year acute rejection rates were comparable between the two groups with no differences in 1-year graft or patient survival nor in infections [10].

Thymoglobulin

Thymoglobulin has replaced horse ATG as the most commonly used polyclonal antilymphocyte antibody in transplantation. It is a very potent immunosuppressive agent, more so compared to the IL-2 receptor blockers, but also has greater side effects. Due to its higher risk-benefit profile, many centers restrict its use for high-risk transplants such as patients with a high panel reactive antibody (PRA) or poorer HLA matching, younger recipients, African American recipients, prolonged cold ischemic times, and in the setting of delayed graft function (DGF) to maintain effective immunosuppression while at the same time delay initiation of CNIs [4]. Additionally, thymoglobulin is often used as the induction agent in corticosteroid-free immunosuppression protocols, although the recent HARMONY trial did not demonstrate any benefit afforded by thymoglobulin compared to basiliximab in low-risk recipients on a corticosteroid-minimization regimen [10].

Thymoglobulin is a polyclonal antibody that causes very rapid T-cell depletion. In addition, it modulates the expression of a variety of T-cell surface markers causing functional T-cell impairment. Although the half-life of thymoglobulin is only about 3 days after the first dose, the half-life progressively increases with a longer treatment course, such that after a 10–14-day course, levels of thymoglobulin are detectable in the serum for 40–50 days after the last dose. Surprisingly, long-lasting effects of thymoglobulin on T cells have been noted such as the persistence of lymphopenia for as long as 1-year after treatment and a reversal in the CD4 to CD8 ratio for as long as 4–5 years. The majority of patients treated with thymoglobulin develop anti-rabbit antibodies (70%), but this has not been shown to be of any clinical significance in determining response to treatment. Other side effects are the frequent development of fever and chills (60% of patients), leukopenia (50%), thrombocytopenia (40%), and rarely anaphylaxis. The dosing regimens for thymoglobulin vary considerably. The usual dose is 1.5 mg/kg/day administered as a slow intravenous infusion for a duration as short as 3–7 days when used as an induction agent or in the setting of DGF to as long as 10–14 days for reversal of acute rejection episodes. During therapy, some centers monitor the CD3 count and modify treatment to achieve a target CD3 count (absolute) of <20 (or 40) cells/mm^3 or a CD3% <15%; many centers have stopped dosing thymoglobulin based on CD3 counts when used as an induction agent. Due to the frequent occurrence of systemic side effects, premedication with steroids, antihistamines, and acetaminophen is recommended at least for the initial few doses.

Campath1H

Campath 1H (alemtuzumab) is a humanized anti-CD 52 T- and B-cell depleting monoclonal antibody that has been used for induction therapy and also for the reversal of acute cellular and humoral rejection in renal transplant recipients. Alemtuzumab is the most potent T-cell depleting antibody available to date and depletes lymphocytes not only from the peripheral blood but also in the lymphoid tissue and bone marrow. After a very short course (1–3 days) of therapy, patients develop prolonged and profound T-cell (as long as 12 months) and B-cell (6 months) depletion; moreover, although T-cell recovery does take place by 12 months, the total counts remain low (2/3rd of baseline levels) in the vast majority of patients even as far out as 3 years. The depleting effects of alemtuzumab are less persistent for B cells and monocytes. Randomized controlled trials of alemtuzumab induction have been small and not well controlled for other immunosuppressive agents making their interpretation difficult. A 2017 Cochrane Database Systematic Review determined that in the setting of steroid minimization regimens, alemtuzumab is more effective than antithymocyte globulin in preventing acute rejection but at the cost of increased CMV infection and without any clear benefit in graft or patient survival [5]. Studies have also shown that, unlike what had been initially hoped for, alemtuzumab by itself is not sufficient as the sole immunosuppression after transplant since the vast majority of patients so treated experience acute rejection [11]. It has been shown that the use of alemtuzumab allows the use of less maintenance immunosuppression and may therefore enable the successful use of CNI-free and/or steroid-free immunosuppressive approaches [12] and may also have a role in highly sensitized patients [13]. Pediatric experience with the use of alemtuzumab is even more limited; more study will be needed before this agent gains wider acceptance in standard immunosuppressive regimens in children [14–16].

Side effects commonly seen are similar to other antibodies (leukopenia, thrombocytopenia, and the cytokine release syndrome). Many investigators have found that compared to conventional immunosuppression, acute rejection episodes that do occur in alemtuzumab-treated patients may happen much later in the posttransplant period; on histology, these rejections appear different, in that the cellular infiltrate is composed predominantly of monocytes. In fact, an increase in the absolute monocyte count in the peripheral blood in alemtuzumab-treated patients may herald the development of acute rejection.

Maintenance Immunosuppression

CNIs

Along with steroids, the CNIs (cyclosporine [CyA] and tacrolimus) have been the cornerstone of all immunosuppressive regimens in renal transplantation for several decades. Both drugs are mechanistically very similar although structurally quite different. After binding to their cytosolic receptors (cyclophilin for CyA and FKBP-12 for tacrolimus), these agents inhibit the activity of the enzyme calcineurin, which then results in reduced IL-2 transcription and subsequent prevention of T-cell proliferation in response to antigenic stimulation. Due to the greater immunosuppressive potency of tacrolimus and the lower incidence of cosmetic side effects such as hirsutism and gingival hyperplasia, tacrolimus has superseded CyA as the CNI of choice in most pediatric transplant centers [3]. Both the microemulsion preparation of CyA (Neoral) and tacrolimus have a low bioavailability (30–40%) due to extensive metabolism in the gastrointestinal tract by the intestinal P-glycoprotein and the cytochrome P450 systems. Interindividual variations in these metabolic pathways lead to considerable variation in pharmacokinetic handling of these drugs between patients, making therapeutic drug monitoring essential, especially since these drugs have a narrow therapeutic index. Moreover, since many other drugs share these metabolic pathways with the CNIs, the potential for drug interactions leading to adverse events is considerable. Both are highly protein bound (90%), Neoral to the lipoprotein and tacrolimus to the α 2-glycoprotein compartment; both are metabolized in the liver and excreted in bile with little drug being found in the urine. Their terminal half-life is about 12 h, so that they are most often dosed in a twice-daily regimen. Dosing regimens and practices vary based on the transplant center and on the concomitant immunosuppression being used. For Neoral, some centers' dose are based on body surface area (500 mg/m^2/day in three divided doses) especially for children <6 years, with weight-based dosing for older children (10–15 mg/kg/day in two divided doses). The dose is then reduced with time to aim for lower target levels [either trough levels or 2-h post-dose (C2) levels]. For tacrolimus, we use a starting dose of 0.1 mg/kg/day in two divided doses to aim for an initial target trough level of 10–15 ng/ml. With increasing time after transplantation, the dose is reduced to achieve lower target trough levels. Unlike Neoral, tacrolimus trough levels correlate reasonably well with overall drug exposure for most patients. However, for determining accurate exposure to Neoral, either a C2 level needs to be monitored [17] or abbreviated pharmacokinetics need to be performed [18]. The results of a randomized pediatric trial comparing Neoral to tacrolimus in renal transplantation confirmed the advantage of tacrolimus over Neoral in reducing the risk of acute rejection (by 20%) with better renal function in the tacrolimus arm at 1 year while at the same time being associated with fewer cosmetic side effects [19].

Prolonged-release tacrolimus, allowing once-daily dosing of the medication, has garnered recent attention in the transplant literature because of its potential to simplify and improve medication adherence. In 2009, an open-label randomized trial comparing the two formulations of tacrolimus in adult renal transplant recipients demonstrated comparability in short-term efficacy (at 6 weeks) and drug exposure [20]. A subsequent randomized phase 3 study in a similar cohort of patients, comparing once-daily and twice-daily tacrolimus (with the same total daily dose of tacrolimus) in conjunction with maintenance steroids and mycophenolate mofetil (MMF), but without antibody induction, showed that the incidence of biopsy-proven acute rejection at 24 weeks was slightly higher in the once-daily dosing arm (20.4% versus 15.8%); 12-month patient and graft survival, graft function, and adverse events were comparable [21]. Conversion of stable adult recipients from a twice-daily to a once-daily regimen of tacrolimus has been shown to result in improved adherence and patient satisfaction without any adverse consequences [22] and, in fact, an improvement in lipid profiles and markers of insulin resistance [23]. Two prolonged-release tacrolimus preparations are now available in the USA; pharmacokinetics of these preparations vary, compared to the traditional shorter-acting tacrolimus formulation, which needs to be taken into consideration when initiating them [24]. Pediatric data are very limited, and in the absence of robust studies assessing outcomes in pediatric patients, especially younger patients who may have different pharmacokinetic profiles, prolonged-release tacrolimus preparations must be used with caution and with close monitoring [25].

The major concern with the use of CNIs is nephrotoxicity, both acute and chronic, the latter being a major contributor to long-term graft loss. Acute CNI toxicity is caused by afferent renal arteriolar vasoconstriction causing ischemia to the kidney. This can be reduced by the use of calcium channel blockers. Over time, the prolonged ischemia causes upregulation of the fibrogenic cytokine, transforming growth factor-β, leading to interstitial fibrosis and tubular atrophy [26]. The mechanism of CNI-induced arteriolar vasoconstriction continues to be debated with some investigators implicating angiotensin-II while others attributing it to the vasoconstrictive prostanoids such as thromboxane A2. Reduction of CNI-induced nephrotoxicity has been achieved with the use of calcium channel blockers [27], angiotensin blockade, and also by the use of biologic oils such as fish oil and juniper oil, the latter in experimental models [28]. The most effective way to prevent CNI nephrotoxicity, however, is by CNI avoidance or withdrawal, which will be discussed later.

Antimetabolites

Azathioprine

Although azathioprine was one of the earliest immunosuppressive agents to be utilized in renal transplantation, its use has declined considerably since MMF was introduced. According to the 2014 NAPRTCS report, by day 30 after transplantation, only 3–5% of pediatric recipients were receiving azathioprine in recent years. Azathioprine is an imidazolyl derivative of 6-MP. It is well absorbed after oral administration and gets extensively metabolized in the liver to the active compounds 6-MP and 6-thionosinic acid monophosphate (TIMP), which are eventually converted to inactive metabolites by xanthine oxidase. TIMP inhibits an enzyme involved in the de novo pathway of purine synthesis. In addition the metabolites of azathioprine are also incorporated into cellular DNA as fraudulent bases, causing chromosomal breaks. Both of these mechanisms impair nucleotide synthesis and prevent T- and B-lymphocyte proliferation. The dose of azathioprine ranges from 1 to 3 mg/kg/day in a single-daily dose. Until the past decade, no drug exposure monitoring was available or recommended for azathioprine, in spite of the fact that there are significant interindividual variations in the levels of thiopurine metabolites that can be achieved for a given dose. Tissue levels rather than blood levels of the thiopurine derivatives of azathioprine are indicative of therapeutic efficacy; more recent data suggest that drug monitoring by measuring the red blood cell levels of the metabolites of azathioprine, now commercially available, accurately reflects tissue levels of the thiopurines and may help improve graft outcomes [29]. The main side effects of the drug are bone marrow suppression, hepatotoxicity, pancreatitis, and the development of neoplasms due to the mutagenicity of this agent. Due to the greater potency of MMF in preventing acute rejection, it has all but replaced azathioprine in clinical practice. One setting in which azathioprine may still be of value is as a substitute for MMF in children who develop intolerable side effects, including allergic reactions, when receiving MMF.

MMF

MMF is the 2-morpholinoethyl ester of mycophenolic acid (MPA), the active immunosuppressive compound which is derived from the fungus *Penicillium*. MPA is a noncompetitive reversible inhibitor of the eukaryotic enzyme inosine monophosphate dehydrogenase (IMPDH), which is a key enzyme in the de novo pathway of purine synthesis. Like azathioprine, MMF inhibits the proliferation of T and B cells which are dependent on the de novo pathway for nucleotide synthesis. MMF also has the theoretical benefit of reducing tubulointerstitial atrophy and fibrosis by inhibiting smooth muscle and mesangial cell proliferation [30]. Retrospective and uncontrolled trials have shown a benefit of MMF in retarding the rate of decline of glomerular filtration rate (GFR) in patients with established chronic changes [31] and perhaps in improving long-term graft survival [32]. After absorption from the gastrointestinal tract, MMF is rapidly hydrolyzed to MPA. The bioavailability of this drug is extremely high (>95%) unlike most other immunosuppressive agents. MPA gets metabolized by the liver to the inactive metabolite, MPA glucuronide (MPAG), and to the active MPA acyl glucuronide, both of which, like MPA, are highly protein bound (80–97%). Since so much of the active drug is bound, measuring free MPA is important since this is the component of the drug that is metabolically active. The drug metabolites of MPA are excreted in the urine (93%). There is also some enterohepatic circulation of the drug causing secondary peaks in the serum level of the drug (at around 6–12 h). Dosing of MMF in children needs to be based on the concomitant immunosuppression being used. Pharmacokinetic studies have shown that patients receiving tacrolimus should receive MMF at a dose of 300 mg/m^2 surface area twice daily, while those receiving CyA need twice that dose (since CyA increases the metabolism of MMF). In children on a CNI-free protocol, the recommended dose of MMF is 500 mg/m^2 twice daily [33]. Even when following these guidelines, it is imperative to realize that there are large interindividual variations in MMF kinetics and also that MPA, free MPA, and MPAG levels, and degree of protein binding are affected by the serum albumin level and the renal function of the patient so that these factors need be taken into consideration. Some issues of drug dosing can be solved by monitoring the serum trough levels of MPA and MPAG. However measuring the trough level may not be enough since MPA trough levels have been shown to correlate poorly with the area under the time-concentration curve (AUC). Nevertheless, drug level monitoring of MPA and MPAG is becoming more common in the USA and Europe. Recent studies have indicated that 50% suppression of IMPDH is critical for preventing acute rejection and that this corresponds to an MPA trough level of 2–5 mcg/ml. Some pediatric and adult studies have shown value to kinetic monitoring in predicting acute rejection and toxicity. The total MPA, AUC, and MPA trough have been shown to correlate with acute rejection, although not with a high enough predictive value to be of universal clinical use. An MPA AUC >34 (and up to 60) mg.h/L has a sensitivity of 75% and a specificity of 64% in ruling out acute rejection, while an MPA trough >1.3 (up to 3.5) mg/L has a sensitivity of 83% and a specificity of 64% in ruling out acute rejection. For toxicity, a high free MPA AUC has been shown to correlate with the development of leukopenia and infectious complications [34, 35]. Since obtaining a complete kinetic profile in all patients on a routine basis is impractical, abbreviated kinetic formulae have been derived and determined to have a high correlation with a complete AUC profile [35].

Prospective controlled trials in adult renal transplant recipients, comparing MMF to azathioprine, have demonstrated a 35% reduction in acute rejection and a reduced need for the use of antilymphocyte agents [36]. Similarly, pediatric trials using historical controls treated with azathioprine have shown 20% reduction in acute rejection and a better 3-year graft survival with the use of MMF [37]. The main toxicities of MMF are hematologic such as leukopenia, neutrophil dysplasia, and anemia, when used in patients with advanced renal insufficiency without dose modification

[38]. Other important side effects are gastrointestinal (GI) (diarrhea, gastric ulcers, and bleeds), increased risk of infections (including urinary tract infections [UTIs], CMV, and varicella), and posttransplant lymphoproliferative disorders (PTLD). The former, which seem to be more common in the younger children, often need to be managed by dose reduction or even temporary cessation of MMF.

Enteric-coated mycophenolate sodium is a preparation that was developed in an attempt to reduce the incidence of upper GI side effects of MMF since its release occurs in the duodenum, bypassing contact of the active agent with the gastric mucosa. Prospective and retrospective studies have demonstrated better tolerability of the enteric-coated preparation and the need for fewer dose reductions, while showing comparable efficacy [39, 40]. Pediatric data are much more limited. In children, the peak concentration of MPA occurs approximately 2.5 h after the administration of the enteric-coated preparation compared to 1–2 h with MMF [41]. Small single-center studies have described the use of this preparation in de novo pediatric renal transplant recipients who can swallow the enteric-coated tablets, without any significant unexpected problems; larger studies are needed to replicate these findings [42]. Of note, studies have not shown any convincingly significant decrease in the incidence of GI adverse side effects with myfortic acid compared to MMF [43].

Sirolimus

Sirolimus is one of the newer immunosuppressive agents added to the armamentarium of transplant nephrologists. The greatest benefit of sirolimus is its lack of nephrotoxicity, making it a very attractive substitute for the CNIs. Sirolimus, a macrocyclic lactone, although structurally different from the CNIs, binds to the same binding protein as tacrolimus (FKBP 12). Sirolimus was first isolated from *Streptomyces hygroscopicus* found in a soil sample on Easter Island (also known as Rapa Nui by its native inhabitants) and hence its initial name "rapamycin." The target on which sirolimus acts has been termed m-TOR or mammalian target of rapamycin. After T-cell activation, m-TOR activates a protein kinase that leads to DNA synthesis. Sirolimus works by inhibiting m-TOR and thereby causing the cell cycle arrest of T and B cells during the G1 to S phase. Compared to the CNIs, sirolimus has a 70-fold greater efficacy in inhibiting B-cell proliferation. In addition, in vitro, sirolimus also inhibits smooth muscle cell, mesenchymal cell, and neointimal cell proliferation. The oral absorption of sirolimus is very poor with a bioavailability of only 15%. Potential drug interactions are similar to the CNIs since sirolimus is also a cytochrome P450 substrate. Sirolimus is hepatically metabolized and predominantly (>90%) fecally excreted so that dose modifications are not required for patients in renal failure. The average half-life of excretion of sirolimus in adults is 60 h, but like most other drugs, there are marked interindividual variations in its kinetics. Trough levels of sirolimus correlate very well with the AUC ($r = 0.96$) both in adults and in children, making therapeutic drug monitoring much easier. It has been recognized that the kinetics of sirolimus are very different in children, mainly in that the half-life of excretion of the drug is much shorter in pediatric patients. The first report found that the half-life of sirolimus in nonrenal transplant recipients was only 11 h at 1 month with an increase to 20 h by 3 months, indicating that perhaps at least in the early posttransplant period, children should be dosed twice daily (unlike the once-daily dosing recommended for adults) [44]. The second report, in renal transplant recipients on a CNI-free protocol, also found a similarly short half-life, but both early and late in the posttransplant period [45], and an even shorter half-life in the children less than 6 years of age.

Trials using sirolimus as a substitute for azathioprine show it to be superior in reducing the risk of rejection [46]. Shortly after it became available, sirolimus was increasingly used along with low-dose CNIs [47], in CNI-free regimens (along with MMF) [48] and in steroid-free protocols, although in more recent years its use, at least in children, has declined considerably [3]. A variety of dosing regimens and target trough levels have been recommended in adult recipients based on the concomitant immunosuppression used. In general when used with low-dose CNIs, lower target trough levels (8–12 ng/nl) are considered acceptable as compared to trough levels of 15–30 ng/ml when used without any CNI. For older pediatric patients, the manufacturer recommends a 3 mg/m^2 loading dose followed by a maintenance dose of 1 mg/m^2 in a single-daily dose. However, as mentioned earlier there is some suggestion in the literature that twice-daily dosing may be more appropriate in children. In any event, irrespective of the starting dose, therapeutic drug monitoring is essential to achieve target trough levels.

The most well-recognized toxicities of sirolimus are the development of leukopenia, thrombocytopenia, and hyperlipidemia. The hematologic toxicities are very common, are dose related, and usually appear soon after starting sirolimus (63% incidence after 1 week, with a peak cumulative incidence of around 80% by 1 month). The majority of the time (90%) they resolve spontaneously after a median interval 3–4 days, although some patients may need temporary dose reduction or discontinuation of the drug [49]. Similarly the incidence of hyperlipidemia is very common, occurring in about 75% of treated patients and necessitating the frequent use of the statins. As the use of sirolimus became more common, a variety of previously unrecognized complications were encountered, which likely has led to a decline in its use, at least in de novo renal transplant recipients. These include poor wound healing (especially when used in conjunction with steroids), interstitial pneumonitis, massive proteinuria, and testosterone deficiency in males. In addition, although non-nephrotoxic by itself, sirolimus worsens preexisting renal injury and thereby prolongs recovery from acute tubular necrosis and DGF, potentiates CNI nephrotoxicity, and may even increase the incidence of DGF [50, 51]. Unlike most other immunosuppressive agents, animal and human data seems to indicate that sirolimus has an antitumor activity, which may prove to be protective against the development of EBV-driven malignancies and other cancers [52–54]. However, this comes at a cost of increased cardiovascular events, mortality, and acute rejection (when compared to CNIs) [53, 54]. CNI withdrawal, at various time points after transplantation, under cover of sirolimus may preserve long-term graft function but with a higher risk of acute rejection [55, 56].

Everolimus is a newer derivative of sirolimus that has very similar properties except for a somewhat higher bioavailability and a shorter half-life of about 30 h, both in adults and in children [57]. This allows faster steady-state levels to be achieved without the need for a loading dose; however, due to its short half-life, twice-daily dosing is needed. The recommended pediatric dose for everolimus is 0.8 mg/m^2 twice daily, with the target trough level being 3.0 ng/ml. The efficacy and toxicity of everolimus are otherwise identical to that of sirolimus, and it has a similar risk-benefit profile.

Newer Immunosuppressive Strategies

Steroid Minimization Immunosuppression

In order to mitigate the profound metabolic and bone-related complications of chronic steroid therapy, the past two decades have seen an increased interest directed toward steroid-free immunosuppression. Following several small single-center uncontrolled trials that demonstrated the safety and efficacy of steroid minimization in adults and children, randomized controlled trials in children have confirmed that steroid minimization is feasible in immunologically low-risk children, using an IL-2 receptor blocker as induction and with MMF and tacrolimus for maintenance therapy. Compared to regimens using maintenance steroids, such an approach is associated with comparable long-term graft survival and function [58], with similar acute rejection rates [58], and with better growth [59, 60], lower incidence of diabetes, and improved cholesterol and blood pressure [58]. Based on biopsy data, subclinical rejection and chronic renal injury are also comparable between the groups on long-term follow-up [61]. Thymoglobulin has been proposed as an alternative induction agent in the setting of steroid minimization [62, 63], although it is unclear if it adds any additional benefit [10]; head to head comparisons between thymoglobulin and an IL-2 receptor blocker in children are lacking.

CNI-Free Protocols or Rapid CNI Withdrawal

In addition to steroid-free immunosuppression, there is also a push to eliminate the CNIs from immunosuppressive protocols in order to limit nephrotoxicity to the graft [64, 65]. This has become feasible today as a consequence of the discovery of potent non-nephrotoxic immunosuppressive medications such as sirolimus and MMF, potent T-cell depleting agents such as thymoglobulin and alemtuzumab, and most recently the costimulatory blockers, all of which have made CNI avoidance safer [66].

Costimulatory Blockade

Belatacept is a fusion protein composed of the Fc fragment of human IgG linked to the extracellular domain of cytotoxic T-lymphocyte-associated antigen 4 (CTLA-4) that inhibits T-cell activation through costimulation blockade. Following T-cell stimulation by an antigenic signal, there is upregulation of CD 154 (or CD 40 ligand) on the T cell. This then interacts with CD40 which is constitutively expressed on the antigen-presenting cell and causes upregulation of B7-2 (and later of B7-1) on the antigen-presenting cell. B7-2 and B7-1 in turn interact with CD28 which is expressed on the T cell to deliver a second signal. This signal works in several ways. It enables the T cell to respond to lower levels of IL-2 (by stabilizing the IL-2 transcript) and by inducing increasing expression of IL-2 and γ-IF and tumor necrosis factor. Moreover, the costimulation induces the expression of the anti-apoptotic *bcl* gene and also inhibits Fas-mediated cell death. Prevention of the costimulation allows T-cell death once cytokine levels, induced by the first signal, have waned. The CD 40/CD 154 interaction also serves other purposes. It directly provides an anti-apoptotic signal to B cells and augments immunoglobulin synthesis. After T-cell costimulation has occurred, there are natural inhibitory processes that take place to reduce over-activation of the immune response. Within 48–72 h, CTLA-4 gets upregulated on activated T cell. This displaces CD 28 from its binding both with B7-1 and B7-2, thereby giving a negative signal to the T cell.

Belatacept functions by binding both to B7-1 and B7-2 with a stronger affinity compared to CD 28 and thereby provides a negative T-cell signal. Data from the BENFIT trial, a phase 3 trial in adults comparing two belatacept-based regimens with a CyA-based regimen, showed that at 12 months both belatacept arms had similar patient and graft survival but better renal function compared to the CyA arm [67]. The incidence of acute rejection, however, was higher in the belatacept-treated patients as were PTLDs, especially in the high-intensity group. Final long-term data were recently published and demonstrated a 43% reduction in risk of death or graft loss at 7 years for both belatacept regimens compared to the cyclosporine regimen [68]. Equally impressive was the observation that the GFR increased over the 7-year period with both belatacept regimens but declined with the CyA regimen. Rates of development of donor specific antibodies were lower for each of the belatacept cohorts, compared to the CyA group. There is very limited experience with belatacept in children; the need for frequent infusions and the great concern in using it in EBV seronegative patients (due to the higher risk of PTLD) may limit its applicability to this population [69].

Individualizing Immunosuppressive Therapy

Based on registry data and from prospective trials, transplant physicians have the ability, albeit limited, to identify donor-recipient combinations that are expected to be at high and low risk for acute rejection and graft loss. This, expectedly, would and should influence the choice of immunosuppressive therapy, although clear distinctions between low- and high-risk category patients are not easily made. Moreover, the use of demographic information on the donor and recipient only gives generic information on probabilities of graft failure and does not take into account individual differences such as might exist in the immune system and with metabolic pathways. The search still continues to identify reliable and clinically useful markers for tailoring of immunosuppression such that individual tailoring of therapy can be done for patients, to reduce the risk of complications and adverse events, while maintaining optimal graft function and maximizing quality of life.

References

1. Hricik DE, Almawi WY, Strom TB. Trends in the use of glucocorticoids in renal transplantation. Transplantation. 1994;57(7):979–89.
2. Hricik DE, Whalen CC, Lautman J, Bartucci MR, Moir EJ, Mayes JT, et al. Withdrawal of steroids after renal transplantation – clinical predictors of outcome. Transplantation. 1992;53(1):41–5.
3. NAPRTCS Annual Report. [Internet]. 2014. [Cited March 18, 2017]. Available from: https://web.emmes.com/study/ped/annlrept/annlrept.html.
4. Kidney Disease: Improving Global Outcomes Transplant Work G. KDIGO clinical practice guideline for the care of kidney transplant recipients. Am J Transplant. 2009;9(Suppl 3):S1–155.
5. Hill P, Cross NB, Barnett AN, Palmer SC, Webster AC. Polyclonal and monoclonal antibodies for induction therapy in kidney transplant recipients. Cochrane Database Syst Rev. 2017;1:CD004759.
6. Baron PW, Ojogho ON, Yorgin P, Sahney S, Cutler D, Ben-Youssef R, et al. Comparison of outcomes with low-dose anti-thymocyte globulin, basiliximab or no induction therapy in pediatric kidney transplant recipients: a retrospective study. Pediatr Transplant. 2008;12(1):32–9.
7. Vincenti F, Kirkman R, Light S, Bumgardner G, Pescovitz M, Halloran P, et al. Interleukin-2-receptor blockade with daclizumab to prevent acute rejection in renal transplantation. Daclizumab Triple Therapy Study Group. N Engl J Med. 1998;338(3):161–5.
8. Sollinger H, Kaplan B, Pescovitz MD, Philosophe B, Roza A, Brayman K, et al. Basiliximab versus antithymocyte globulin for prevention of acute renal allograft rejection. Transplantation. 2001;72(12):1915–9.
9. Clark G, Walsh G, Deshpande P, Koffman G. Improved efficacy of basiliximab over antilymphocyte globulin induction therapy in paediatric renal transplantation. Nephrol Dial Transplant. 2002;17(7):1304–9.
10. Thomusch O, Wiesener M, Opgenoorth M, Pascher A, Woitas RP, Witzke O, et al. Rabbit-ATG or basiliximab induction for rapid steroid withdrawal after renal transplantation (Harmony): an open-label, multicentre, randomised controlled trial. Lancet. 2016;388(10063):3006–16.
11. Kirk AD, Hale DA, Mannon RB, Kleiner DE, Hoffmann SC, Kampen RL, et al. Results from a human renal allograft tolerance trial evaluating the humanized CD52-specific monoclonal antibody alemtuzumab (CAMPATH-1H). Transplantation. 2003;76(1):120–9.
12. Calne R, Moffatt SD, Friend PJ, Jamieson NV, Bradley JA, Hale G, et al. Campath IH allows low-dose cyclosporine monotherapy in 31 cadaveric renal allograft recipients. Transplantation. 1999;68(10):1613–6.
13. Kim IK, Choi J, Vo AA, Kang A, Patel M, Toyoda M, et al. Safety and efficacy of alemtuzumab induction in highly sensitized pediatric renal transplant recipients. Transplantation. 2017;101(4):883–9.
14. Supe-Markovina K, Melquist JJ, Connolly D, DiCarlo HN, Waltzer WC, Fine RN, et al. Alemtuzumab with corticosteroid minimization for pediatric deceased donor renal transplantation: a seven-yr experience. Pediatr Transplant. 2014;18(4):363–8.
15. Serrano OK, Friedmann P, Ahsanuddin S, Millan C, Ben-Yaacov A, Kayler LK. Outcomes associated with steroid avoidance and alemtuzumab among kidney transplant recipients. Clin J Am Soc Nephrol. 2015;10(11):2030–8.
16. Sung J, Barry JM, Jenkins R, Rozansky D, Iragorri S, Conlin M, et al. Alemtuzumab induction with tacrolimus monotherapy in 25 pediatric renal transplant recipients. Pediatr Transplant. 2013;17(8):718–25.

17. Cole E, Maham N, Cardella C, Cattran D, Fenton S, Hamel J, et al. Clinical benefits of neoral C2 monitoring in the long-term management of renal transplant recipients. Transplantation. 2003;75(12):2086–90.
18. Meier-Kriesche HU, Bonilla-Felix MA, Ferris ME, Swinford R, Kahan BD, Brannan P, et al. A limited sampling strategy for the estimation of neoral AUCs in pediatric patients. Pediatr Nephrol. 1999;13(9):742–7.
19. Trompeter R, Filler G, Webb NJ, Watson AR, Milford DV, Tyden G, et al. Randomized trial of tacrolimus versus cyclosporin microemulsion in renal transplantation. Pediatr Nephrol. 2002;17(3):141–9.
20. Wlodarczyk Z, Squifflet JP, Ostrowski M, Rigotti P, Stefoni S, Citterio F, et al. Pharmacokinetics for once- versus twice-daily tacrolimus formulations in de novo kidney transplantation: a randomized, open-label trial. Am J Transplant. 2009;9(11):2505–13.
21. Kramer BK, Charpentier B, Backman L, Silva HT Jr, Mondragon-Ramirez G, Cassuto-Viguier E, et al. Tacrolimus once daily (ADVAGRAF) versus twice daily (PROGRAF) in de novo renal transplantation: a randomized phase III study. Am J Transplant. 2010;10(12):2632–43.
22. Guirado L, Cantarell C, Franco A, Huertas EG, Fructuoso AS, Fernandez A, et al. Efficacy and safety of conversion from twice-daily to once-daily tacrolimus in a large cohort of stable kidney transplant recipients. Am J Transplant. 2011;11(9):1965–71.
23. Sessa A, Esposito A, Iavicoli G, Lettieri E, Ragosta G, Rossano R, et al. Cardiovascular risk factors in renal transplant patients after switch from standard tacrolimus to prolonged-release tacrolimus. Transplant Proc. 2012;44(7):1901–6.
24. Tremblay S, Nigro V, Weinberg J, Woodle ES, Alloway RR. A steady-state head-to-head pharmacokinetic comparison of all FK-506 (tacrolimus) formulations (ASTCOFF): an open-label, prospective, randomized, two-arm, three-period crossover study. Am J Transplant. 2017;17(2):432–42.
25. Zhao W, Fakhoury M, Baudouin V, Storme T, Maisin A, Deschenes G, et al. Population pharmacokinetics and pharmacogenetics of once daily prolonged-release formulation of tacrolimus in pediatric and adolescent kidney transplant recipients. Eur J Clin Pharmacol. 2013;69(2):189–95.
26. Shihab FS, Bennett WM, Tanner AM, Andoh TF. Mechanism of fibrosis in experimental tacrolimus nephrotoxicity. Transplantation. 1997;64(12):1829–37.
27. Midtvedt K, Hartmann A, Foss A, Fauchald P, Nordal KP, Rootwelt K, et al. Sustained improvement of renal graft function for two years in hypertensive renal transplant recipients treated with nifedipine as compared to lisinopril. Transplantation. 2001;72(11):1787–92.
28. Butani L, Afshinnik A, Johnson J, Javaheri D, Peck S, German JB, et al. Amelioration of tacrolimus-induced nephrotoxicity in rats using juniper oil. Transplantation. 2003;76(2):306–11.
29. Bergan S, Rugstad HE, Bentdal O, Sodal G, Hartmann A, Leivestad T, et al. Monitored high-dose azathioprine treatment reduces acute rejection episodes after renal transplantation. Transplantation. 1998;66(3):334–9.
30. Dubus I, Vendrely B, Christophe I, Labouyrie JP, Delmas Y, Bonnet J, et al. Mycophenolic acid antagonizes the activation of cultured human mesangial cells. Kidney Int. 2002;62(3):857–67.
31. Henne T, Latta K, Strehlau J, Pape L, Ehrich JH, Offner G. Mycophenolate mofetil-induced reversal of glomerular filtration loss in children with chronic allograft nephropathy. Transplantation. 2003;76(9):1326–30.
32. Ojo AO, Meier-Kriesche HU, Hanson JA, Leichtman AB, Cibrik D, Magee JC, et al. Mycophenolate mofetil reduces late renal allograft loss independent of acute rejection. Transplantation. 2000;69(11):2405–9.
33. Filler G, Zimmering M, Mai I. Pharmacokinetics of mycophenolate mofetil are influenced by concomitant immunosuppression. Pediatr Nephrol. 2000;14(2):100–4.
34. Weber LT, Shipkova M, Armstrong VW, Wagner N, Schutz E, Mehls O, et al. The pharmacokinetic-pharmacodynamic relationship for total and free mycophenolic acid in pediatric renal transplant recipients: a report of the German study group on mycophenolate mofetil therapy. J Am Soc Nephrol. 2002;13(3):759–68.

35. Filler G, Feber J, Lepage N, Weiler G, Mai I. Universal approach to pharmacokinetic monitoring of immunosuppressive agents in children. Pediatr Transplant. 2002;6(5):411–8.
36. Mycophenolate mofetil in cadaveric renal transplantation. US Renal Transplant Mycophenolate Mofetil Study Group. Am J Kidney Dis. 1999;34(2):296–303.
37. Jungraithmayr T, Staskewitz A, Kirste G, Boswald M, Bulla M, Burghard R, et al. Pediatric renal transplantation with mycophenolate mofetil-based immunosuppression without induction: results after three years. Transplantation. 2003;75(4):454–61.
38. Butani L, Palmer J, Baluarte HJ, Polinsky MS. Adverse effects of mycophenolate mofetil in pediatric renal transplant recipients with presumed chronic rejection. Transplantation. 1999;68(1):83–6.
39. Sollinger HW, Sundberg AK, Leverson G, Voss BJ, Pirsch JD. Mycophenolate mofetil versus enteric-coated mycophenolate sodium: a large, single-center comparison of dose adjustments and outcomes in kidney transplant recipients. Transplantation. 2010;89(4):446–51.
40. Salvadori M, Holzer H, de Mattos A, Sollinger H, Arns W, Oppenheimer F, et al. Enteric-coated mycophenolate sodium is therapeutically equivalent to mycophenolate mofetil in de novo renal transplant patients. Am J Transplant. 2004;4(2):231–6.
41. Ettenger R, Bartosh S, Choi L, Zhu W, Niederberger W, Campestrini J, et al. Pharmacokinetics of enteric-coated mycophenolate sodium in stable pediatric renal transplant recipients. Pediatr Transplant. 2005;9(6):780–7.
42. Niaudet P, Charbit M, Loirat C, Lapeyraque AL, Tsimaratos M, Cailliez M, et al. Enteric-coated mycophenolate sodium in de novo pediatric renal transplant patients. Pediatr Nephrol. 2009;24(2):395–402.
43. Budde K, Curtis J, Knoll G, Chan L, Neumayer HH, Seifu Y, et al. Enteric-coated mycophenolate sodium can be safely administered in maintenance renal transplant patients: results of a 1-year study. Am J Transplant. 2004;4(2):237–43.
44. Schubert M, Venkataramanan R, Holt DW, Shaw LM, McGhee W, Reyes J, et al. Pharmacokinetics of sirolimus and tacrolimus in pediatric transplant patients. Am J Transplant. 2004;4(5):767–73.
45. Schachter AD, Meyers KE, Spaneas LD, Palmer JA, Salmanullah M, Baluarte J, et al. Short sirolimus half-life in pediatric renal transplant recipients on a calcineurin inhibitor-free protocol. Pediatr Transplant. 2004;8(2):171–7.
46. Kahan BD. Efficacy of sirolimus compared with azathioprine for reduction of acute renal allograft rejection: a randomised multicentre study. The Rapamune US Study Group. Lancet. 2000;356(9225):194–202.
47. McAlister VC, Gao Z, Peltekian K, Domingues J, Mahalati K, MacDonald AS. Sirolimus-tacrolimus combination immunosuppression. Lancet. 2000;355(9201):376–7.
48. Kreis H, Cisterne JM, Land W, Wramner L, Squifflet JP, Abramowicz D, et al. Sirolimus in association with mycophenolate mofetil induction for the prevention of acute graft rejection in renal allograft recipients. Transplantation. 2000;69(7):1252–60.
49. Hong JC, Kahan BD. Sirolimus-induced thrombocytopenia and leukopenia in renal transplant recipients: risk factors, incidence, progression, and management. Transplantation. 2000;69(10):2085–90.
50. Stallone G, Di Paolo S, Schena A, Infante B, Battaglia M, Ditonno P, et al. Addition of sirolimus to cyclosporine delays the recovery from delayed graft function but does not affect 1-year graft function. J Am Soc Nephrol. 2004;15(1):228–33.
51. Smith KD, Wrenshall LE, Nicosia RF, Pichler R, Marsh CL, Alpers CE, et al. Delayed graft function and cast nephropathy associated with tacrolimus plus rapamycin use. J Am Soc Nephrol. 2003;14(4):1037–45.
52. Majewski M, Korecka M, Joergensen J, Fields L, Kossev P, Schuler W, et al. Immunosuppressive TOR kinase inhibitor everolimus (RAD) suppresses growth of cells derived from post-transplant lymphoproliferative disorder at allograft-protecting doses. Transplantation. 2003;75(10):1710–7.
53. Dharnidharka VR, Schnitzler MA, Chen J, Brennan DC, Axelrod D, Segev DL, et al. Differential risks for adverse outcomes 3 years after kidney transplantation based on initial immunosuppression regimen: a national study. Transpl Int. 2016;29(11):1226–36.

54. Knoll GA, Kokolo MB, Mallick R, Beck A, Buenaventura CD, Ducharme R, et al. Effect of sirolimus on malignancy and survival after kidney transplantation: systematic review and meta-analysis of individual patient data. BMJ. 2014;349:g6679.
55. Weir MR, Pearson TC, Patel A, Peddi VR, Kalil R, Scandling J, et al. Long-term follow-up of kidney transplant recipients in the spare-the-nephron-trial. Transplantation. 2017;101(1):157–65.
56. Mulay AV, Hussain N, Fergusson D, Knoll GA. Calcineurin inhibitor withdrawal from sirolimus-based therapy in kidney transplantation: a systematic review of randomized trials. Am J Transplant. 2005;5(7):1748–56.
57. Hoyer PF, Ettenger R, Kovarik JM, Webb NJ, Lemire J, Mentser M, et al. Everolimus in pediatric de nova renal transplant patients. Transplantation. 2003;75(12):2082–5.
58. Sarwal MM, Ettenger RB, Dharnidharka V, Benfield M, Mathias R, Portale A, et al. Complete steroid avoidance is effective and safe in children with renal transplants: a multicenter randomized trial with three-year follow-up. Am J Transplant. 2012;12(10):2719–29.
59. Tsampalieros A, Knoll GA, Molnar AO, Fergusson N, Fergusson DA. Corticosteroid use and growth after pediatric solid organ transplantation: a systematic review and meta-analysis. Transplantation. 2017;101(4):694–703.
60. Webb NJ, Douglas SE, Rajai A, Roberts SA, Grenda R, Marks SD, et al. Corticosteroid-free kidney transplantation improves growth: 2-year follow-up of the TWIST randomized controlled trial. Transplantation. 2015;99(6):1178–85.
61. Naesens M, Salvatierra O, Benfield M, Ettenger RB, Dharnidharka V, Harmon W, et al. Subclinical inflammation and chronic renal allograft injury in a randomized trial on steroid avoidance in pediatric kidney transplantation. Am J Transplant. 2012;12(10):2730–43.
62. Li L, Chaudhuri A, Chen A, Zhao X, Bezchinsky M, Concepcion W, et al. Efficacy and safety of thymoglobulin induction as an alternative approach for steroid-free maintenance immunosuppression in pediatric renal transplantation. Transplantation. 2010;90(12):1516–20.
63. Lau KK, Berg GM, Schjoneman YG, Perez RV, Butani L. Extended experience with a steroid minimization immunosuppression protocol in pediatric renal transplant recipients. Pediatr Transplant. 2010;14(4):488–95.
64. Weir MR, Anderson L, Fink JC, Gabregiorgish K, Schweitzer EJ, Hoehn-Saric E, et al. A novel approach to the treatment of chronic allograft nephropathy. Transplantation. 1997;64(12):1706–10.
65. Nankivell BJ, Borrows RJ, Fung CL, O'Connell PJ, Allen RD, Chapman JR. The natural history of chronic allograft nephropathy. N Engl J Med. 2003;349(24):2326–33.
66. Kreis H, Oberbauer R, Campistol JM, Mathew T, Daloze P, Schena FP, et al. Long-term benefits with sirolimus-based therapy after early cyclosporine withdrawal. J Am Soc Nephrol. 2004;15(3):809–17.
67. Vincenti F, Charpentier B, Vanrenterghem Y, Rostaing L, Bresnahan B, Darji P, et al. A phase III study of belatacept-based immunosuppression regimens versus cyclosporine in renal transplant recipients (BENEFIT study). Am J Transplant. 2010;10(3):535–46.
68. Vincenti F, Rostaing L, Grinyo J, Rice K, Steinberg S, Gaite L, et al. Belatacept and long-term outcomes in kidney transplantation. N Engl J Med. 2016;374(4):333–43.
69. Lerch C, Kanzelmeyer NK, Ahlenstiel-Grunow T, Froede K, Kreuzer M, Drube J, et al. Belatacept after kidney transplantation in adolescents: a retrospective study. Transpl Int. 2017;30:494–501.

Chapter 15
Acute and Chronic Kidney Transplant Rejection in Adolescents: Causes and Treatment

Jonathan H. Pelletier, Emeraghi E. David, Annabelle N. Chua, and Eileen Tsai Chambers

Introduction

During adolescence, a child undergoes considerable changes in emotions, behavior, pubertal development, and immunobiology. It is not surprising that adolescent recipients sustain the highest risk for poor kidney transplant outcomes including allograft rejection [1–3] and loss [4–6]. Multiple factors may contribute to this increased risk of allograft rejection and failure in adolescence and early adulthood. These include medication non-adherence [1–3, 5], risk-taking behaviors associated with adolescence [5], influence of pubertal changes [7], and the capacity to produce a dynamic immune cell repertoire in response to environmental antigen exposure [8]. This chapter focuses on aspects of acute and chronic rejection that are unique to adolescent and young adult kidney transplant recipients with emphasis on mechanism, classification, and treatment strategies.

Factors Predisposing Adolescents to Acute and Chronic Kidney Transplant Rejection

The Relationship Between Age and the Immune System in Allograft Rejection

As children grow into adolescents, they develop an immune repertoire that is a unique product of their prior and ongoing environmental exposures, resulting in a gradual change from a predominantly naïve to a memory phenotype [9]. Indeed,

J. H. Pelletier (✉) · E. E. David · A. N. Chua · E. T. Chambers
Department of Pediatrics, Duke University Medical Center, Durham, NC, USA
e-mail: jonathan.pelletier@duke.edu; emeraghi.david@duke.edu; annabelle.chua@duke.edu; eileen.chambers@duke.edu

M. N. Haddad et al. (eds.), *Adolescents with Chronic Kidney Disease*,
https://doi.org/10.1007/978-3-319-97220-6_15

adolescents experience a peak in both their CD4 and CD8 T cells [8] and have a more adult-like repertoire with 50–60% of their T cells expressing memory characteristics [9]. Additionally, beginning in early childhood, the peripheral B cell compartment expands with an increase in the absolute number of B cells and antigen-experienced memory B cells [8, 10]. This primed and more mature immune repertoire may contribute to the increased rates of allograft rejection seen during adolescence.

Adolescent Brain Development, Behavior, and Allograft Rejection

During adolescence, many transplant recipients gain more autonomy, including management of their own healthcare, irrespective of their ability to take on this responsibility. Most caregivers base the decision to transfer medical care responsibility upon chronological age, not developmental age. The adolescent brain is still undergoing continual development, which does not reach completion until mid to late 20s. Moreover, the last step to brain development involves the prefrontal cortex, responsible for higher, executive functions including foresight, planning, and evaluation of risk and reward. Therefore, most transplanted adolescents do not have the organizational or cognitive capacity to manage their own healthcare [11]. Furthermore, MRI studies of adolescent brains show that regions associated with reward are completely developed at age 15–17, while adequate control systems mature later at age 18–21 [12–15]. This might explain the peak of risk-taking behavior in mid-adolescence between age 14 and 17. Additionally, patients with chronic kidney disease (CKD) have neurocognitive deficits, independent from the physiological changes associated with adolescence. Increased CKD severity, duration of CKD, and CKD associated with significant proteinuria have been associated with lower IQ, memory function, and executive function [11, 16]. Altogether, these factors may help explain why adolescent transplant recipients are predisposed to medication nonadherence.

The Relationship Between Adolescent Sex Hormones and the Immune System in Allograft Rejection

Pubertal growth and the development of secondary sexual characteristics are somewhat delayed in patients with CKD and improve after patients have undergone renal transplantation [17–21]. During puberty, adolescents experience a marked increase in sex hormone production that drives development of secondary sexual characteristics [7, 22]. Puberty and response to sex hormones are known to alter the inflammatory response; women are at higher risk for development of autoimmune conditions such as rheumatoid arthritis, autoimmune hepatitis, and dermatomyositis during their reproductive years [7]. Additionally, earlier age of menarche has been associated with higher risk of development of multiple sclerosis [23]. Animal studies and in vitro models have also confirmed a role for sex hormones in immunomodulation [24]. In mouse models, male mice are less susceptible to autoimmune encephalitis and have higher IL-10 and IL-4 than female mice. Treating female mice with testosterone increases IL-10 production and decreases IL-12 [25]. In vitro experiments have shown that testosterone acts directly on the dihydrotestosterone receptor of CD4 T cells to increase IL-10 expression [25]. IL-10 can suppress autoimmunity, T cell alloimmunity, and class switching in humoral immunity [26–28]. These findings may explain the small, but statistically significant, superior renal allograft survival among male compared to female recipients [29]. However, at this time, these links are merely speculative.

The Immunology of Acute and Chronic Kidney Transplant Rejection

Ischemia and Reperfusion Injury

By nature of kidney transplantation process, organs are oftentimes procured from donors at outside centers and transported prior to implantation into recipients. During this period, the transplanted kidney frequently undergoes both periods of cold ischemia (transit outside of the human body) and warm ischemia (both while in the deceased donor and after rewarming prior to implantation into the recipient) [30–32]. Thus, the allograft develops an ischemia and reperfusion injury of variable severity during the transplant process [30–32].

Subsequently, the donor tissue develops acidosis and increased production of reactive oxygen species during transplantation [33]. This results in direct cellular injury and caspase-mediated apoptosis [34, 35]. Additionally, the injury causes the release of inflammatory mediators, including IL-6, TNF-α, and IFN-γ, and activation of the complement cascade with production of C3a and C5a immediately following transplantation that, in the absence of immunosuppression, makes rejection nearly inevitable [32, 36–42]. From the moment of recipient-graft blood vessel anastomosis, graft capillaries are infused with circulating recipient leukocytes. Ischemia within the allograft results in upregulation of selectins, ICAMs, and VCAMs on the endothelium [43]. These facilitate recipient leukocyte adhesion, rolling, extravasation, and infiltration into graft tissue [43].

Augmented leukocyte adhesion is coupled with increased expression of donor antigens on major histocompatibility complexes (MHC) on the surface of donor antigen-presenting cells induced by the ischemic insult; these antigens are, in turn, presented to recipient lymphocytes, resulting in T cell activation and production of donor-specific human leukocyte antigen (HLA) antibodies by activated B cells [32,

36–39]. Additionally, ischemia-reperfusion injury causes increased whiexpression of toll-like receptor ligands by the transplanted cells, thereby inducing a pro-inflammatory state [44]. Furthermore, tissue damage from ischemia-reperfusion can lead to the exposure of cryptic autoantigens and the development of non-HLA auto-antibodies which can bind to the vasculature and cause further injury [45]. Clinically, ischemia-reperfusion predisposes the renal allograft to acute kidney injury, delayed graft function, as well as acute and chronic rejection, which are discussed in the following sections. Methods to prevent ischemia-reperfusion have focused on organ perfusion solutions, optimizing deceased donor management prior to kidney implantation, and organ perfusion devices [46]. Promising research for intervention include perfusion of donor organs with small interfering RNA cocktails [47] or approaches to epithelial cell repair and regeneration [48].

T Cell Allorecognition in Rejection

Transplantation provides a milieu whereby T cell recognition of an alloantigen can arise through pathways that operate outside of conventional responses to traditional protein antigens [49]. Antigens are presented to lymphocytes by MHC encoded on chromosomes 6p and 15q (for beta-2-microglobulin) [50]. Humans have two categories of MHC; MHC class I (with associated beta-2-microglobulin) is found on nucleated cells and presents intracellular peptides to T cell receptors on CD8 T lymphocytes [30, 32]. MHC class II is found on antigen-presenting cells (e.g., dendritic cells, macrophages, and B cells) and presents digested extracellular peptides to T cell receptors on CD4 T lymphocytes [30, 32]. The activation of lymphocytes in response to antigens presented by MHC occurs in an antigen-specific manner, such that a very small proportion of T lymphocytes are activated at any given time [30]. The pathways by which T cells are able to recognize MHC alloantigen include direct allorecognition [51], indirect allorecognition, and semi-direct allorecognition [53] as outlined in Fig. 15.1. Each of these pathways will be described in the following sections.

In response to the myriad of inflammatory mediators released from tissue ischemia-reperfusion injury, donor antigen-presenting cells from the renal allograft migrate through the blood stream and present antigen through MHC to recipient T lymphocytes of secondary lymphoid organs including lymph nodes (Fig. 15.1a [54]). The direct T cell alloresponse is polyclonal, contributes to acute allograft rejection, and surprisingly involves 1–10% of the T cell repertoire [30, 54, 55]. There are two theories to explain this phenomenon. In the “high determinant density” model, it is proposed that structural differences between donor and recipient MHC cause recipient T cells to bind donor MHC in a low-affinity, antigen-independent manner and that the high density of MHC on the donor antigen-presenting cell increases the avidity of the interaction and causes recipient T cell activation [30, 54, 56, 57]. In the “multiple binary complex model,” donor antigens

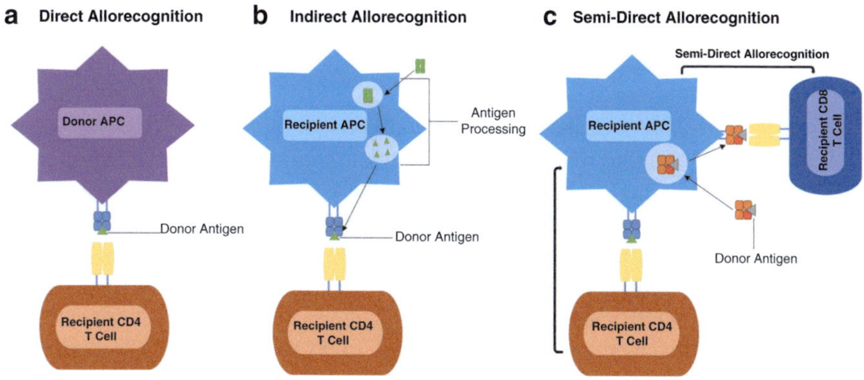

Fig. 15.1 Three pathways by which recipient T cells can recognize donor antigen are direct, indirect, and semi-direct allorecognition and mediate kidney transplant rejection. (**a**) Direct allorecognition: donor APC presents donor antigen to recipient T cell. (**b**) Indirect allorecognition: recipient APC recognizes donor antigen, processes it, and presents it to recipient T cell. (**c**) Semi-direct allorecognition: recipient APC internalizes donor antigen and presents it intact on cell surface without processing to recipient T cell, *APC* antigen-presenting cell

simultaneously present multiple donor-self antigens to the recipient T cells that are recognized as foreign, each inciting a classical antigen-dependent T cell response [30, 54, 58]. It is possible that both of these mechanisms exist, either in multiple patients or simultaneously within the same patient [54].

The indirect pathway of the alloimmune response follows the conventional mechanism of antigen-specific immunity (Fig. 15.1b [30]). In this pathway, as donor allograft cells undergo lysis or apoptosis, their antigens are engulfed and processed by recipient antigen-presenting cells bound to recipient MHC [30, 54], which trigger a recipient T lymphocyte response against the donor [30, 54, 59]. Whether antigen processing by recipient cells occurs in response to circulating donor antigens, destruction of donor antigen-presenting cells in recipient lymphoid tissue, migration of donor antigen-presenting cells into the allograft, or a combination of these three mechanisms remains to be elucidated [54]. The initial activity of the indirect pathway is significantly less than that of the direct pathway (as it is comparable to a typical antigen-specific response); however, it is thought to play a more significant role in chronic rejection after donor antigen-presenting cells have dwindled [30].

A third pathway, referred to as semi-direct allorecognition, has been suggested [52, 53], whereby alloantigen is internalized by the recipient antigen-presenting cell and instead of being processed is presented intact on the cell surface. As shown in Fig. 15.1c, a recipient antigen-presenting cell acquires donor MHC class I and presents this intact on its surface to recipient CD8 T lymphocyte through semi-direct allorecognition [60]. Simultaneously, recipient MHC class II within the same antigen-presenting cell stimulates the recipient CD4 T lymphocyte via the indirect pathway, which in turn activates CD8 T cell response.

Modulating the Three-Signal Model of Alloimmunity to Prevent Rejection in Adolescents

T cell receptor binding to MHC is essential, but not sufficient for T cell activation and mediation of allograft rejection [32]. In order to trigger an alloimmune response, three signals within the T cell are necessary and will be the focus of this section. An emphasis on immunomodulation of the three-signal model as a method of potentially preventing rejection in adolescent transplant recipients will be addressed. In addition to the binding of the MHC-antigen-T cell receptor complex termed "signal 1," extensive research has shown that simultaneous costimulatory "signal 2" is required for T cell activation as outlined in Fig. 15.2 [30, 32, 54, 61]. This simultaneous interaction has been termed the immunological synapse [32, 62]. Costimulatory signals can potentiate or inhibit the downstream signaling pathways of the T cell receptor and the resultant lymphocyte response [30, 32, 54]. One well-characterized costimulatory molecule on the surface of T cells is CD28, which binds to CD80 and CD86 on the surface of antigen-presenting cells and potentiates T cell activation [30, 32, 54]. Competitive antagonism of this signal decreases rejection and prolongs allograft survival [63, 64]. Cytotoxic T lymphocyte-associated antigen 4 (CTLA4) is another coregulatory molecule on the surface of T cells that also binds to CD80 and CD86 but exerts an inhibitory effect on lymphocyte activation, both by limiting cell-cell contact between the antigen-presenting cell and lymphocyte and by reducing intracellular signaling from the TCR [30, 32, 54, 65, 66]. CD154 on T lymphocytes, which binds to CD40 on antigen-presenting cells, is another example of a costimulatory interaction, which has a role in activation of both T and B cell responses [54, 67].

Costimulatory molecules involved with "signal 2" have emerged as ideal targets for immunomodulatory maintenance therapy in adolescent transplant recipients (Fig. 15.2). As adolescents struggle with taking their medications, a monthly infusion given by the transplant center allows the medical provider to have more control over medication administration. Abatacept, a bioengineered CTLA4 mimetic fused with immunoglobulin designed to competitively inhibit CD80/86 and block the costimulation mediated by CD28 [68], failed to prevent kidney transplant rejection in nonhuman primates [69, 70]. Belatacept, a derivative of abatacept with better binding avidity for both CD80 and CD86, has demonstrated improvement in long-term renal function, graft survival, patient mortality, and development of de novo donor-specific antibody when compared to cyclosporine A in multiple clinical trials [71–74]. Additionally, belatacept has been shown to stabilize/improve renal function in nonadherent, EBV-seropositive adolescent recipients [75]. The patients who were nonadherent with their oral immunosuppressive medications were 100% adherent with their monthly infusions. Of importance, belatacept is contraindicated in EBV seronegative patients due to an increased risk of posttransplant lymphoproliferative disease [76, 77]. Another promising costimulatory blockade agent is a fully humanized antibody against CD40 (ASKP1240 and CFZ533) which is currently in phase 2 clinical trials [78, 79].

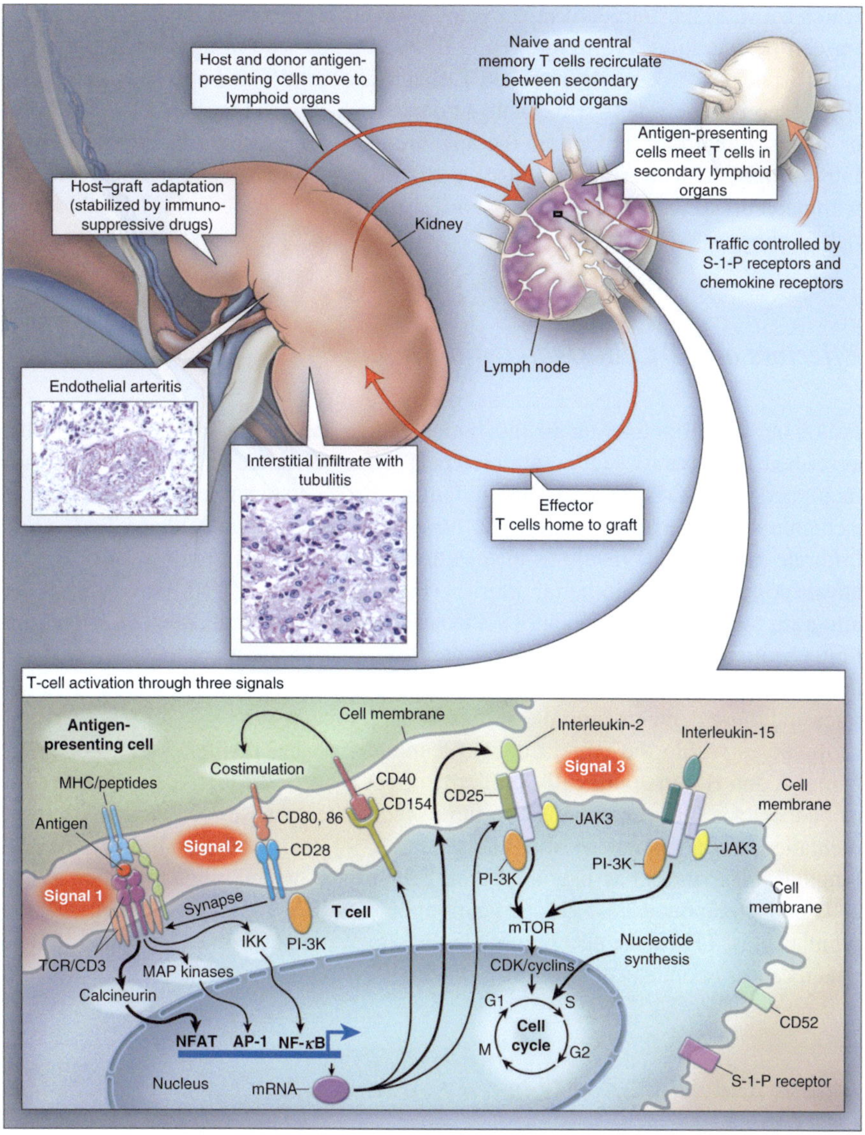

Fig. 15.2 T cell-mediated rejection. T cells migrate to lymph nodes where they interact with APCs. T cells are activated through the three signaling model, home to the allograft, and infiltrate the renal parenchyma causing tubulitis and interstitial infiltrate, or in severe cases damage the renal blood vessels, APC antigen-presenting cell. (From Halloran [61], with permission)

The combination of signal 1 and signal 2 activates three-signal transduction pathways: the calcium-calcineurin pathway, the RAS-mitogen-activated protein (MAP) kinase pathway, and the nuclear factor-KB pathway [80] (Fig. 15.2). These pathways stimulate transcription factors that trigger the expression of interleukin-2 (IL-2) which activates the "target of rapamycin" pathway to provide "signal 3," the trigger for cell proliferation. Proliferation and differentiation lead to numerous effector T cells. Strategies to decrease activated T effectors or total T cell number using either IL-2 receptor blockade (basiliximab) or depletional agents (antithymocyte globulin or alemtuzumab) as induction therapy are used to prevent rejection [81–86]. Interestingly, African American black pediatric kidney transplant recipients treated with depletional therapies compared to IL2 receptor blockade had a 1.5-fold lower risk of allograft rejection [87].

Effectors and T Cell-Mediated Rejection

Following T cell activation in the lymph nodes and spleen by the mechanisms described in previous sections, recipient T effectors home to the renal allograft facilitated by ICAMs, VCAMs, and inflammatory mediators released in response to ischemia and reperfusion injury [32, 36–43, 62]. Subsequently these T effectors infiltrate the allograft resulting in rejection lesions such as tubulitis and in more advanced rejection, endothelial arteritis (Fig. 15.2, [61, 88, 89]). Once within the allograft, recipient T lymphocytes act in several pathways to mediate tissue destruction. Cytotoxic CD8 T lymphocytes contain cytoplasmic granules that hold perforin and granzymes; when activated, they degranulate in a calcium-dependent manner, releasing these contents onto the surface of target donor cells [62, 90, 91]. Perforin forms pores within the target donor cell membrane and facilitates entry of granzymes A and B into donor cells, either by direct passage through membranes pores or endocytosis [90]. Granzymes, in turn, precipitate caspase-mediated DNA fragmentation and apoptosis of allograft cells [62, 90, 91]. Additionally, cytotoxic T lymphocytes express Fas-ligand on their cell surface, which binds to Fas on donor cells and precipitates caspase-mediated apoptosis [62, 90, 91]. A subset of CD4 lymphocytes, TH1 cells, also migrate to the allograft and secrete TNF-α and IFN-γ, which causes apoptosis of allograft cells [62, 92].

B Cells and Antibody-Mediated Rejection

Three signaling pathways exist that result in T cell-dependent activation of B cells and the formation of donor-specific antibodies (DSA) against the renal allograft [93, 94], as shown in Fig. 15.3. This process occurs within germinal centers of secondary lymphoid organs such as the spleen or lymph nodes, as well as within the kidney itself [95, 96]. First, naïve mature B cells become activated through alloantigen engagement of the B cell receptor. Consequently, primed B cells are translocated into T cell-rich areas of the germinal center where the interaction between T helper CD4 lymphocytes and B cells through MHC class II provides multiple costimulation signals (CD40L-CD40; CD28-CD80/CD86) for B cell activation. After

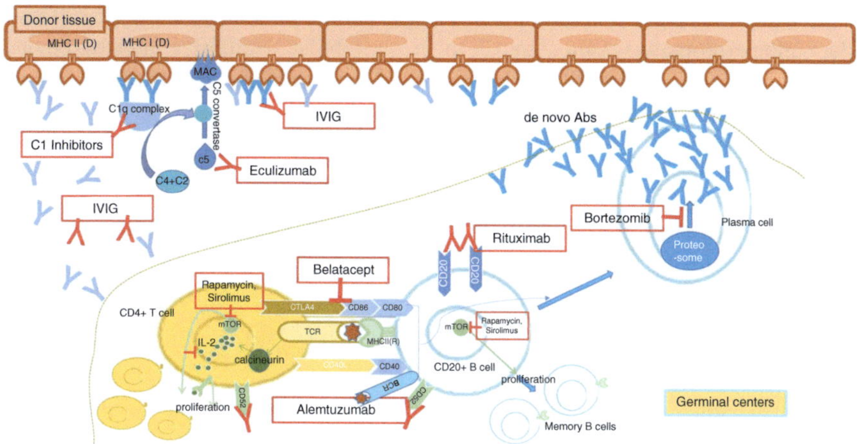

Fig. 15.3 Antibody-mediated rejection pathways and therapeutic targets. In germinal centers, B cells are activated by CD4+ T cells and become plasma cells in turn producing DSA. DSA bind to the renal allograft endothelium, activate complement, and cause damage to the renal blood vessels. Current therapeutic strategies target various steps of this pathway, *DSA* donor-specific antibody. (From Ng et al. [94], with permission)

alloantigen recognition and costimulation, B cell activation requires cytokines, including IL-4, IL-5, IL-10, and IL-13, which are produced by various helper T cells [32, 54, 67]. B cells then differentiate into memory B cells and plasma cells that produce DSA [30, 32]. These antibodies bind to donor cell membranes and can result in complement fixation with deposition of complement end product (C4d), formation of the membrane attack complex (C5b-C9), cell membrane damage, and endothelial cell death within the allograft [62, 97]. Damaged endothelial cells release inflammatory mediators, von Willebrand factor, and P-selectin, resulting in coagulation and microthrombosis within the allograft [62, 97]. Finally, the role of humoral immunity is not limited to antibody production [98]. B lymphocytes have also been shown to migrate into renal allografts and act as antigen-presenting cells to T lymphocytes by the indirect pathway discussed above [98].

Chronic Rejection

Chronic rejection refers to ongoing immune injury to the allograft, which results from an inability to maintain adequate immunosuppression. Thus, residual anti-graft lymphocytes and/or DSA persist leading to eventual decline in renal function. Chronic T cell-mediated rejection (TCMR) is characterized by invasion of the renal parenchyma by T cells and persistent T cell and macrophage infiltration. Occasionally, this involves the renal vessels and is associated with proliferation, hyperplasia, and vascular occlusion [62]. In chronic antibody-mediated rejection (ABMR), DSA induce persistent endothelial injury to glomerular and peritubular capillaries resulting in duplication of the glomerular basement membrane (transplant glomerulopathy), C4d deposition in peritubular capillaries, and basement-membrane multilamination [40]. Unfortunately, chronic rejection is often difficult to treat with a poor clinical outcome [99].

T Cell-Mediated Rejection: Epidemiology, Classification, and Treatment

Epidemiology

With advancements in immunosuppression, the frequency of acute TCMR has markedly decreased by transplantation era from 69.6% of children transplanted from 1987 to 1991 having at least one rejection to 16.1% in children transplanted between 2007 and 2013 [29]. Despite this improvement, adolescents are at the highest risk for acute TCMR and are less likely to fully recover from rejection episodes than younger children [29]. Under immunosuppression from continual medication, nonadherence in adolescent recipients has been implicated in refractory T cell-mediated rejection episodes, leading to ongoing chronic rejection and increased allograft loss [96, 100, 101].

Clinical Presentation and Classification

The majority of adolescents will be clinically asymptomatic and only present after a rise in serum creatinine on serial laboratory assessments [102, 103]. Adolescents who are clinically symptomatic may present with fever, malaise, hypertension, decreased urine output, and/or pain over the graft site [103]. Additional laboratory findings may include gross hematuria, proteinuria, or pyuria [103]. Although biomarker development to diagnose TCMR is ongoing [104], kidney biopsy remains the gold standard for diagnosis. The pathologic type and severity of rejection are classified according to the Banff Criteria, originally developed in 1991 [105]. The criteria merged with the Collaborative Clinical Trials in Transplantation (CCTT) to create the Banff 1997 Working Classification of Renal Allograft Pathology [106]. Since that time, the criteria have undergone a number of revisions. Table 15.1 provides the most updated Banff 2015 criteria for acute and chronic TCMR [107]. The spectrum of acute TCMR includes borderline changes with focal tubulitis and minor interstitial inflammation, type I T cell-mediated rejection (significant interstitial inflammation and tubulitis), and type II/III TCMR (mild to severe intimal arteritis). Chronic TCMR now includes mononuclear infiltration in arterial intimal fibrosis in addition to areas of tubular atrophy [107].

Table 15.1 Banff 2015 classification of T cell-mediated rejection in renal allografts

	Borderline TCMR/ suspicious for acute TCMR	Acute/active TCMR	Chronic/active TCMR
Tissue injury	Foci of tubulitis (t1, t2, or t3) with minor interstitial inflammation (i0 or i1) or interstitial inflammation (i2, i3) with mild (t1) tubulitis	IA. Significant interstitial inflammation (>25% of nonsclerotic cortical parenchyma, i2 or i3) and foci of moderate tubulitis (t2)	Fibrosis with mononuclear cell infiltration in the arterial intima (neointima formation) or tubulointerstitial compartment
	No intimal arteritis ($v = 0$)	IB. Significant interstitial inflammation (>25% of nonsclerotic cortical parenchyma, i2 or i3) and foci of severe tubulitis (t3)	
		IIA. Mild to moderate intimal arteritis (v1) with or without interstitial inflammation and tubulitis	
		IIB. Severe intimal arteritis comprising >25% of the luminal area (v2) with or without interstitial inflammation and tubulitis	
		III. Transmural arteritis and/or arterial fibrinoid change and necrosis of medial smooth muscle cells with accompanying lymphocytic inflammation (v3)	

Treatment

Therapy for TCMR is guided by biopsy findings. High-dose corticosteroid pulses are the first line of treatment of acute TCMR, and approximately 75% of the episodes are responsive to treatment. Intravenous methylprednisolone is given in doses that range from 5 to 10 mg/kg per day for 3–5 days [108, 109]. Lymphocyte-depleting antibodies, such as antithymocyte globulin and alemtuzumab, reverse up to 90% of the acute rejection episodes that do not respond to steroids but have a higher rate of adverse events [110–113]. These agents can be used to treat episodes that do not respond to corticosteroids within 7–10 days, are classified as type II/III, or are recurrent/ongoing. Additionally for persistent or chronic TCMR, augmented maintenance immunosuppression must be considered. The majority of ongoing chronic rejection, however, is antibody-mediated.

Antibody-Mediated Rejection: Epidemiology, Classification, and Treatment

Epidemiology

As previously discussed, ABMR involves the production of alloantibodies directed toward antigens from the donor allograft (DSA). DSA can be preformed leading to sensitization or develop de novo after kidney transplantation. Approximately 30% of patients on the waiting list are sensitized with a panel reactive antibody of >20%. Factors that contribute to sensitization in adolescence and young adulthood include blood transfusions, previous transplants, infections, and pregnancy/miscarriages. Fifteen to 22% of children develop de novo posttransplant DSA with adolescents being at the highest risk [114–116]. Risk factors for the development of de novo posttransplant DSA are infection usually concurrent with a decrease in immunosuppression and medication nonadherence [2, 3, 116].

Most centers utilize single antigen beads (Luminex®) to detect antibodies against HLA class I (HLA A, B, C) and HLA class II (HLA DR, DP, DQ) [94]. Luminex-based assays for C3d and C1q antibody binding may be helpful to differentiate more pathogenic antibodies, stratify patients according to risk, and determine who may benefit from complement inhibition [117, 118]. Although non-HLA antibodies against endothelial cell targets such as angiotensin II type 1 receptor, endothelin-1 type A receptor, major histocompatibility complex class 1-related chain A, and perlecan are gaining recognition for their pathogenesis in ABMR [119, 120], testing is currently not standardized. Further investigation is warranted to determine the utility of incorporating non-HLA antibody monitoring into routine clinical practice.

Classification

ABMR can be categorized clinically by the timing of rejection in relationship to transplantation [102, 121]. Rejection due to preformed DSA within the first 24 h following transplantation is termed hyperacute ABMR. With the advent of complement-dependent cytotoxicity and flow cytometry crossmatch to detect preformed DSA prior to renal transplantation [102], the incidence of hyperacute rejection has improved to 0.6% [29]. Rejection involving DSA and sudden deterioration in graft function any time after the first 24 h is termed acute ABMR. Finally, DSA leading to chronic vascular damage and fibrosis is termed chronic ABMR [121] and accounts for approximately two thirds of late allograft loss [115].

Similar to T cell-mediated rejection, histological classification of acute and chronic ABMR by renal biopsy remains critical to the diagnosis. ABMR requires all three of the following: evidence of tissue injury, presence of recent interaction between antibody and vascular endothelium, and circulating HLA or non-HLA DSA. The Banff criteria includes categorization for ABMR, which were published

Table 15.2 Banff 2015 classification of antibody-mediated rejection in renal allografts

	Acute/active ABMR	Chronic/active ABMR	C4d staining without ABMR
Tissue injury	Evidence of acute tissue injury with 1 or more of:	Evidence of chronic tissue injury with 1 or more of:	$g = 0$, ptc = 0, cg = 0 (by light and EM, if available), $v = 0$; no TMA, no ptc basement membrane multilayering, no acute tubular injury
	1. Microvascular inflammation ($g > 0$ and/or ptc > 0)	1. Transplant glomerulopathy (cg > 0), if no evidence of chronic TMA	
	2. Acute TMA with no other cause	2. Severe peritubular capillary basement membrane multilayering by EM	
	3. Acute tubular injury with no other cause	3. New-onset arterial intimal fibrosis without any other causes	
Vascular endothelial injury/ C4d staining	Evidence of current/ recent antibody interaction with vascular endothelium with 1 or more of:	Evidence of current/ recent antibody interaction with vascular endothelium with 1 or more of:	Linear C4d staining in peritubular capillaries (C4d2+ by IF on frozen sections or C4d > 0 by IHC on paraffin sections)
	1. Linear C4d staining in peritubular capillaries (C4d2+ by IF on frozen sections or C4d > 0 by IHC on paraffin sections)	1. Linear C4d staining in peritubular capillaries (C4d2+ by IF on frozen sections or C4d > 0 by IHC on paraffin sections)	
	2. Moderate microvascular inflammation (g + ptc) ≥ 2	2. Moderate microvascular inflammation (g + ptc) ≥ 2	
	3. Increased expression of thoroughly validated gene transcripts in the biopsy tissue consistent with endothelial injury	3. Increased expression of thoroughly validated gene transcripts in the biopsy tissue consistent with endothelial injury	
Serology/other findings	Serologic evidence of DSAs (HLA or other antigens)	Serologic evidence of DSAs (HLA or other antigens)	No acute cell-mediated rejection (Banff type 1A or greater) or borderline changes

From Ng et al. [94], with permission

in 2003 [122, 123]. The Banff criteria has been updated to include C4d-negative acute and chronic ABMR, which involves DSA-mediated vascular and microvascular injury in the absence of C4d staining as shown in Table 15.2 [107, 124]. Additionally, histological evidence of transplant glomerulopathy and/or arterial intimal fibrosis denotes chronic ABMR and distinguishes it from the acute process (Table 15.2, [94, 107, 124]).

Treatment

Unlike TCMR, there is varying efficacy for the treatment of acute and chronic ABMR. Several challenges remain which include resistance to corticosteroids, repeated episodes and resurgence of DSA despite therapy, and eventual progression to allograft failure [94, 115]. Although current treatments for ABMR will be reviewed, the optimal therapy is to avoid the development of DSA. Studies in both adults and children have shown that DR and DQ matching may help prevent DSA formation [125, 126]. Moreover, the use of belatacept-based maintenance regimens shows a reduction in de novo DSA to 0–5% [74, 127, 128] compared to calcineurin-based regimens. Of note, concomitant use of alemtuzumab and belatacept eliminated DSA production [127, 128]. Additionally, as medication nonadherence has been strongly associated with DSA [2, 3, 116], potential strategies to reduce nonadherence may decrease the development of DSA. These methods include the use of structured transition programs from pediatric to adult nephrology care, the use of an electronic medication-dispensing device, or the utilization of alarm/medication app on mobile phones to assist in remembering medications [129–131].

The final sections of this chapter will concentrate on the various therapies for ABMR, as shown in Fig. 15.3 [94]. Therapeutic strategies focus on (1) the elimination of DSA, (2) immunomodulation of B cells, and/or (3) the inhibition of complement. Removal of DSA with plasmapheresis is the most common first-line therapy for acute ABMR and has been shown to be beneficial in one randomized controlled trial [132]. Used as monotherapy, the response rate for plasmapheresis is approximately 50% and increases to 80–90% when combined with intravenous immunoglobulin (IVIG) [133, 134].

B cell immunomodulation has also been employed to treat ABMR with mixed results. Rituximab, a humanized chimeric anti-CD20 antibody, depletes mature antigen-presenting B cells from the circulation and allows reconstitution of the naïve B cell population. Thus, rituximab may reprogram the B cell repertoire, which becomes less capable of developing an immune response to the alloantigen. While some studies have shown that the addition of rituximab improves graft function in children [135, 136], others have shown limited efficacy [137–139]. Rituximab is hindered by its inability to deplete terminal differentiated plasma cells, which continue to produce DSA, as well as memory B cells residing in secondary lymphoid organs. Additionally, in some studies, the use of rituximab has been associated with increased BK nephropathy and other infections [140, 141]. Bortezomib, a proteasome inhibitor, targets plasma cells and may more effectively decrease antibody production and stabilize renal function in children and nonadherent adolescents [137, 142]. However, it is more efficacious in treating acute ABMR when used as an adjunct therapy in combination with plasmapheresis, steroids, rituximab, and IVIG [137, 138]. Clinical trials are currently under way to assess the utility of bortezomib to treat chronic ABMR, which often times is refractory and results in allograft loss (TRIBUTE, NCT02201576). A promising therapy for chronic ABMR is tocilizumab, which prevents binding of IL 6 to its respective receptor and modulates T cells, B cells, and plasma cells, resulting in decreased DSA production [143, 144]. Patients with persistent DSA and transplant glomerulopathy who failed IVIG, rituximab, and plasmapheresis had stabilization of renal function, 80% graft survival at 6 years, and significant reduction of DSA with the addition of tocilizumab [143].

Lastly, inhibiting the complement pathway is another strategy to treat acute ABMR. IVIG is pooled immunoglobulin that fix DSA at low dose (1 g/kg) preventing complement activation. At higher doses (2 g/kg), it can modulate B and T cells and reduce DSA production [145]. As previously stated, it is most effective when combined with other therapies such as plasmapheresis and rituximab. Eculizumab is a humanized antibody that inhibits C5 component of the complement pathway, the formation of membrane attack complex, and tissue destruction. It has been used as rescue therapy ABMR with varying results [146–148]. However, eculizumab does not prevent chronic ABMR, especially when used in desensitization regimens [149]. By contrast, C1 esterase inhibitor, which also prevents complement activation, may prevent chronic ABMR when used in combination with plasmapheresis and IVIG [150]. C1q and C3d binding assays may guide management and responsiveness to complement inhibition, although data is limited.

Nevertheless, acute and chronic ABMR requires multiple therapies. Data in children and adolescents are primarily driven by either case reports/series rather than randomized controlled trials or extrapolated from larger adult studies. Unfortunately, ABMR is an indolent disease that can be mitigated, but not entirely eliminated. Large randomized controlled trials are greatly needed and central to the advancement of the field.

References

1. Fernandez HE, Gjertson D, Date C, Choi IK, Ettenger RB, Tsai EW. Tacrolimus percent coefficient of variation as a marker of acute rejection associated with nonadherence in adolescent renal transplant recipients. Pediatr Transplant. 2011;15:135.
2. Sellares J, de Freitas DG, Mengel M, Reeve J, Einecke G, Sis B, et al. Understanding the causes of kidney transplant failure: the dominant role of antibody-mediated rejection and nonadherence. Am J Transplant. 2012;12(2):388–99.
3. Wiebe C, Nevins TE, Robiner WN, Thomas W, Matas AJ, Nickerson PW. The synergistic effect of class II HLA epitope-mismatch and nonadherence on acute rejection and graft survival. Am J Transplant. 2015;15(8):2197–202.
4. Foster BJ, Dahhou M, Zhang X, Platt RW, Samuel SM, Hanley JA. Association between age and graft failure rates in young kidney transplant recipients. Transplantation. 2011;92(11):1237–43.
5. Smith JM, Ho PL, McDonald RA. Renal transplant outcomes in adolescents: a report of the North American Pediatric Renal Transplant Cooperative Study. Pediatr Transplant. 2002;6(6):493–9.
6. Van Arendonk KJ, James NT, Boyarsky BJ, Garonzik-Wang JM, Orandi BJ, Magee JC, et al. Age at graft loss after pediatric kidney transplantation: exploring the high-risk age window. Clin J Am Soc Nephrol. 2013;8(6):1019–26.
7. Gubbels Bupp MR. Sex, the aging immune system, and chronic disease. Cell Immunol. 2015;294(2):102–10.

8. Shearer WT, Rosenblatt HM, Gelman RS, Oyomopito R, Plaeger S, Stiehm ER, et al. Lymphocyte subsets in healthy children from birth through 18 years of age: the Pediatric AIDS Clinical Trials Group P1009 study. J Allergy Clin Immunol. 2003;112(5):973–80.
9. Gourley TS, Wherry EJ, Masopust D, Ahmed R. Generation and maintenance of immunological memory. Semin Immunol. 2004;16(5):323–33.
10. IJspeert H, van Schouwenburg PA, van Zessen D, Pico-Knijnenburg I, Driessen GJ, Stubbs AP, et al. Evaluation of the antigen-experienced B-cell receptor repertoire in healthy children and adults. Front Immunol. 2016;7:410.
11. Hooper SR, Gerson AC, Butler RW, Gipson DS, Mendley SR, Lande MB, et al. Neurocognitive functioning of children and adolescents with mild-to-moderate chronic kidney disease. Clin J Am Soc Nephrol. 2011;6(8):1824–30.
12. Galvan A, Hare TA, Parra CE, Penn J, Voss H, Glover G, et al. Earlier development of the accumbens relative to orbitofrontal cortex might underlie risk-taking behavior in adolescents. J Neurosci. 2006;26(25):6885–92.
13. Galvan A, Hare T, Voss H, Glover G, Casey BJ. Risk-taking and the adolescent brain: who is at risk? Dev Sci. 2007;10(2):F8–F14.
14. Somerville LH, Hare T, Casey BJ. Frontostriatal maturation predicts cognitive control failure to appetitive cues in adolescents. J Cogn Neurosci. 2011;23(9):2123–34.
15. Silverman MH, Jedd K, Luciana M. Neural networks involved in adolescent reward processing: an activation likelihood estimation meta-analysis of functional neuroimaging studies. NeuroImage. 2015;122:427–39.
16. Gipson DS, Hooper SR, Duquette PJ, Wetherington CE, Stellwagen KK, Jenkins TL, et al. Memory and executive functions in pediatric chronic kidney disease. Child Neuropsychol. 2006;12(6):391–405.
17. Haffner D, Nissel R. Growth and puberty in chronic kidney disease. In: Geary DF, Schaefer F, editors. Comprehensive pediatric nephrology. 1st ed. Philadelphia: Mosby Elsevier; 2008. p. 709–32.
18. Rizzoni G, Broyer M, Brunner FP, Brynger H, Challah S, Kramer P, et al. Combined report on regular dialysis and transplantation of children in Europe, XIII, 1983. Proc Eur Dial Transplant Assoc Eur Ren Assoc. 1985;21:66–95.
19. Haffner D, Zivicnjak M. Molecular and functional noninvasive immune monitoring in the ESCAPE study for prediction of subclinical renal allograft rejection. Pediatr Nephrol. 2017;32(6):949–64.
20. Nissel R, Brazda I, Feneberg R, Wigger M, Greiner C, Querfeld U, et al. Effect of renal transplantation in childhood on longitudinal growth and adult height. Kidney Int. 2004;66(2):792–800.
21. Tainio J, Qvist E, Vehmas R, Jahnukainen K, Holtta T, Valta H, et al. Pubertal development is normal in adolescents after renal transplantation in childhood. Transplantation. 2011;92(4):404–9.
22. Low MJ. Neuroendocrinology. In: Melmed S, Polonsky KS, Larsen PR, Kronenberg HM, editors. Williams textbook of endocrinology. 13th ed. Philadelphia: Elsevier; 2016. p. 109–75.
23. Ahn JJ, O'Mahony J, Moshkova M, Hanwell HE, Singh H, Zhang MA, et al. Puberty in females enhances the risk of an outcome of multiple sclerosis in children and the development of central nervous system autoimmunity in mice. Mult Scler. 2015;21(6):735–48.
24. Brenhouse HC, Schwarz JM. Immunoadolescence: neuroimmune development and adolescent behavior. Neurosci Biobehav Rev. 2016;70:288–99.
25. Liva SM, Voskuhl RR. Testosterone acts directly on CD4+ T lymphocytes to increase IL-10 production. J Immunol. 2001;167(4):2060–7.
26. Mingomataj EC, Bakiri AH. Regulator versus effector paradigm: interleukin-10 as indicator of the switching response. Clin Rev Allergy Immunol. 2016;50(1):97–113.
27. McDaniel DO, Rigney DA, McDaniel KY, Windham WJ, Redmond P, Williams B, et al. Early expression profile of inflammatory markers and kidney allograft status. Transplant Proc. 2013;45(4):1520–3.
28. Sabat R, Grutz G, Warszawska K, Kirsch S, Witte E, Wolk K, et al. Biology of interleukin-10. Cytokine Growth Factor Rev. 2010;21(5):331–44.

29. Studies NAPRTaC. North American Pediatric Renal Trials and Collaborative Studies 2014 Annual transplant report. 2014.
30. Male D, Brostoff J, Roth DB, Roitt IM. Transplantation and rejection. In: Hyde M, Vosburgh A, editors. Immunology. Philadelphia: Saunders Elsevier; 2013. p. 341–2.
31. Dharnidharka VR, Fiorina P, Harmon WE. Kidney transplantation in children. N Engl J Med. 2014;371(6):549–58.
32. Tse G, Marson L. Immunology of graft rejection. In: Forsythe JL, editor. Transplantation. Philadelphia: Saunders Elsevier; 2014. p. 34–53.
33. Carden DL, Granger DN. Pathophysiology of ischaemia-reperfusion injury. J Pathol. 2000;190(3):255–66.
34. Land W. Postischemic reperfusion injury to allografts – a case for 'innate immunity'? Eur Surg Res. 2002;34(1–2):160–9.
35. Lopez-Neblina F, Toledo AH, Toledo-Pereyra LH. Molecular biology of apoptosis in ischemia and reperfusion. J Investig Surg. 2005;18(6):335–50.
36. Tilney NL, Guttmann RD. Effects of initial ischemia/reperfusion injury on the transplanted kidney. Transplantation. 1997;64(7):945–7.
37. Lu CY, Winterberg PD, Chen J, Hartono JR. Acute kidney injury: a conspiracy of toll-like receptor 4 on endothelia, leukocytes, and tubules. Pediatr Nephrol. 2012;27(10):1847–54.
38. Briscoe DM, Alexander SI, Lichtman AH. Interactions between T lymphocytes and endothelial cells in allograft rejection. Curr Opin Immunol. 1998;10(5):525–31.
39. Kim IK, Bedi DS, Denecke C, Ge X, Tullius SG. Impact of innate and adaptive immunity on rejection and tolerance. Transplantation. 2008;86(7):889–94.
40. Colvin RB. Antibody-mediated renal allograft rejection: diagnosis and pathogenesis. J Am Soc Nephrol. 2007;18(4):1046–56.
41. Linfert D, Chowdhry T, Rabb H. Lymphocytes and ischemia-reperfusion injury. Transplant Rev (Orlando). 2009;23(1):1–10.
42. Boros P, Bromberg JS. New cellular and molecular immune pathways in ischemia/reperfusion injury. Am J Transplant. 2006;6(4):652–8.
43. Mitchell P, Afzali B, Lombardi G, Lechler RI. The T helper 17-regulatory T cell axis in transplant rejection and tolerance. Curr Opin Organ Transplant. 2009;14(4):326–31.
44. Alegre ML, Leemans J, Le Moine A, Florquin S, De Wilde V, Chong A, et al. The multiple facets of toll-like receptors in transplantation biology. Transplantation. 2008;86(1):1–9.
45. Cardinal H, Dieude M, Hebert MJ. The emerging importance of non-HLA autoantibodies in kidney transplant complications. J Am Soc Nephrol. 2017;28(2):400–6.
46. Dikdan GS, Mora-Esteves C, Koneru B. Review of randomized clinical trials of donor management and organ preservation in deceased donors: opportunities and issues. Transplantation. 2012;94(5):425–41.
47. Zheng X, Zang G, Jiang J, He W, Johnston NJ, Ling H, et al. Attenuating ischemia-reperfusion injury in kidney transplantation by perfusing donor organs with siRNA cocktail solution. Transplantation. 2016;100(4):743–52.
48. Rogers NM, Zhang ZJ, Wang JJ, Thomson AW, Isenberg JS. CD47 regulates renal tubular epithelial cell self-renewal and proliferation following renal ischemia reperfusion. Kidney Int. 2016;90(2):334–47.
49. Benichou G, Thomson AW. Direct versus indirect allorecognition pathways: on the right track. Am J Transplant. 2009;9(4):655–6.
50. NCBI. NIH. 2016. Available from: https://www.ncbi.nlm.nih.gov/gene/.
51. Benichou G, Valujskikh A, Heeger PS. Contributions of direct and indirect T cell alloreactivity during allograft rejection in mice. J Immunol. 1999;162(1):352–8.
52. Marino J, Paster J, Benichou G. Allorecognition by T lymphocytes and allograft rejection. Front Immunol. 2016;7:582.
53. Herrera OB, Golshayan D, Tibbott R, Ochoa FS, James MJ, Marelli-Berg FM, et al. A novel pathway of alloantigen presentation by dendritic cells. J Immunol. 2004;173(8):4828–37.
54. Ingulli E. Mechanism of cellular rejection in transplantation. Pediatr Nephrol. 2010;25(1):61–74.

55. Bach F, Hirschhorn K. Lymphocyte interaction: a potential histocompatibility test in vitro. Science. 1964;143(3608):813–4.
56. Kaye J, Hedrick SM. Analysis of specificity for antigen, Mls, and allogenic MHC by transfer of T-cell receptor alpha- and beta-chain genes. Nature. 1988;336(6199):580–3.
57. Daniel C, Horvath S, Allen PM. A basis for alloreactivity: MHC helical residues broaden peptide recognition by the TCR. Immunity. 1998;8(5):543–52.
58. Weber DA, Terrell NK, Zhang Y, Strindberg G, Martin J, Rudensky A, et al. Requirement for peptide in alloreactive CD4+ T cell recognition of class II MHC molecules. J Immunol. 1995;154(10):5153–64.
59. Lechler RI, Batchelor JR. Restoration of immunogenicity to passenger cell-depleted kidney allografts by the addition of donor strain dendritic cells. J Exp Med. 1982;155(1):31–41.
60. Ali JM, Bolton EM, Bradley JA, Pettigrew GJ. Allorecognition pathways in transplant rejection and tolerance. Transplantation. 2013;96(8):681–8.
61. Halloran PF. Immunosuppressive drugs for kidney transplantation. New Engl J Med. 2004;351(26):2715–29.
62. Nankivell BJ, Alexander SI. Rejection of the kidney allograft. N Engl J Med. 2010;363(15):1451–62.
63. Baliga P, Chavin KD, Qin L, Woodward J, Lin J, Linsley PS, et al. CTLA4Ig prolongs allograft survival while suppressing cell-mediated immunity. Transplantation. 1994;58(10):1082–90.
64. Linsley PS, Bradshaw J, Greene J, Peach R, Bennett KL, Mittler RS. Intracellular trafficking of CTLA-4 and focal localization towards sites of TCR engagement. Immunity. 1996;4(6):535–43.
65. Schneider H, Downey J, Smith A, Zinselmeyer BH, Rush C, Brewer JM, et al. Reversal of the TCR stop signal by CTLA-4. Science. 2006;313(5795):1972–5.
66. Schneider H, Smith X, Liu H, Bismuth G, Rudd CE. CTLA-4 disrupts ZAP70 microcluster formation with reduced T cell/APC dwell times and calcium mobilization. Eur J Immunol. 2008;38(1):40–7.
67. Garside P, Ingulli E, Merica RR, Johnson JG, Noelle RJ, Jenkins MK. Visualization of specific B and T lymphocyte interactions in the lymph node. Science. 1998;281(5373):96–9.
68. Linsley PS, Wallace PM, Johnson J, Gibson MG, Greene JL, Ledbetter JA, et al. Immunosuppression in vivo by a soluble form of the CTLA-4 T cell activation molecule. Science. 1992;257(5071):792–5.
69. Kirk AD, Harlan DM, Armstrong NN, Davis TA, Dong Y, Gray GS, et al. CTLA4-Ig and anti-CD40 ligand prevent renal allograft rejection in primates. Proc Natl Acad Sci U S A. 1997;94(16):8789–94.
70. Linsley PS, Greene JL, Brady W, Bajorath J, Ledbetter JA, Peach R. Human B7-1 (CD80) and B7-2 (CD86) bind with similar avidities but distinct kinetics to CD28 and CTLA-4 receptors. Immunity. 1994;1(9):793–801.
71. Larsen CP, Pearson TC, Adams AB, Tso P, Shirasugi N, Strobert E, et al. Rational development of LEA29Y (belatacept), a high-affinity variant of CTLA4-Ig with potent immunosuppressive properties. Am J Transplant. 2005;5(3):443–53.
72. Charpentier B, Medina Pestana JO, Del CRM, Rostaing L, Grinyo J, Vanrenterghem Y, et al. Long-term exposure to belatacept in recipients of extended criteria donor kidneys. Am J Transplant. 2013;13(11):2884–91.
73. Rostaing L, Vincenti F, Grinyo J, Rice KM, Bresnahan B, Steinberg S, et al. Long-term belatacept exposure maintains efficacy and safety at 5 years: results from the long-term extension of the BENEFIT study. Am J Transplant. 2013;13(11):2875–83.
74. Vincenti F, Rostaing L, Grinyo J, Rice K, Steinberg S, Gaite L, et al. Belatacept and long-term outcomes in kidney transplantation. N Engl J Med. 2016;374(4):333–43.
75. Lerch C, Kanzelmeyer NK, Ahlenstiel-Grunow T, Froede K, Kreuzer M, Drube J, et al. Belatacept after kidney transplantation in adolescents: a retrospective study. Transpl Int. 2017;30(5):494–501.
76. Chopra B, Sureshkumar KK. Co-stimulatory blockade with belatacept in kidney transplantation. Expert Opin Biol Ther. 2014;14(5):563–7.

77. Grinyo J, Charpentier B, Pestana JM, Vanrenterghem Y, Vincenti F, Reyes-Acevedo R, et al. An integrated safety profile analysis of belatacept in kidney transplant recipients. Transplantation. 2010;90(12):1521–7.
78. Okimura K, Maeta K, Kobayashi N, Goto M, Kano N, Ishihara T, et al. Characterization of ASKP1240, a fully human antibody targeting human CD40 with potent immunosuppressive effects. Am J Transplant. 2014;14(6):1290–9.
79. Ma A, Dun H, Song L, Hu Y, Zeng L, Bai J, et al. Pharmacokinetics and pharmacodynamics of ASKP1240, a fully human anti-CD40 antibody, in normal and renal transplanted Cynomolgus monkeys. Transplantation. 2014;97(4):397–404.
80. Wang D, Matsumoto R, You Y, Che T, Lin XY, Gaffen SL, et al. CD3/CD28 costimulation-induced NF-kappaB activation is mediated by recruitment of protein kinase C-theta, Bcl10, and IkappaB kinase beta to the immunological synapse through CARMA1. Mol Cell Biol. 2004;24(1):164–71.
81. Shapiro R, Zeevi A, Basu A, Tan HP, Kayler LK, Blisard DM, et al. Alemtuzumab preconditioning with tacrolimus monotherapy-the impact of serial monitoring for donor-specific antibody. Transplantation. 2008;85(8):1125–32.
82. Tan HP, Kaczorowski D, Basu A, McCauley J, Marcos A, Donaldson J, et al. Steroid-free tacrolimus monotherapy after pretransplantation thymoglobulin or Campath and laparoscopy in living donor renal transplantation. Transplant Proc. 2005;37(10):4235–40.
83. Shapiro R, Basu A, Tan H, Gray E, Kahn A, Randhawa P, et al. Kidney transplantation under minimal immunosuppression after pretransplant lymphoid depletion with Thymoglobulin or Campath. J Am Coll Surg. 2005;200(4):505–15. quiz A59–61
84. Sung J, Barry JM, Jenkins R, Rozansky D, Iragorri S, Conlin M, et al. Alemtuzumab induction with tacrolimus monotherapy in 25 pediatric renal transplant recipients. Pediatr Transplant. 2013;17(8):718–25.
85. Supe-Markovina K, Melquist JJ, Connolly D, DiCarlo HN, Waltzer WC, Fine RN, et al. Alemtuzumab with corticosteroid minimization for pediatric deceased donor renal transplantation: a seven-yr experience. Pediatr Transplant. 2014;18(4):363–8.
86. Kaabak MM, Babenko NN, Samsonov DV, Sandrikov VA, Maschan AA, Zokoev AK. Alemtuzumab induction in pediatric kidney transplantation. Pediatr Transplant. 2013;17(2):168–78.
87. Crowson CN, Reed RD, Shelton BA, MacLennan PA, Locke JE. Lymphocyte-depleting induction therapy lowers the risk of acute rejection in African American pediatric kidney transplant recipients. Pediatr Transplant. 2017;21(1):e12823.
88. Akalin E, Hendrix RC, Polavarapu RG, Pearson TC, Neylan JF, Larsen CP, et al. Gene expression analysis in human renal allograft biopsy samples using high-density oligoarray technology. Transplantation. 2001;72(5):948–53.
89. Hoffmann SC, Hale DA, Kleiner DE, Mannon RB, Kampen RL, Jacobson LM, et al. Functionally significant renal allograft rejection is defined by transcriptional criteria. Am J Transplant. 2005;5(3):573–81.
90. Barry M, Bleackley RC. Cytotoxic T lymphocytes: all roads lead to death. Nat Rev Immunol. 2002;2(6):401–9.
91. Bradley JA, Mason DW, Morris PJ. Evidence that rat renal allografts are rejected by cytotoxic T cells and not by nonspecific effectors. Transplantation. 1985;39(2):169–75.
92. Al-Lamki RS, Wang J, Skepper JN, Thiru S, Pober JS, Bradley JR. Expression of tumor necrosis factor receptors in normal kidney and rejecting renal transplants. Lab Investig. 2001;81(11):1503–15.
93. Kwun J, Manook M, Page E, Burghuber C, Hong J, Knechtle SJ. Crosstalk between T and B cells in the germinal center after transplantation. Transplantation. 2017;101(4):704–12.
94. Ng YW, Singh M, Sarwal MM. Antibody-mediated rejection in pediatric kidney transplantation: pathophysiology, diagnosis, and management. Drugs. 2015;75(5):455–72.
95. Sarwal M, Chua MS, Kambham N, Hsieh SC, Satterwhite T, Masek M, et al. Molecular heterogeneity in acute renal allograft rejection identified by DNA microarray profiling. N Engl J Med. 2003;349(2):125–38.

96. Zarkhin V, Kambham N, Li L, Kwok S, Hsieh SC, Salvatierra O, et al. Characterization of intra-graft B cells during renal allograft rejection. Kidney Int. 2008;74(5):664–73.
97. Terasaki PI. Humoral theory of transplantation. Am J Transplant. 2003;3(6):665–73.
98. Alegre ML, Florquin S, Goldman M. Cellular mechanisms underlying acute graft rejection: time for reassessment. Curr Opin Immunol. 2007;19(5):563–8.
99. Bhatti AB, Usman M. Chronic renal transplant rejection and possible anti-proliferative drug targets. Cureus. 2015;7(11):e376.
100. Tsai EW, Rianthavorn P, Gjertson DW, Wallace WD, Reed EF, Ettenger RB. CD20+ lymphocytes in renal allografts are associated with poor graft survival in pediatric patients. Transplantation. 2006;82(12):1769–73.
101. Tsai EW, Wallace WD, Gjertson DW, Reed EF, Ettenger RB. Significance of intragraft CD138+ lymphocytes and p-S6RP in pediatric kidney transplant biopsies. Transplantation. 2010;90(8):875–81.
102. Durkan AM, Robinson LA. Acute allograft dysfunction. In: Geary DF, Schaefer F, editors. Comprehensive pediatric nephrology. 1st ed. Philadelphia: Mosby Elsevier; 2008. p. 931–45.
103. Goldberg RJ, Weng FL, Kandula P. Acute and chronic allograft dysfunction in kidney transplant recipients. Med Clin N Am. 2016;100(3):487–503.
104. Crespo E, Roedder S, Sigdel T, Hsieh SC, Luque S, Cruzado JM, Tran TQ, Grinyó JM, Sarwal MM, Bestard O. Relationship among viremia/viral Infection, alloimmunity, and nutritional parameters in the first year after pediatric kidney transplantation. Transplantation. 2017;101(6):1400–9.
105. Solez K, Axelsen RA, Benediktsson H, Burdick JF, Cohen AH, Colvin RB, et al. International standardization of criteria for the histologic diagnosis of renal allograft rejection: the Banff working classification of kidney transplant pathology. Kidney Int. 1993;44(2):411–22.
106. Racusen LC, Solez K, Colvin RB, Bonsib SM, Castro MC, Cavallo T, et al. The Banff 97 working classification of renal allograft pathology. Kidney Int. 1999;55(2):713–23.
107. Loupy A, Haas M, Solez K, Racusen L, Glotz D, Seron D, et al. The Banff 2015 kidney meeting report: current challenges in rejection classification and prospects for adopting molecular pathology. Am J Transplant. 2017;17(1):28–41.
108. Gray D, Shepherd H, Daar A, Oliver DO, Morris PJ. Oral versus intravenous high-dose steroid treatment of renal allograft rejection. The big shot or not? Lancet. 1978;1(8056):117–8.
109. Vineyard GC, Fadem SZ, Dmochowski J, Carpenter CB, Wilson RE. Evaluation of corticosteroid therapy for acute renal allograft rejection. Surg Gynecol Obstet. 1974;138(2):225–9.
110. Kidney Disease: Improving Global Outcomes Transplant Work G. KDIGO clinical practice guideline for the care of kidney transplant recipients. Am J Transplant. 2009;9(Suppl 3):S1–155.
111. Webster AC, Pankhurst T, Rinaldi F, Chapman JR, Craig JC. Monoclonal and polyclonal antibody therapy for treating acute rejection in kidney transplant recipients: a systematic review of randomized trial data. Transplantation. 2006;81(7):953–65.
112. Upadhyay K, Midgley L, Moudgil A. Safety and efficacy of alemtuzumab in the treatment of late acute renal allograft rejection. Pediatr Transplant. 2012;16(3):286–93.
113. van den Hoogen MW, Hesselink DA, van Son WJ, Weimar W, Hilbrands LB. Treatment of steroid-resistant acute renal allograft rejection with alemtuzumab. Am J Transplant. 2013;13(1):192–6.
114. Ettenger R, Chin H, Kesler K, Bridges N, Grimm P, Reed EF, Sarwal M, Sibley R, Tsai E, Warshaw B, Kirk AD. Relationship among viremia/viral infection, alloimmunity, and nutritional parameters in the first year after pediatric kidney transplantation. Am J Transplant. 2016;17(6):1549–62.
115. Rees L, Kim JJ. HLA sensitisation: can it be prevented? Pediatr Nephrol. 2015;30(4):577–87.
116. Pizzo HP, Ettenger RB, Gjertson DW, Reed EF, Zhang J, Gritsch HA, et al. Sirolimus and tacrolimus coefficient of variation is associated with rejection, donor-specific antibodies, and nonadherence. Pediatr Nephrol. 2016;31(12):2345–52.

117. Sicard A, Ducreux S, Rabeyrin M, Couzi L, McGregor B, Badet L, et al. Detection of C3d-binding donor-specific anti-HLA antibodies at diagnosis of humoral rejection predicts renal graft loss. J Am Soc Nephrol. 2015;26(2):457–67.
118. Sutherland SM, Chen G, Sequeira FA, Lou CD, Alexander SR, Tyan DB. Complement-fixing donor-specific antibodies identified by a novel C1q assay are associated with allograft loss. Pediatr Transplant. 2012;16(1):12–7.
119. Dragun D, Catar R, Philippe A. Non-HLA antibodies against endothelial targets bridging allo- and autoimmunity. Kidney Int. 2016;90(2):280–8.
120. Zhang Q, Reed EF. The importance of non-HLA antibodies in transplantation. Nat Rev Nephrol. 2016;12(8):484–95.
121. Webb NJ, Maxwell H. Chronic renal transplant dysfunction. In: Geary DF, Schaefer F, editors. Comprehensive pediatric nephrology. 1st ed. Philadelphia: Mosby Elsevier; 2008. p. 947–65.
122. Haas M. An updated Banff schema for diagnosis of antibody-mediated rejection in renal allografts. Curr Opin Organ Transplant. 2014;19(3):315–22.
123. Racusen LC, Colvin RB, Solez K, Mihatsch MJ, Halloran PF, Campbell PM, et al. Antibody-mediated rejection criteria – an addition to the Banff 97 classification of renal allograft rejection. Am J Transplant. 2003;3(6):708–14.
124. Haas M, Sis B, Racusen LC, Solez K, Glotz D, Colvin RB, et al. Banff 2013 meeting report: inclusion of c4d-negative antibody-mediated rejection and antibody-associated arterial lesions. Am J Transplant. 2014;14(2):272–83.
125. Wiebe C, Pochinco D, Blydt-Hansen TD, Ho J, Birk PE, Karpinski M, et al. Class II HLA epitope matching-A strategy to minimize de novo donor-specific antibody development and improve outcomes. Am J Transplant. 2013;13(12):3114–22.
126. Gralla J, Tong S, Wiseman AC. The impact of human leukocyte antigen mismatching on sensitization rates and subsequent retransplantation after first graft failure in pediatric renal transplant recipients. Transplantation. 2013;95(10):1218–24.
127. Xu H, Samy KP, Guasch A, Mead SI, Ghali A, Mehta A, et al. Postdepletion lymphocyte reconstitution during belatacept and rapamycin treatment in kidney transplant recipients. Am J Transplant. 2016;16(2):550–64.
128. Kirk AD, Guasch A, Xu H, Cheeseman J, Mead SI, Ghali A, et al. Renal transplantation using belatacept without maintenance steroids or calcineurin inhibitors. Am J Transplant. 2014;14(5):1142–51.
129. Henriksson J, Tyden G, Hoijer J, Wadstrom JA. Prospective randomized trial on the effect of using an electronic monitoring drug dispensing device to improve adherence and compliance. Transplantation. 2016;100(1):203–9.
130. Kreuzer M, Prufe J, Bethe D, Vogel C, Grosshennig A, Koch A, et al. The TRANSNephro-study examining a new transition model for post-kidney transplant adolescents and an analysis of the present health care: study protocol for a randomized controlled trial. Trials. 2014;15:505.
131. Browning RB, McGillicuddy JW, Treiber FA, Taber DJ. Kidney transplant recipients' attitudes about using mobile health technology for managing and monitoring medication therapy. J Am Pharm Assoc (2003). 2016;56(4):450–4. e1
132. Bonomini V, Vangelista A, Frasca GM, Di Felice A, Liviano D'Arcangelo G. Effects of plasmapheresis in renal transplant rejection. A controlled study. Trans Am Soc Artif Intern Organs. 1985;31:698–703.
133. Montgomery RA, Zachary AA, Racusen LC, Leffell MS, King KE, Burdick J, et al. Plasmapheresis and intravenous immune globulin provides effective rescue therapy for refractory humoral rejection and allows kidneys to be successfully transplanted into cross-match-positive recipients. Transplantation. 2000;70(6):887–95.
134. Rocha PN, Butterly DW, Greenberg A, Reddan DN, Tuttle-Newhall J, Collins BH, et al. Beneficial effect of plasmapheresis and intravenous immunoglobulin on renal allograft survival of patients with acute humoral rejection. Transplantation. 2003;75(9):1490–5.

135. Zarkhin V, Li L, Kambham N, Sigdel T, Salvatierra O, Sarwal MM. A randomized, prospective trial of rituximab for acute rejection in pediatric renal transplantation. Am J Transplant. 2008;8(12):2607–17.
136. Gulleroglu K, Baskin E, Bayrakci US, Turan M, Ozdemir BH, Moray G, et al. Antibody-mediated rejection and treatment in pediatric patients: one center's experience. Exp Clin Transplant. 2013;11(5):404–7.
137. Pearl MH. Bortezomib may stabilize pediatric renal transplant recipients with antibody-mediated rejection. Pediatric Nephrology. 2016;31(8):1341–8.
138. Nguyen S, Gallay B, Butani L. Efficacy of bortezomib for reducing donor-specific antibodies in children and adolescents on a steroid minimization regimen. Pediatr Transplant. 2014;18(5):463–8.
139. Sautenet B, Blancho G, Buchler M, Morelon E, Toupance O, Barrou B, et al. One-year results of the effects of rituximab on acute antibody-mediated rejection in renal transplantation: RITUX ERAH, a multicenter double-blind randomized placebo-controlled trial. Transplantation. 2016;100(2):391–9.
140. Delbue S, Ferraresso M, Elia F, Belingheri M, Carloni C, Signorini L, et al. Investigation of polyomaviruses replication in pediatric patients with nephropathy receiving rituximab. J Med Virol. 2012;84(9):1464–70.
141. Gulleroglu K, Baskin E, Moray G, Ozdemir H, Arslan H, Haberal M. Rituximab therapy and infection risk in pediatric renal transplant patients. Exp Clin Transplant. 2016;14(2):172–5.
142. Kizilbash S, Claes D, Ashoor I, Chen A, Jandeska S, Matar RB, et al. Bortezomib in the treatment of antibody-mediated rejection in pediatric kidney transplant recipients: a multicenter Midwest Pediatric Nephrology Consortium study. Pediatr Transplant. 2017;21(3):e12873.
143. Choi J, Aubert O, Vo A, Loupy A, Haas M, Puliyanda D, et al. Assessment of tocilizumab (anti-interleukin-6 receptor monoclonal) as a potential treatment for chronic antibody-mediated rejection and transplant glomerulopathy in HLA-sensitized renal allograft recipients. Am J Transplant. 2017;17:2381–9.
144. Kim I, Wu G, Chai NN, Klein AS, Jordan S. Anti-interleukin 6 receptor antibodies attenuate antibody recall responses in a mouse model of allosensitization. Transplantation. 2014;98(12):1262–70.
145. Jordan SC, Vo AA, Toyoda M, Tyan D, Nast CC. Post-transplant therapy with high-dose intravenous gammaglobulin: applications to treatment of antibody-mediated rejection. Pediatr Transplant. 2005;9(2):155–61.
146. Ghirardo G, Benetti E, Poli F, Vidal E, Della Vella M, Cozzi E, et al. Plasmapheresis-resistant acute humoral rejection successfully treated with anti-C5 antibody. Pediatr Transplant. 2014;18(1):E1–5.
147. Burbach M, Suberbielle C, Brocheriou I, Ridel C, Mesnard L, Dahan K, et al. Report of the inefficacy of eculizumab in two cases of severe antibody-mediated rejection of renal grafts. Transplantation. 2014;98(10):1056–9.
148. Locke JE, Magro CM, Singer AL, Segev DL, Haas M, Hillel AT, et al. The use of antibody to complement protein C5 for salvage treatment of severe antibody-mediated rejection. Am J Transplant. 2009;9(1):231–5.
149. Cornell LD, Schinstock CA, Gandhi MJ, Kremers WK, Stegall MD. Positive crossmatch kidney transplant recipients treated with eculizumab: outcomes beyond 1 year. Am J Transplant. 2015;15(5):1293–302.
150. Montgomery RA, Orandi BJ, Racusen L, Jackson AM, Garonzik-Wang JM, Shah T, et al. Plasma-derived C1 esterase inhibitor for acute antibody-mediated rejection following kidney transplantation: results of a randomized double-blind placebo-controlled pilot study. Am J Transplant. 2016;16:3468–78.

Chapter 16
Transitioning Care of the Adolescent Patient with Chronic Kidney Disease to Adult Providers

Mina Matsuda-Abedini

Introduction

Advances in the care of children with chronic kidney disease (CKD) and the possibility of successful pediatric renal replacement therapies, dialysis and renal transplantation, have resulted in improved life expectancy of this patient population [1]. This in turn has led to many adolescents and young adults (AYA) with childhood-onset CKD whose care needs to be transitioned to adult nephrologists. In the United States, AYA make up approximately 3% of the end-stage renal disease (ESRD) population [2], which reflects a threefold increase since 1980, with majority of this AYA population being between the ages of 20 and 29 years [2]. Without adequate support during a critical transition period, AYA with CKD and ESRD are at an increased risk of poor health outcomes.

This chapter will address how gaps in care exist as adolescents with CKD transition to adult care, and given the neurocognitive deficits that may be present and under-recognized in this patient population, implementation of a transition care program is critically important.

Gaps in Care During Transition

There are gaps in the care of AYA with CKD as they transition from pediatric to adult health systems, with costly consequences. Poor health outcomes are thought to be multifactorial, including lapses in adherence [3–6], loss to follow-up [7], and changes in health insurance coverage [8]. The exact prevalence of

M. Matsuda-Abedini
Hospital for Sick Children, Toronto, ON, Canada
e-mail: mina.matsuda-abedini@sickkids.ca

M. N. Haddad et al. (eds.), *Adolescents with Chronic Kidney Disease*,
https://doi.org/10.1007/978-3-319-97220-6_16

nonadherence among AYA with CKD and ESRD is unknown, but nonadherence rates as high as 75% have been reported among adolescent transplant recipients [6], with increases in graft failure rates between ages 17 and 24 years [9]. One UK study showed that 35% (7 of 20) of young adult renal transplant recipients had unexpectedly lost their graft by 36 months after transfer of care from pediatric to adult renal transplant unit [5]. A similar finding was reported in a Canadian study, where three deaths (9%) and seven graft losses (21%) occurred within 2 years of transfer to adult renal transplant programs [10]. These data indicate that gaps in care exist. In another Canadian study, where patients have access to universal health insurance, Samuel et al. analyzed a national database to examine health service use of patients with ESRD during adolescence and after transfer to adult care [7]. In this study, the investigators used avoidable hospitalizations as a surrogate for lapses in outpatient primary or specialty care, given that these conditions could have been managed in an ambulatory clinic. They found that among the 92 patients transferred to adult care during their study period, compared with the year before transfer, the proportion of avoidable hospitalizations was threefold to fourfold higher during the period 3 to <4 years after transfer [7].

An additional challenge for some CKD and ESRD patients is the nonrenal care that also requires long-term follow-up and, therefore, transitioning to an adult specialist. Registry data shows that the main cause of CKD in children is congenital anomalies of the kidney and urinary tract (CAKUT) followed by hereditary nephropathies and glomerulonephritis [11]. Many AYA with CAKUT would benefit from an adult urologist involvement once their care has been transferred; however, an adult urologist with expertise in bladder management associated with some CAKUT is not always readily available [12]. Furthermore, some individuals with congenital genitourinary anomalies may face challenges related to sexuality and fertility as they enter adulthood and require interdisciplinary care from adult urologists and gynecologists with expertise in congenital genitourinary anomalies [12]. And, in patients with rare hereditary conditions, such as cystinosis, there are late, nonrenal complications that require long-term monitoring and treatment, and it would be critical to plan a proper transition to an adult specialist who is familiar with rare genetic diseases [13–15].

The transition of healthcare from pediatric to adult nephrology is only one of several transitions that occur during adolescence [16, 17]. As the adolescent matures to a young adult, he or she may start post-secondary education or start a vocation and may move out of the family home to live independently. At this time, parental involvement and support may decrease [6, 9]. In addition, there may be underrecognized anxiety or depression, making this transition period even more challenging for a young adult with CKD. Both pediatric and adult nephrologists need to be aware of all these concurrent transitions and its potential effect on the health of the AYA. Identifying various resources (e.g., social workers, school counselors, youth workers, mental health specialists) in the community who can provide support and facilitating a referral to the appropriate services should be considered during the transition process.

Developing Brain and Neurocognitive Impact of CKD

As adolescents transition to adulthood, they are expected to make independent decisions in the face of uncertainty and risks. Brain structural and functional imaging studies are emerging that show differential trajectories of maturation in various brain regions, with the prefrontal cortex being one of the last regions to mature [18]. The prefrontal cortex is involved in cognitive control, regulation of emotion, and gives an individual the capacity to exercise good judgment when making a decision, weighing risks versus reward [19]. Any deficit in judgment, risk perception, and logical reasoning would be problematic for an AYA with CKD and ESRD and can result in nonadherence to prescribed medications and decreased engagement with healthcare providers at a time that parental supervision may be decreasing.

In addition to the normal brain maturation processes that are not yet complete until young adulthood, children and adolescents with CKD can also have under-recognized cognitive deficits, including impaired executive function and lower memory [20–23]. These neurocognitive deficits can further contribute to nonadherence to treatments in AYA with CKD. In a recently published comprehensive review of neuroimaging studies in adults and children with kidney disease spanning over 35 years, only 13 studies involved children, and most of the pediatric studies were from the 1980s and early 1990s using CT scans [24]. In the 1980s, brain CT imaging studies in children with CKD showed cerebral atrophy, a sign of chronic brain injury, or abnormal brain development in many affected children [25–27]. In the past three decades, the care of children with CKD has changed dramatically. Improved renal nutrition, elimination of aluminum as a phosphate binder, use of erythropoietin for the management of anemia, and better dialysis treatment and timely transplantation have all contributed to improve neurological outcomes [28]. Despite these advances in treatment, emerging studies continue to suggest the presence of neurocognitive impairments in children with CKD [20, 29–31]. In a recent study of 368 children with mild-to-moderate CKD, up to 40% of children scored at least one standard deviation below the mean on measures of intelligence quotient, working memory, academic achievement, attention regulation, or executive functioning [23]. As we look at the entire life span of a child with CKD, these deficits may impact their disease self-management, their health outcomes, as well as their education and vocational attainment. The only contemporary pediatric neuroimaging studies in children with CKD using brain MRI are those from a relatively homogeneous Finnish cohort, affected predominantly by congenital nephrotic syndrome of the Finnish type [32, 33]. Brain MRI showed high rates of stroke, with characteristics that suggested episodes of brain hypoperfusion. Many of the changes were chronic, predominantly in the brain white matter [32, 33]. Together, all these data suggest that (a) brain abnormalities can be associated with CKD and ESRD and (b) recognition of any associated neurocognitive deficits would be important in planning a successful transition.

Acknowledging the gaps in care and the potential presence of neurocognitive deficits in AYA with CKD highlights the need for a properly designed transition care.

Transition Care

One definition of transition in the medical setting is "the purposeful, planned movement of adolescents and young adults with chronic physical and medical conditions from child-centered to adult-oriented health care systems [34]." The aim of a transition program would be to empower adolescents and their families such that they are ready for the transfer of care, resulting in successful integration into the adult healthcare system in an uninterrupted manner. Transfer is only one component of the transition process [17]. A successful transition requires an integrated effort from both the pediatric and the adult healthcare programs [35].

The "triple aim" [36] – a framework developed by the Institute for Health Care Improvement – of a CKD transition care program would be to improve the health of AYA with CKD, optimize their experience of care, and reduce or control the per capita healthcare cost [36, 37]. Recently, a healthcare delivery innovation lab, tasked with designing a transition care model based on the "triple aim" framework, identified three main areas of focus that can be applied to any patient population with a chronic illness [38], including CKD:

1. *Establishing and supporting self-management during the transition period* [38]

Adolescents with progressing CKD often need to follow a prescribed diet and daily fluid intake and learn their medication names, doses, indications, and side effects while developing strategies to remember to take their medications on time, as prescribed. They may be asked to monitor blood pressures at home, and some need to do daily intermittent bladder catheterizations. As the parents shift the responsibility of care to the adolescent, the adolescent needs to learn how to best problem solve, communicate with the healthcare team, self-advocate, as well as manage the stress that can be associated with the increased responsibility. This shift of the responsibility of care needs to occur gradually, and it can take longer for some than others, which is why the transition process needs to start as early as 12 years of age. Self-management does not mean leaving the adolescent patient to cope on their own but rather providing appropriate support to allow the adolescent to develop the confidence and skills needed to manage their CKD through the transition period. The anticipated impact of establishing and supporting self-management is better adherence, decreased visits to the emergency department and less hospitalizations, and, therefore, lower healthcare cost [38].

2. *Engaging the receiving adult healthcare team* [38]

As mentioned earlier in this chapter, the transition process does not end with transfer of care. It is essential to engage key providers from the adult nephrology team early in transition planning. Whether members of the adult team join the pediatric team or vice versa, creating a sense of familiarity and continuity of care would certainly enhance the experience of care for the AYA and their family.

3. *Using a checklist-driven guide during the transition process* [38]

Adolescents should reach a series of milestones as the responsibility of care is gradually shifted from the parent to the AYA [39]. There are a number of tools that have been developed for tracking the transition progress, assessing individual readiness, and facilitating communication of medical information (e.g., Fig. 16.1. MyHealth Passport – https://www.sickkids.ca/myhealthpassport/). Several validated self-care assessment tools, such as the Transition Readiness Assessment Questionnaire (TRAQ) [40], ON TRAC [http://www.ontracbc.ca], and the TRxANSITION Scale [41, 42], can help providers identify key areas that the patient may require additional education and support and come up with a plan of action.

Timing of Transition

In 2011, the International Pediatric Nephrology Association and the International Society of Nephrology jointly published a consensus statement [43], where they highlighted the need for a transition plan that should be individualized. Furthermore,

Name	Kid Ney
DOB	Jan 1, 1999
Diagnosis	CKD Stage 4, PUV
Med Hx	Asthma
Meds	Darbepoietin, Sodium Bicarb
Other meds	Iron, Calcium carbonate, Calcitriol
Drug allergies	Penicillin
Immunization	DPTP, MMR, HIB, Varicella, Mening., Pneumovax, Prevnar, Hep B, Annual Flu
Devices	CIC during day, Indwelling at night
Dialysis	No
Transplant	Assessed
Labs	eGFR: 23 ml/min/1.73m2
Diet	Low Potassium, Low Phosphorus
Blood group	O+
Bloodwork	Monthly
Coverage	Ontario Health Insurance Plan
Ped Neph	Dr. Glomerulus
Adult provider	Dr. Transplant
Family Doctor	Dr. General
Pharmacy	Shoppers Drug Mart
Emergency contact	Mom and Dad
Date Created	5/3/2017www.sickkids.ca/myhealthpassport

Fig. 16.1 An example of MyHealth Passport for an AYA with CKD that can be folded and laminated to fit in a wallet. (https://www.sickkids.ca/myhealthpassport/)

they stated that transfer should take place during a period without crises [43]. Two years after the publication, transition practices of 15 pediatric units across Europe were surveyed, and majority of the units were aware of the guidelines, and one third had integrated them into their transition practice [44]. It is advocated that the exact timing of transfer should depend on factors other than the chronological age of the patient, such as maturity and readiness, disease activity, and availability of adult specialty services [43]. Currently, majority of pediatric units are required by their institution to transfer their patients' care by a certain age. Ideally, there should be some flexibility in times of crises such as disease flares or progression or family or societal instability [45] to delay the transfer. Similarly, it would be reasonable for the adult program to have some flexibility in accepting the care of an adolescent patient who may need to be transferred sooner than anticipated, for example, for the management of a pregnancy in an adolescent with CKD. The key is to implement a transition program that starts as early as 12 years of age and is designed to optimize the adolescents' readiness for uninterrupted integration into an adult practice by the age of 18–22 years. The "Six Core Elements of Health Care Transition (2.0)" [http://www.gottransition.org] include establishing a policy, tracking progress, administering transition readiness assessments, planning for adult care, transferring, and integrating into an adult practice. The recommended timeline is [46]:

Age 12: Discuss the transition policy of the institution with the adolescent and family.
Ages 13–15: Initiate transition planning. Establish and support self-management skills following a checklist as a guide to assess readiness.
Ages 16–18: Prepare youth and family for adult model of care, engage the receiving adult healthcare team, and discuss upcoming transfer.
Ages 18–22: Transfer care to adult nephrology team with transfer package.
Ages 23–26: Integrate young adult into adult nephrology care program.

Implementation of a Transition Program

There are a number of nephrology transition programs that have been implemented at different institutions that have applied the core elements of transition outlined above. Most programs involve joint efforts of transition champions from the pediatric nephrology as well the adult nephrology teams. The actual integrated clinic structure differs depending on the local geography and available resources, but regardless of the actual clinic design, the goal is an integrated transition pathway that allows the AYA with CKD and his or her family to progressively gain trust in the adult healthcare program before the final transfer [10, 47].

One example of a transition clinic was developed at B.C. Children's Hospital in Canada. Starting at the age of 12 years, families were introduced to the transition policy of the institution. During their regular clinic visits, ON TRAC [http://www.ontracbc.ca] would be used as a guideline to build and support self-management skills and track transition progress. Around the age of 16 years, the adolescent patients were assessed by a multidisciplinary transition team, consisting of their pediatric nephrologist, renal nurse, adolescent medicine specialist, renal pharmacist, dietitian, and social worker. Specific individualized educational goals were to be achieved by adolescents during the transition visits to optimize their readiness for adult model of care. An adult nephrology program in geographic proximity to the patient's home would then be selected and engaged in the transition preparation and eventual transfer of care. This particular transition model was evaluated in terms of its efficacy, as well as its cost [10]. The investigators compared patient and allograft survival in renal transplant recipients who received care since the establishment of the transition clinic to a cohort of patients transferred prior to the introduction of a transition clinic. In the pre-transition clinic era, there had been a combined poor outcome (death or allograft loss) incidence of 24% within 2 years post-transfer, compared with no death or graft loss in the transition clinic cohort with at least 2 years of follow-up in an adult transplant unit [10]. The cost estimate analysis showed that the operating cost of this transition clinic was much less than the cost associated with graft loss and return to dialysis, and this did not even include the cost attributed to loss of work for patients and family members or the cost of untimely death of a young person [10]. This is one of many transition programs that have demonstrated improved health outcomes and reduced per capita healthcare cost [10, 47]. Continued research is needed to compare the efficacy of the different transition models, and it requires achieving consensus on a core set of transition measures in order to compare outcomes.

Conclusion

A comprehensive planned transition care program is essential to provide the necessary skills to the adolescents with CKD and ESRD to navigate changes in healthcare settings and successfully integrate in an adult program. With neurocognitive deficits [20, 23, 29-31], and brain abnormalities [32, 33, 48] still present in children and youth with CKD despite modern renal care, transition programs that address the particular needs of AYA should be a component of CKD clinical programs. A well-designed transition program is anticipated to improve the health outcome of young adults with CKD and ESRD, positively influence their experience of care, and reduce or control the per capita healthcare cost.

References

1. Groothoff JW. Long-term outcomes of children with end-stage renal disease. Pediatr Nephrol. 2005;20(7):849–53.
2. Ferris ME, et al. Self-management and transition among adolescents/young adults with chronic or end-stage kidney disease. Blood Purif. 2015;39(1–3):99–104.

3. Aujoulat I, et al. Non-adherence in adolescent transplant recipients: the role of uncertainty in health care providers. Pediatr Transplant. 2011;15(2):148–56.
4. Jarzembowski T, et al. Impact of non-compliance on outcome after pediatric kidney transplantation: an analysis in racial subgroups. Pediatr Transplant. 2004;8(4):367–71.
5. Watson AR. Non-compliance and transfer from paediatric to adult transplant unit. Pediatr Nephrol. 2000;14(6):469–72.
6. Fredericks EM, Dore-Stites D. Adherence to immunosuppressants: how can it be improved in adolescent organ transplant recipients? Curr Opin Organ Transplant. 2010;15(5):614–20.
7. Samuel SM, et al. Avoidable hospitalizations in youth with kidney failure after transfer to or with only adult care. Pediatrics. 2014;133(4):e993–1000.
8. Goudie A, Carle AC. Ohio study shows that insurance coverage is critical for children with special health care needs as they transition to adulthood. Health Aff (Millwood). 2011;30(12):2382–90.
9. Foster BJ, et al. The TAKE-IT study: aims, design, and methods. BMC Nephrol. 2014;15:139.
10. Prestidge C, et al. Utility and cost of a renal transplant transition clinic. Pediatr Nephrol. 2012;27(2):295–302.
11. Harambat J, et al. Epidemiology of chronic kidney disease in children. Pediatr Nephrol. 2012;27(3):363–73.
12. Hsieh MH, et al. Research needs for effective transition in lifelong care of congenital genitourinary conditions: a workshop sponsored by the National Institute of Diabetes and Digestive and Kidney Diseases. Urology. 2017;103:261–71.
13. Nesterova G, Gahl WA. Cystinosis: the evolution of a treatable disease. Pediatr Nephrol. 2013;28(1):51–9.
14. Emma F, et al. Nephropathic cystinosis: an international consensus document. Nephrol Dial Transplant. 2014;29(Suppl 4):iv87–94.
15. Ariceta G, et al. A coordinated transition model for patients with cystinosis: from pediatrics to adult care. Nefrologia. 2016;36(6):616–30.
16. American Academy of Pediatrics Committee on Children With, D. The role of the pediatrician in transitioning children and adolescents with developmental disabilities and chronic illnesses from school to work or college. American Academy of Pediatrics. Committee on Children With Disabilities. Pediatrics. 2000;106(4):854–6.
17. Rosen DS. Transition from pediatric to adult-oriented health care for the adolescent with chronic illness or disability. Adolesc Med. 1994;5(2):241–8.
18. Somerville LH, Jones RM, Casey BJ. A time of change: behavioral and neural correlates of adolescent sensitivity to appetitive and aversive environmental cues. Brain Cogn. 2010;72(1):124–33.
19. Giedd JN, Rapoport JL. Structural MRI of pediatric brain development: what have we learned and where are we going? Neuron. 2010;67(5):728–34.
20. Gipson DS, et al. Memory and executive functions in pediatric chronic kidney disease. Child Neuropsychol. 2006;12(6):391–405.
21. Fennell RS, et al. A longitudinal study of the cognitive function of children with renal failure. Pediatr Nephrol. 1990;4(1):11–5.
22. Warady BA, et al. Optimal care of the pediatric end-stage renal disease patient on dialysis. Am J Kidney Dis. 1999;33(3):567–83.
23. Hooper SR, et al. Neurocognitive functioning of children and adolescents with mild-to-moderate chronic kidney disease. Clin J Am Soc Nephrol. 2011;6(8):1824–30.
24. Moodalbail DG, et al. Systematic review of structural and functional neuroimaging findings in children and adults with CKD. Clin J Am Soc Nephrol. 2013;8(8):1429–48.
25. Schnaper HW, et al. Cerebral cortical atrophy in pediatric patients with end-stage renal disease. Am J Kidney Dis. 1983;2(6):645–50.
26. Steinberg A, et al. Computerized tomography of the brain in children with chronic renal failure. Int J Pediatr Nephrol. 1985;6(2):121–6.

27. Trompeter RS, et al. Neurological complications of arterial hypertension. Arch Dis Child. 1982;57(12):913–7.
28. Warady BA, Neu AM, Schaefer F. Optimal care of the infant, child, and adolescent on dialysis: 2014 update. Am J Kidney Dis. 2014;64(1):128–42.
29. Gipson DS, et al. The nervous system and chronic kidney disease in children. Pediatr Nephrol. 2004;19(8):832–9.
30. Gerson AC, et al. Neurocognitive outcomes in children with chronic kidney disease: current findings and contemporary endeavors. Ment Retard Dev Disabil Res Rev. 2006;12(3):208–15.
31. Gipson DS, et al. The central nervous system in childhood chronic kidney disease. Pediatr Nephrol. 2007;22(10):1703–10.
32. Qvist E, et al. Neurodevelopmental outcome in high-risk patients after renal transplantation in early childhood. Pediatr Transplant. 2002;6(1):53–62.
33. Valanne L, et al. Neuroradiologic findings in children with renal transplantation under 5 years of age. Pediatr Transplant. 2004;8(1):44–51.
34. Blum RW, et al. Transition from child-centered to adult health-care systems for adolescents with chronic conditions. A position paper of the Society for Adolescent Medicine. J Adolesc Health. 1993;14(7):570–6.
35. Callahan ST, Winitzer RF, Keenan P. Transition from pediatric to adult-oriented health care: a challenge for patients with chronic disease. Curr Opin Pediatr. 2001;13(4):310–6.
36. Institute for Healthcare, I. The triple aim. Optimizing health, care and cost. Healthc Exec. 2009;24(1):64–6.
37. Prior M, et al. Measuring the "triple aim" in transition care: a systematic review. Pediatrics. 2014;134(6):e1648–61.
38. Vaks Y, et al. Better health, less spending: redesigning the transition from pediatric to adult healthcare for youth with chronic illness. Healthc (Amst). 2016;4(1):57–68.
39. Bell LE, Sawyer SM. Transition of care to adult services for pediatric solid-organ transplant recipients. Pediatr Clin N Am. 2010;57(2):593–610. table of contents
40. Wood DL, et al. The Transition Readiness Assessment Questionnaire (TRAQ): its factor structure, reliability, and validity. Acad Pediatr. 2014;14(4):415–22.
41. Javalkar K, et al. Socioecologic factors as predictors of readiness for self-management and transition, medication adherence, and health care utilization among adolescents and young adults with chronic kidney disease. Prev Chronic Dis. 2014;11:E117.
42. Javalkar K, et al. Ecological factors predict transition readiness/self-management in youth with chronic conditions. J Adolesc Health. 2016;58(1):40–6.
43. Watson AR, et al. Transition from pediatric to adult renal services: a consensus statement by the International Society of Nephrology (ISN) and the International Pediatric Nephrology Association (IPNA). Pediatr Nephrol. 2011;26(10):1753–7.
44. Forbes TA, et al. Adherence to transition guidelines in European paediatric nephrology units. Pediatr Nephrol. 2014;29(9):1617–24.
45. Ingelfinger JR, Kalantar-Zadeh K, Schaefer F. World kidney day 2016: averting the legacy of kidney disease – focus on childhood. Am J Kidney Dis. 2016;67(3):349–54.
46. Paone MC, Wigle M, Saewyc E. The ON TRAC model for transitional care of adolescents. Prog Transplant. 2006;16(4):291–302.
47. Harden PN, et al. Bridging the gap: an integrated paediatric to adult clinical service for young adults with kidney failure. BMJ. 2012;344:e3718.
48. Mina Matsuda-Abedini, et al. Brain abnormalities in children and adolescents with chronic kidney disease. Pediatric Research 2018. http://doi.org/10.1038/s41390-018-0037-5. [Epub ahead of print]

Index

M. N. Haddad et al. (eds.), *Adolescents with Chronic Kidney Disease*,
https://doi.org/10.1007/978-3-319-97220-6

MIX
Papier aus verantwortungsvollen Quellen
Paper from responsible sources
FSC® C105338
FSC
www.fsc.org

If you have any concerns about our products,
you can contact us on
ProductSafety@springernature.com

In case Publisher is established outside the EU,
the EU authorized representative is:
Springer Nature Customer Service Center GmbH
Europaplatz 3, 69115 Heidelberg, Germany

Printed by Libri Plureos GmbH
in Hamburg, Germany